The End of Physiotherapy

Physiotherapy is arriving at a critical point in its history. Since World War I, physiotherapy has been one of the largest allied health professions and the established provider of orthodox physical rehabilitation. But ageing populations of increasingly chronically ill people, a growing scepticism towards biomedicine and the changing economy of healthcare threaten physiotherapy's long-held status. Paradoxically, physiotherapy's affinity for treating the 'body-as-machine' has resulted in an almost complete inability to identify the roots of the profession's present problems, or define possible ways forward. Physiotherapists need to engage in critically informed theoretical discussion about the profession's past, present and future – to explore their practice from economic, philosophical, political and sociological perspectives.

The End of Physiotherapy aims to explain how physiotherapy has arrived at this critical point in its history, and to point to a new future for the profession. The book draws on critical analyses of the historical and social conditions that have made present-day physiotherapy possible. Nicholls examines some of the key discourses that have had a positive impact on the profession in the past, but now threaten to derail it. This book makes it possible for physiotherapists to think otherwise about their profession and their day-to-day practice. It will be essential reading for scholars and students of physiotherapy, interprofessional and community rehabilitation, as well as appealing to those working in medical sociology, the medical humanities, medical history and health care policy.

David A. Nicholls is Associate Professor in the School of Clinical Sciences, Auckland University of Technology, New Zealand.

Routledge Advances in Health and Social Policy

The End of Physiotherapy

David A. Nicholls

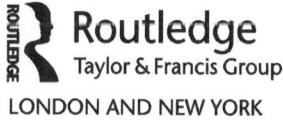

Routledge
Taylor & Francis Group

LONDON AND NEW YORK

First published 2018 by Routledge

2 Park Square, Milton Park, Abingdon, Oxfordshire OX14 4RN

52 Vanderbilt Avenue, New York, NY 10017

Routledge is an imprint of the Taylor & Francis Group, an informa business

First issued in paperback 2019

British Library Cataloguing-in-Publication Data
A catalogue record for this book is available from the British Library

Library of Congress Cataloging-in-Publication Data
Names: Nicholls, David (David A.), author.
Title: The end of physiotherapy/David Nicholls.
Other titles: Routledge advances in health and social policy.
Description: Abingdon, Oxon; New York, NY: Routledge, 2017. |
Series: Routledge advances in health and social policy
Identifiers: LCCN 2017007963 | ISBN 9781138673557 (hardback) |
ISBN 9781315561868 (ebook)
Subjects: | MESH: Physical Therapy Specialty–history | Physical Therapy
Specialty–trends | Physical Therapy Modalities–history | Physical Therapy
Modalities–trends | Philosophy, Medical | Professional Role | Physical
Therapists–psychology
Classification: LCC RM700 | NLM WB 460 | DDC 615.8/2–dc23
LC record available at https://lccn.loc.gov/2017007963

ISBN: 978-1-138-67355-7 (hbk)
ISBN: 978-0-367-22451-6 (pbk)

Typeset in Times New Roman
by Sunrise Setting Ltd, Brixham, UK

For Tom and Ali

Contents

Acknowledgements

The End of Physiotherapy has been years in the making. For more years than I care to remember, I have been arguing for the profession to break out of its self-imposed shackles and reach its full potential. Along the way, I have been fortunate to have had the advice and support of countless colleagues and students who have shown admirable patience and kindness in sharing their thoughts and ideas, comments and supportive criticisms. I am particularly indebted here to Martin Chadwick, Erik Dombroski, Dave Holmes, Peter Larmer, Jo Fadyl, Filip Maric, Debbie Payne, Amélie Perron, Trudy Rudge, Todd and Caroline Stretton, Rachel Vickery and my friends and co-conspirators in the In Sickness and In Health community. Many thanks go to Richard Horwood, Gwyn Owen, Jenny Setchell and Kate Waterworth, who offered valuable comments, critique and suggestions on various parts of the book. And to my colleagues and friends in the Critical Physiotherapy Network, especially those on the CPN Executive, who prove every day that there is a growing and passionate community of practitioners looking for some new ways to think about our profession. Thanks go to the superb team at Routledge who have supported this book from the outset, especially Emily Briggs and Carolina Antunes. Most especially, I would like to acknowledge and thank Barbara Gibson, whose critique, inspirations, exemplary scholarship, friendship and influence is woven into every line of this book. And finally, to my family, who have walked every step of the way with me. To Sue, my constant companion and partner in everything, this book is ours. To my mother, Irene, and the memory of my father, Michael, and, of course, to Tom and Ali. You are precious beyond measure.

Abbreviations

APA	Australian Physiotherapy Association
APTA	American Physical Therapy Association
CPA	Canadian Physiotherapy Association
CSP	Chartered Society of Physiotherapy
ISTM	Incorporated Society of Trained Masseuses
STM	Society of Trained Masseuses
WCPT	World Confederation for Physical Therapy

Part I

1   Introduction

Physiotherapy – or Physical Therapy[1] – is one of the largest and most successful professions allied to medicine. There are more than 250,000 physiotherapists practicing around the world today and there are physiotherapists practicing in almost every country. Physiotherapy is also one of the oldest organised health professions, originating in the late 19th century and predating most of the other allied health professions, including dietetics, occupational therapy, podiatry, radiography and speech and language therapy. It draws its inspiration from a set of techniques that may be the oldest therapies known to humankind and it has been an important feature in the development of modern 'Westernised' medical care. Physiotherapists have partnered with doctors and nurses during some of the most significant human events of the 20th century. Physiotherapists – or masseurs and masseuses as they were known then – played an important part in the rehabilitation of injured servicemen in both world wars; they developed rehabilitation systems to help people recover from epidemics of influenza, tuberculosis and polio; and they established themselves as *the* provider of orthodox rehabilitation services under the welfare reforms that dominated much of the last century. Today, you will find physiotherapists working in private practices and large hospitals, community clinics and specialist rehabilitation units. They are educators, practitioners and researchers, and they work in acute and chronic cardiorespiratory care, exercise-based rehabilitation, mental health, acute musculoskeletal injury, neurology, orthopaedics, pain management, sports, women's health and workplace health, and they work across the entire lifespan from newborn to a person's last days.

Physiotherapists have been trusted and reliable servants of the state, and have been rewarded with status and privilege. Most developed countries offer protection of title to physiotherapists, codifying their role and purpose in law. With this comes secure access to patients within the public health system. They are trusted by the public and respected by governments for doing work that often involves highly sensitive and intimate contact with people in a manner that rarely causes any suspicion or concern. Physiotherapy carries with it a high level of occupational prestige (Turner 2001), and through its increasingly significant role within higher education, is beginning to provide critical commentary on the nature of its own practice and its future as a health provider. So, while it might be exaggeration to suggest that physiotherapy has been the backbone of the orthodox healthcare system during the 20ᵗʰ century, it is probably not unreasonable to claim that the profession has at least represented one of its limbs. Alongside medicine and nursing, physiotherapy has provided one of the principal mechanisms for people to restore movement and function, reduce pain and stiffness, return to fitness and regain their health.

How can it be then, that at the very point where physiotherapists should be congratulating themselves on a job well done, a book can be written that predicts the end of physiotherapy? How can it be, given the seeming health of the profession, its appeal to students and its status within the orthodox health system, that someone might suggest that physiotherapy is facing the most significant crisis of its long and distinguished history? How is it even remotely possible that someone could argue that everything that the profession has achieved may be undone in the years to come? These are the questions that this book attempts to address.

•

Many physiotherapists may find this book uncomfortable reading: not because it is highbrow or pessimistic (my sincere hope is that it is quite the opposite), but because it deliberately asks question that practitioners would prefer not to ask and it does so in a manner that may be confronting, challenging and provocative. The book may be uncomfortable reading because it challenges physiotherapists to think differently about their profession, and it runs counter to much of the perceived wisdom emanating from teachers, researchers, policy makers and practitioners about the future direction for the physiotherapy. It has been written primarily for practitioners, students, teachers, researchers and those who work to shape the profession's future, and so the very people it is directed towards are the very people who may find it most challenging. I hope other readers who know something of physiotherapy's history, or work with practitioners on a daily basis, will gain a new appreciation for some of the profession's present tensions, however, and that these readers may find something valuable to apply to their own work. Many of the issues tackled in this book are common to other health professions.

The purpose of the book is to provide the first critical overview of the historical and social conditions that have contributed to physiotherapy's present problems and to open a space for a different future. Let me be clear, after 25 years of practising, teaching and researching physiotherapy practice, I have come to the conclusion that the profession must change. If we continue to practice physiotherapy in the manner that has seemingly worked so well in the past, the profession – as we know it today – will become increasingly obsolete in the future. The evidence is all around – from the encroachment of other professions to the declining legislative protections and difficulties being seen as an essential part of healthcare reforms. Physiotherapists are being shown daily that they need to find new ways to think and new ways to 'be'. What they are not being shown, however, is how to do it. It seems there is no route map, no path to follow, no new philosophy of practice that we can marshal their forces behind. This is not because there are no new philosophies of practice in healthcare or a lack of new ideas, but that these seem to be a little removed from the 'essence' of physiotherapy practice and they are often couched in pseudo-philosophical language that is far too 'fluffy' for many practitioners with a traditional physiotherapy training.

Physiotherapy is in a uniquely paradoxical situation in that it cannot easily develop a new future precisely *because* of its past. No other health profession experiences this paradox in the same way, and so clinicians, educators and researchers cannot easily look to others for help. What is more, if the physiotherapy paradox prevents the profession from seeing itself more clearly, then reform is going to be very hard, not least because it demands that we challenge some of the principles that define the very essence of what physiotherapists do and who they are. This paradox must be confronted, therefore, if the profession is going to begin the process of reform. And so, it is to this that we must turn if we are to begin the process of seeing physiotherapists' ways of thinking and practicing more clearly.

The physiotherapy paradox

Physiotherapy is, by anyone's estimation, a strong profession. In most countries, it is well respected by the public and government, it has legal protection of title and access to the public health system, it is considered orthodox and so benefits from years of close association with other well-established professions like medicine and nursing, and its training courses are often some of the most oversubscribed and popular programmes in the university. Physiotherapists have a reputation for being bold, energetic, positive people often with 'Type-A' personalities and a pragmatic drive to get things done. But for all these positive traits, physiotherapy can also be seen as quite an exclusive profession that has a very limited biomedical view of the body, movement, function and health, and a rather unsophisticated view of a profession's role within society. Physiotherapists are rarely asked to think about their own individual or collective culture, or are trained to see themselves as being connected to broader societal questions. Because of physiotherapy's history, it can also be seen as somewhat elitist – inferring superiority over other similar professions (like masseurs, chiropractors and personal trainers) through its longstanding association with medicine. It is, in many ways, a profession that mirrors dominant white, European culture in that it assumes culture is something others have and that there is an objective 'truth' to the biomedical – or more accurately biomechanical – basis to the profession's practice that does not need to be questioned. It just *is*.

New Zealand General Practitioner and poet Glenn Colquhoun makes this point very well in the opening quote when he says that 'The most difficult thing about majorities is not that they cannot see minorities but that they cannot see themselves' (Colquhoun 2012). Colquhoun was writing about the tensions that persist between New Zealand Europeans and Māori, but he might just as easily have been speaking about physiotherapy and other established health professions, where there is a degree of cultural myopia brought on by the profession's elevated status in society. But some health professions do more than others to examine their status in society, and do much more than physiotherapy has done to understand its elite social status. As Lauren Williams wrote in 2005:

> Much has been written from a sociological or political perspective about medicine and, increasingly, nursing. This is not surprising since doctors largely control the health system and nurses comprise approximately two-thirds of the health workforce. By contrast, allied health professions have been largely overlooked in the literature, which reflects their relatively small numbers and less than powerful position within the health system . . . Perhaps more surprising, is the fact that the allied health professions themselves have not demonstrated a critical perspective . . . most of the professions align themselves with medical science, largely neglecting to develop a culture that encourages criticism of their own development.
>
> (Williams 2005, p. 350)

Medicine and nursing, but also professions like occupational therapy, and psychology have all developed sophisticated historical and social critiques both from within their professions and without over the last century[2]. In medicine, for example, discrete branches of history, humanities and sociology exist, each with their own publications and special interest groups, all directed at casting a critical eye over the profession. Elliot Freidson, Thomas Osborne, Nikolas Rose, David Armstrong, Mike Saks, Deborah Lupton and hundreds of others have written about medicine; where it comes from; what it does and does not do; its past, present and future and identified more clearly the ideas and principles that are ever changing in the profession (Lupton 2012; Saks 1995; Armstrong 1983; Rose 1994; Osborne 1993; Freidson 1970). The same is true in nursing, occupational therapy, psychology and many of the alternative and complementary professions, despite their significantly reduced resources. So why does physiotherapy lag so far behind in critical self-scrutiny? It clearly cannot be simply because the profession is elite or orthodox or it would surely have followed the example of medicine and the other professions in developing critical approaches to its practice. And it cannot be said to lack resources because there are many other smaller professions who have been far more active in this field. There must be something specific to physiotherapy culture itself that discourages practitioners from examining their own culture. This is the nature of the physiotherapy paradox.

•

One of the principal arguments in this book is that physiotherapy's longstanding approach towards the body underpins its relative ignorance of itself. Physiotherapists are trained to think of the body in terms of its physical form and function at the exclusion of other ways of thinking. The evidence for this is very clear. In recent years, there has been an explosion of interest in the philosophy and sociology of the body, for example, but little of this penetrates the physiotherapy literature. Physiotherapists are rarely exposed to writings on embodiment, or work that distinguishes the biological from the social, gendered or the post-human body.

There is little room in physiotherapy curricula for the writings of Nicholas Fox (Fox 2012), Bryan Turner (Turner 2008) or Chris Shilling (Shilling 2012) even though these are completely contemporary and highly relevant to physiotherapy practice. There is little overt engagement with the vast volumes of disability theory (although this is improving); the science of haptics, physical geography; sensuality or spirituality; the ethics of bodily practices or bodies in a cultural context. Compare perhaps the contents of journals like *Body & Society* (http://bod.sagepub.com/) with any of the mainstream physiotherapy journals and it will be clear that physiotherapy thinking is and has always been focused on the physical functioning on the biomechanical body[3].

This is not a negative statement, however. Every profession has to draw its boundaries somewhere, and anyone who knows anything about the history of physiotherapy will know that its biomechanical approach has been a vital component of the profession's success over the last century. But just as an approach can open doors to make some things possible, it can also deny other things, and what physiotherapy's approach has done has opened the door to the problems now faced by the profession while restricting its ability to respond.

My contention is that adopting a specifically 'biomechanical' view of the body may have been not just desirable but vital to the success of the profession in the past, but it has now become problematic. It may have been necessary, for example, for the founders of the profession to adopt a biomechanical view of the body to prove their legitimacy in the late 19th century, which, in turn, led to physiotherapy becoming trusted by government and the public. It may also have been necessary for the women who founded the profession to maintain this dispassionate approach to the body during World War I when female masseuses began treating male patients, and after the war as orthodox rehabilitation for returned servicemen became a vital part of their work. Although training men to massage – many of whom were blind – remained hugely problematic, not least because 'it was still considered unseemly for lay women to teach men anything involving physical contact' (Barclay 1994, p. 59). The profession's ability to set aside its heteronormative social attitudes, however, may have subsequently placed the profession in an enviable position when the welfare reforms of the 1930s and 1940s established physiotherapy as *the* orthodox provider of rehabilitation services. Security of state protection led to the professionalisation and regulation of physiotherapy around some quite restrictive definitions of its scope, but the move towards university-based education in the latter part of the 20th century created opportunities for critical analysis of these restrictions. Still, physiotherapists sought to perfect its view of the body-as-machine through clinical trials and evidence-based practice. The profession's research capacity has grown, but only really in the area of the clinical sciences that most physiotherapists believe to be the cornerstone of its practice. And why would they think otherwise? Throughout this entire period, physiotherapy has flourished. Its purpose clear, its distinguishing characteristics obvious, its status the envy of other similar allied and complementary professions.

At no point in its history has the profession been seriously challenged to think otherwise. From its inception in the 1890s in England to the present day – a point

I will return to in much more depth later – physiotherapy has been on a course of incremental growth and so has never seen the need to challenge its long history of success. Clearly, there have been threats to the profession's dominance from the horizontal and vertical encroachment of other professions, but nothing to make physiotherapy seriously question its identity or the theoretical and philosophical basis of its knowledge. Indeed, if you asked physiotherapists to define the theoretical and philosophical basis of the profession, they would be hard pressed to tell you. This lack of insight leads to the paradoxical situation where physiotherapists generally believe that their professional identity is opaque and vague and that the public does not understand what they do, while all along their professional identity, knowledge base and beliefs about what is real could not be more straightforward.

Rather than physiotherapy having an opaque and vague notion of itself, the argument I set down here is that physiotherapy is, in fact, quite straightforward. The problem is that physiotherapists have no training in how to 'read' it, and so it can appear more complicated and confusing than it actually is. This is the true nature of the physiotherapy paradox: the fundamental principles that underpin physiotherapy prevent its practitioners from viewing health in other ways that might, in turn, help the profession to see itself more clearly. Where other professions require their practitioners to have a more rounded appreciation for the complexities of health and illness, disability and disorder, physiotherapists typically concentrate only on the body-to-hand and work with the physical form and function of the person in front of them. To explain this with reference to two other allied health professions, one only has to look at nursing and occupational therapy to see how their approach to health is so very different.

Both nursing and occupational therapy have what are lazily called 'holistic' approaches to the health. Both are concerned not only with the physical body, but also the broader personal, cultural, environmental, spiritual and social dimensions of what it is to be human. One only has to look at two of the commonly used models of occupational performance and science to see this. The Canadian Model of Occupational Performance and Engagement (CMOP-*e*) and the Model of Human Occupation (MOHO) (Townsend & Polataiko 2007; Kielhofner 2008), each looks to emphasise different dimensions of human occupation but neither only considers the person's physical performance as their sole interest. Similarly, the nursing profession has spent years debating the true nature of nursing (Dahlke & Stahlke Wall 2016). Drawing on critical theory, philosophy and sociology, it is implicit in nursing that there is a diversity of approaches to practice, all underpinned by a robust engagement in science. These skills of critical analysis are necessary for nursing and occupational therapy practitioners if they are to understand the complexities of the patients they serve, but they are also easily applied back to the profession itself and critical self-analysis has been a longstanding hallmark of these professions.

No such breadth and depth of scholarship exists in physiotherapy. There are a mere handful of tentative models of physiotherapy practice, and these are rarely debated (Trede 2006). Helen Hislop's call for a pathokinesiological model of practice in 1975 (Hislop 1975), and Cheryl Cott et al's 1995 Movement Continuum Theory of Physical Therapy (Cott et al 1995) remain unchallenged, as does Catharina

Broberg and colleagues' 2003 conceptual 'corkscrew' (Broberg et al 2003) and Noronen and Wikström-Grotell's paradigmatic approach from 1999 (Noronen & Wikström-Grotell 1999). Lacking the solid grounding in critical social studies and philosophy that are implicit to other health professionals, physiotherapy lacks the ability to see how straightforward its professional identity is or how complex the world of healthcare has become. The physiotherapy paradox is, itself, relatively simple then. Physiotherapists cannot see themselves because the very approach that has afforded it the status and security it now enjoys, actively discourages it from seeing the 'bigger picture'. Over the last century, physiotherapy has not been asked to change. It has not needed to examine itself in the way that other professions have. It has been secure in its tenure, growing into one of the largest health professions in the world.

Something, therefore, must have changed to now awaken the profession to the possibility that the future for the profession may not be secure. Unfortunately, one does not have to look far to find evidence of this and it is in the real world of everyday practice that practitioners have started to appreciate the physiotherapy paradox, even if they cannot easily define its boundaries. Physiotherapists are experiencing increasing pressure from other health professions who are encroaching on what was once physiotherapy territory. They have experienced job cuts and rationalisation. They have heard that healthcare is moving away from traditional models of practice, and they have seen a healthcare marketplace emerge. They know that patients want something more these days than just a skilled clinician and that patients – now patients – have greater opportunities to explore alternatives to orthodox practice. And they have felt the incessant march of technology and seen what might be possible for people in the future. For these reasons, and many others besides, there cannot be a physiotherapist in practice today who feels completely secure in their position, safe in the knowledge that physiotherapy will never have to change or adapt to the times. All physiotherapists feel the pressure and the need to change, but who knows how?

The new economy of healthcare

Feeling pressured to change may be a reality for physiotherapists but it hardly counts as the objective basis for a belief that we are experiencing the 'end of physiotherapy'. Just because practitioners feel ill at ease does not prove that there is something fundamentally wrong with the profession. Besides, physiotherapists can hardly be said to have a monopoly on feeling ill at ease. In today's postmodern world, nothing seems stable anymore and it is increasingly difficult to know who is right and who is wrong. Not so long ago, the public placed its trust in authority figures like priests, judges and doctors to tell it what was good and what was bad; what was normal and abnormal; who was healthy and who was sick. Can we say that we still believe the same today? What is more, we are constantly assailed by doom-laden messages about climate change, global financial crisis, food security, international unrest, antibiotic resistant bugs, Internet security and social isolation. So, it seems that it is not just physiotherapists that are feeling a sense of unease.

Everything, it seems, that we once held to be true, now seems to be in doubt. One could be forgiven for thinking that this book represented just one more pessimistic analysis of something that we once thought would be here forever.

One of the positive features of today's postmodern worldview is that people are more open to the idea of thinking differently. Our scepticism, however, makes us less easy to convince. So, anyone proclaiming the 'end of physiotherapy' must be able to base their arguments on more than just feelings of disquiet. Unfortunately, there is now ample justification for physiotherapists' concern and much of this book is devoted to this. There are conditions that are inherent to physiotherapy itself and these will be explored over the course of the next few chapters. There are also conditions that appear to be external to the profession – cultural, economic, political and social forces – that are having a profound effect on the way the public and the State now view the profession and may, ultimately, determine its fate. These conditions are having their most significant influence in the new economy of healthcare.

Taken in no particular order, people living in developed countries are now experiencing:

1   Demographic shifts towards an increasingly ageing population, many of whom will be living with chronic illnesses that affect their ability to participate in health-promoting activity.
2   Greater costs of care for these people and a growing number of people dependent on others for support. We are seeing not only an increasing number of informal carers (daughters, sons, neighbours and friends) who are, themselves, often struggling to work, raise families, enjoy their own healthy leisure time while looking after an ageing relative, but also rising costs of social welfare services.
3   The need to reduce public funding for healthcare. Governments in the developed world have been trying to find ways of reducing public funding for healthcare since the 1970s. As the population of dependent people increases in proportion to the working population, the amount of income from taxation slowly diminishes.
4   The epidemic in lifestyle disorders among the working age populations and the distance between the affluent 'worried well' and those with 'traditional' biomedical health problems. The growing social gradient between those who can afford personalised health and those who are dependent on traditional health services creates its own problems; with people using State-subsidised emergency services, for example, to avoid having to pay for a visit to their general practitioner.
5   The growing perception that the healthcare system is inefficient and ineffective. Tertiary care in large centralised hospitals is thought to be inefficient and not patient-centred, and so the focus is moving towards community-based primary care, health promotion and population health. Traditional healthcare structures and systems are being dismantled and replaced with new diversified networks of providers and support services.

6   Scepticism towards orthodox healthcare. Years of reports of medical misadventure added to the sense that the trillions of dollars spent on the established healthcare system have not reduced people's ill health and instead have fuelled a scepticism for the present healthcare system. At the same time, people are much more willing to try an alternative or complementary therapy before going to an orthodox professional for health advice.

7   Increasingly complex understandings of health. People are much less certain about the traditional distinction between health and sickness, such that we are now all committed to the unobtainable idea of optimal health. At one time, sickness was an occasional state that warranted specialist attention. Now none of us is ever optimally healthy, so must always be engaged in 'body projects' to improve ourselves. This has given people much more choice, but opened an enormous market for 'soft' healthcare services, from nutritional supplements and herbal medicine, to beauty 'therapies' and reconstructive surgery, gym memberships and healthy eating plans.

8   The growth in the importance of individual responsibility. Pivotal in the shift towards greater personal choice has been the economic and social drive towards greater individual responsibility. Based on the common logic that everyone wants to be healthy, we are all increasingly encouraged to take care of ourselves and take advantage of the avalanche of personal health and wellness information that is now available to us, such that we now have very little excuse but to be healthy.

9   The democratisation of knowledge. In the past, one of the defining characteristics of a profession was the possession of an extensive body of specialist knowledge that took years of training to acquire. Nowadays, anyone with a networked computer can have this knowledge at their fingertips. You can find applications for your mobile device that not only shows you the detailed anatomy of the neck, but also how to manipulate it. It is now possible to find detailed information on all common and uncommon diseases and disorders, all the relevant pharmaceutical information and the evidence in support of various claims for their efficacy. This does not mean that people necessarily do the right thing because we also have access to a bewildering array of contrary opinions, but it means people are less likely to trust an orthodox health professional to tell them what to do simply because they say so.

In setting out some of the changes that have taken place in and around healthcare, it is important to note that I am not saying that any of these is necessarily good *or* bad. In fact, it is most likely that they are both good *and* bad. The democratisation of healthcare information, for example, has had many positive effects, not least allowing everyone access to information that was once denied to them by professional hubris or 'boundary protection'. It has placed the spotlight on some orthodox health practices that were unjustified, cruel and unethical, and it has forced practitioners to ask patients for their needs and wants. At the same time, it has dented people's confidence in orthodox healthcare and placed complex and subtle health information in the hands of people who have not benefitted from a training that might help them to discriminate between what they can trust and what they cannot. The key point here is not to try to judge the changes that are taking place in black-and-white terms but rather to see all the changes as the effect of the changing system we are all part of, and therefore worthy of analysis and understanding.

This analysis is particularly prescient when it threatens the fundamental principles upon which a historic profession is based. In the case of physiotherapy, the changes we are seeing in the new economy of healthcare will affect the profession in some quite specific ways because of the way physiotherapy is configured. Traditional physiotherapy services and their attendant ideologies are being rationalised in most developed countries. Hospital-based in-patient care, day hospitals and rehabilitation centres, hydrotherapy services, acute care for anyone other than the most severely ill, long-term neurological rehabilitation, orthopaedic rehabilitation, acute musculoskeletal injury and many other areas of strength in traditional physiotherapy, are all under pressure in the long slow demise of the welfare state. Added to this, it is becoming increasingly difficult to obtain insurance coverage for rehabilitation programmes, and horizontal and vertical encroachment from other health professions is intruding on areas of practice that physiotherapists once had a monopoly over.

In an effort to demonstrate the value of its work and to emphasise, once more, the close bond between physiotherapy and medicine, physiotherapists have turned to evidence-based practice and have conducted a number of significant clinical trials. In many cases, however, the results of these studies are underwhelming, and the profession has been left with the sense that its practice somehow feels more significant than the results of these studies appear to show. For their part, the public seem to care little for these subtleties as we become saturated with health information. Not so long ago, people had little or no choice but to visit an orthodox health professional if they were ill. There was no healthcare marketplace to speak of, and complementary and alternative medicine (CAM) practitioners were few and far between. Now, a significant proportion of the population visit CAM practitioners *before* visiting an orthodox provider (Macartney & Wahlberg 2014). As a result, mainstream medicine is becoming a final destination for many people who have exercised their right to experiment with other options first.

Not surprisingly then, there has been a loss of confidence in the present state of affairs and the future possibilities for physiotherapists. Professional societies are criticised for not marketing the profession to the public and the claim that 'the public does not know what physiotherapists do' is frequently heard. There is a concern that the rapidly changing market in healthcare is escaping the profession's grasp and that physiotherapists are literally and metaphorically 'losing touch'. It seems the profession is aware that the government and the public now want something different from health services. And it should not be that difficult to imagine physiotherapists becoming more engaged in the shift to public health, population health and health promotion, particularly given its long history as the preeminent physical rehabilitation profession. But it seems that others are getting there first and physiotherapists are finding it difficult to understand why the profession is being increasingly marginalised.

If this book has one over-arching purpose then, it would be to address this problem. It is my belief that there are some specific reasons for this tension that can be found in the profession's culture and history and by understanding the profession's political and social past physiotherapists can see how they have arrived at this point and, hopefully, approach the future with more confidence. In this respect, while it may at times seem to be a book with a strongly critical disposition (and a rather distressing title), it is neither nihilistic nor pessimistic, but rather, I hope, a book that creates an opening for a long overdue conversation among physiotherapists about where their profession has come from, where it is now and where it might be going. I hope the book liberates the profession to see that there is a future for its practice, and that this future is vital for the health and wellbeing of the population.

•

So why is the book titled *The End of Physiotherapy*? Without wanting to simplify what are some quite complex arguments, I do not believe the future lies with the profession currently known as physiotherapy. Having read the book – and I sincerely hope you do – you will see that my conclusion is that physiotherapy has ideological foundations that are creating the conditions of the profession's own demise. The fact that there is so little scholarly discussion of these things is evidence in itself of the power of these ideologies to focus on very specific aspects of physical function at the expense of the myriad other ways of understanding health; knowledge that could be so helpful to physiotherapists and the people they serve. Perhaps more significantly because these ideologies discourage self-reflection (preferring instead a pragmatic approach to practice that physiotherapists are famous for), practitioners are largely unaware of their existence and the power they exert over them, despite the fact that these ideologies exert their effects every day in their practice.

My point, therefore, is that physiotherapy as a coherent professional identity is in decline because physiotherapists do not possess the necessary historical, philosophical political and socio-cultural vocabulary to see themselves more clearly and bring about the necessary professional reform. There are too many practitioners who believe that the profession will ride out these latest tribulations as it has done before; that evidence-based practice will eventually prove its worth or, that in the end, people will return to a profession that they trust when they have exhausted their dalliance with alternatives. To some extent, I have sympathy with these suggestions. I believe passionately that people will always want skilled, trusted, empathic, well-rounded practitioners who can assess, diagnose and treat a wide range of physical health problems, and that the current marketplace in healthcare services does not always offer that. People will always want skilled professionals who can touch without fear of licentiousness; analyse movement disorders and identify the source of someone's pain; differentially diagnose and assess functional disorders; treat and rehabilitate with skill and decisiveness. But, it is looking increasingly unlikely that physiotherapy – as it is currently configured – will be the profession to do this. If physiotherapy, with all its inherent advantages, cannot command the market today, it is unlikely to capture it tomorrow. Indeed, as time passes, and the advantages that physiotherapy has accrued over the last century whittle away, it is likely that the profession will become increasingly marginalised. Unless, of course, it is completely in tune with the changes and responsive to the new economy of healthcare. But here the physiotherapy paradox comes in, because the very skills that made physiotherapy so valued in the 20th century are hampering its efforts at change today.

Where does this leave us? As I have said already, one could be forgiven for thinking that this book is nihilistic. On the contrary, there is a very positive message in this book and it is that the future for the profession is in its own hands. Given its skills in assessment and diagnosis, I am confident that a coherent argument will resonate with people across the profession. And given its experience of treatment and rehabilitation, I believe strongly that it can make the changes necessary to have a healthy future. This is a rather clichéd metaphor but physiotherapy is like the patient who comes into the clinic with a longstanding problem that is now causing them problems. They have lived with the problem for so long they do not realise that they are perpetuating it by the way they think and move. What feels natural to them is, in fact, making the matter worse. The job of the physiotherapist has always been to identify the sources of the problem and return the patient to healthy function. You will, no doubt, call on the support of others – family, friends and other clinical colleagues – and the whole process will take time. But the end result will be improved health and wellbeing. Physiotherapists now have to turn this same approach back on itself and apply its skills of rehabilitation to its own practice. To do this, it will need help: help to diagnose what is causing the profession's pain and declining function; help to find new ways to move and the support to see it through.

Obviously, one book can only hope to start this process. Weighed against the library shelves stacked with literature on how physiotherapy *used* to be practiced this text will hardly make a dent. After all, physiotherapists have arrived at this point in their history after millions of hours of collective study and the work of hundreds of thousands of practitioners, so one book cannot hope to turn this around in an instant. But it can make a start and my hope is that it opens the door to some new thinking and some new ways of working that will, in time, see physiotherapy successful in the rehabilitation of itself.

Design and structure of the book

This book has been written to be read by all physiotherapists. It assumes nothing about the reader's particular knowledge of the history of the profession or an in depth understanding of cultural studies, philosophy or sociology. It is my hope that undergraduate and postgraduate students will find the book useful as a resource as they examine aspects of physiotherapy's history and culture. But I also hope the book appeals to everyday practitioners who would, perhaps, be more familiar with a textbook describing a new practice technique. I am most likely to obtain a sympathetic hearing from three groups of readers. The first are the practitioners who have been in practice long enough to feel dissatisfied with their profession but not long enough to be disillusioned. These people are the critical life-blood of the profession. They will fight tooth-and-nail to change their world and they have the vision and perseverance to do it. I hope this book gives them encouragement. The second are the physiotherapy educators and academics who have laboured to try to define physiotherapy for their students and who are increasingly looking to critically evaluate their profession. And the third are practitioners, historians, cultural theorists and sociologists who have an interest in healthcare. I hope this book goes some way towards filling the gap in the literature around the study of the physical therapies. There are few books available that critically analyse the past, present and future of the profession, and so I have drawn on comparable works in medicine, nursing and elsewhere to provide a context in some instances where there is nothing available in physiotherapy. The book cannot hope to address some of the issues raised in this growing body of literature with a great deal of complexity, however, so I would ask readers experienced with some of these concepts to excuse the liberties I take with some ideas in my effort to communicate them to a wider audience.

The book is written in three parts. Part I explores the historical antecedents of the present tensions. Part II unpacks some of the critical discourses that underpin present-day physiotherapy. Part III examines the implications of these discourses for key areas of physiotherapy work. Part I divides physiotherapy history across four chapters. Chapter 2 addresses the period immediately before the formation of the profession and examines the practices that physiotherapists co-opted in defining their professional identity. Chapter 3 looks at the first 20 years of physiotherapy and concentrates on the actions of the founders of the Society of Trained Masseuses (STM) in England. I look closely at *how* the founders of the Society established the legitimacy of their massage practice and laid the cornerstone for many of the present tensions for physiotherapists. Chapter 4 explores the period between 1914 and 1973; a period of consolidation in which physiotherapy established itself as an orthodox health profession par excellence. The chapter ends at the 1973 oil crisis – a pivotal turning point in the economy of healthcare, and the beginning of the end for a significant period of growth and consolidation in physiotherapy and in state-sponsored healthcare more generally. Chapter 5 takes the reader from 1973 to the present and examines the effect that neo-liberal economic reforms have had not only on physiotherapy practice, but also on people's personal freedoms and expectations. The chapter brings us to the present day and the tensions and uncertainties that now surround contemporary healthcare. Part II focuses on key discourses in the construction of contemporary physiotherapy and traces their historical origins. Chapter 6 addresses the body and the very particular way physiotherapists have made sense of its complexities and challenges. Chapters 7 and 8 then develop these ideas, firstly by considering how physiotherapeutic understandings of the body were applied to posture and movement (Chapter 7) and then to function and rehabilitation (Chapter 8). Part III draws these various cultural, historical, philosophical and sociological critiques together and considers what how they are influencing physiotherapy education, practice, regulation and research (Chapter 9). The final substantive chapter involves a detailed discussion of the future, and considers whether we are, indeed, experiencing *The End of Physiotherapy* (Chapter 10). The book concludes with a short 'Epilogue' outlining some of the methodological and philosophical approaches taken in developing the book.

•

Before embarking on the book in earnest, there are one or two qualifying comments I would like to make in order that my intentions in writing the book are made clear. Firstly, this book is intended as a celebration of physiotherapy. Although readers will discover a great deal of critique in the pages that follow, my goal is that this text opens a space for a vast flourishing of new ideas and practices. My belief is that the future of the profession lies in diversity and inclusiveness and I hope that this work goes some way to making that more attainable. Secondly, and in keeping with these ideas, I have assiduously avoided any suggestion that I will be providing 'the answer' to the profession's present predicaments. Readers looking for a formula or prescription for how the profession should proceed may be disappointed. My hope, instead, is that a clearer understanding of the conditions that have made present-day physiotherapy historically and socially possible will make a thousand new physiotherapies possible.

Because no account of a profession can ever be complete, I hope readers will forgive omissions and perspectives that I was either unaware of or unable to incorporate into the text. No history of events can ever be anything but a partial account. And no book based on one person's analysis can ever address all of the elements that go to make up the complex living organism that is physiotherapy. There is only a cursory discussion, for instance, of gendered questions surrounding the profession, which may be the first female-dominated health profession in the world to adopt an androcentric model of practice. Equally, there is little critical discussion of the role that rehabilitation practices have played in the growth of Western capitalism in the 20th century. Given that physiotherapists' stated desire is to return people to normal function, it would seem to be a question worthy of some rigorous discussion. The reader will note the bias towards an Anglocentric history of physiotherapy. One of the principal arguments I make in the book is that physiotherapy has been dominated by British and North American approaches to the body, posture and movement, function and rehabilitation. These approaches have, in their own small way, been colonising influences on other cultures around the world and I have tried to reflect that in the data I used to populate my analyses. Because these approaches have been so effective in colonising other physiotherapy curricula and scopes of practice, I believe many readers – wherever they are based – will recognise at least some of the tensions set out in the pages that follow. I do, at the same time, acknowledge that some may feel that the book does not adequately address their particular practice experience.

Finally, I realise that readers may find themselves strongly disagreeing with some of the arguments made in the book. Some will see the work as unorthodox and dissenting, others may see it as overly critical or deprecating. Physiotherapists are naturally protective of their profession and may not take kindly to the kinds of prolonged critique set down here. But I would argue that a book like this is both a reflection of the profession's growing self-confidence, and a necessary step if it is to remain relevant and valued in the decades to come. Only if physiotherapists can see themselves more clearly will they know if and how they may need to adapt to the changing economy of healthcare in the future. I hope this book goes some way to meeting that goal.

Notes

1 The term *physiotherapy* will be used throughout the book to refer to the profession as it has developed in Commonwealth countries and parts of Europe, but also to the term *physical therapy*, which is more common in North America.
2 For nursing, see *Nursing Philosophy* or *Nursing Inquiry* journals and Alligood (2014); for occupational therapy see Boniface & Seymour (2012) or Kronenberg et al (2005); and for psychology see Jarvis (2005) and Burke (2006).
3 When I refer to physiotherapy's 'biomechanical' view of the body, I am not referring to a body made up of levers, fulcrums and physical forces, but rather a more philosophical way of viewing the body that draws on biomedical principles of reductionism, mind vs body dualism and objectivity, and excludes other cultural, environmental, humanistic, spiritual or social understandings of the body. It is synonymous with the notion of the body-as-machine that is explored in more depth in Chapter 2.

References

Alligood, M.R., 2014, *Nursing theory: Utilization & application*, Elsevier, St Louis, Missouri.

Armstrong, D., 1983, *Political anatomy of the body: Medical knowledge in Britain in the twentieth century*, Cambridge University Press, Cambridge.

Barclay, J., 1994, *In good hands: The history of the Chartered Society of Physiotherapy 1894–1994*, Butterworth Heinemann, Oxford.

Boniface, G. & Seymour, A., 2012, *Using occupational therapy theory in practice*, Wiley-Blackwell, Chichester, UK.

Broberg, C., Aars, M., Beckmann, K., Emaus, N., Lehto, P., Lähteenmäki, M.-L., Thys, W. & Vandenberghe, R., 2003, A conceptual framework for curriculum design in physiotherapy education – an international perspective, *Advances in Physiotherapy*, 5(4), pp. 161–8.

Burke, P.J., 2006, *Contemporary social psychological theories*, Stanford Social Sciences, Stanford, CA.

Colquhoun, G., 2012, *Jumping ship and other essays*, Steele Roberts, Wellington, New Zealand.

Cott, C.A., Finch, E., Gasner, D., Yoshida, K., Thomas, S.G. & Verrier, M.C., 1995, The movement continuum theory of physical therapy, *Physiotherapy Canada*, 47(2), pp. 87–95.

Dahlke, S. & Stahlke Wall, S., 2016, Does the emphasis on caring within nursing contribute to nurses' silence about practice issues?, *Nursing Philosophy*. doi: 10.1111/nup.12150.

Fox, N.J., 2012, *The body*, Polity, London.

Freidson, E., 1970, *Profession of medicine: A study of the sociology of applied knowledge*, Dodd Mead, New York.

Hislop, H.J., 1975, The not-so-Impossible Dream, *Physical Therapy*, 55(10), pp. 1069–80.

Jarvis, M., 2005, *Theoretical approaches in psychology*, Routledge, London.

Kielhofner, G., 2008, *Model of human occupation: Theory and application*, Lippincott Williams & Wilkins, Baltimore, MD.

Kronenberg, F., Simó, A.S. & Pollard, N., 2005, *Occupational therapy without borders: Learning from the spirit of survivors*, Elsevier/Churchill Livingstone, Edinburgh; New York.

Lupton, D., 2012, *Medicine as culture: Illness, disease and the body in western society*. Sage, London.

Macartney, J.I. & Wahlberg, A., 2014, The problem of complementary and alternative medicine use today: Eyes half closed?, *Qualitative Health Research*, doi: 10.1177/1049732313518977.

Noronen, L. & Wikström-Grotell, C., 1999, Towards a paradigm-oriented approach in physiotherapy, *Physiotherapy Theory and Practice*, 15(3), pp. 175–84.

Osborne, T., 1993, On liberalism, neo-liberalism and the 'iberal profession' of medicine, *Economy and Society*, 22(3), pp. 345–56.

Rose, N., 1994, Medicine, history and the present, in C. Jones & R. Porter (eds.), *Reassessing Foucault: Power, medicine and the body*, Routledge, London, pp. 48–72.

Saks, M., 1995, *Professions and the public interest*, Routledge, London.

Shilling, C., 2012, *The body and social theory*, Sage, London.

Townsend, E.A. & Polataiko, J., 2007, *Enabling occupation II: Advancing an occupational therapy vision for health, well-being & justice through occupation*, Canadian Association of Occupational Therapists, Ottawa, Canada.

Trede, F., 2006, *A critical practice model for physiotherapy*, doctoral thesis, University of Sydney, Australia.

Turner, B.S., 2008, *The body and society: Explorations in social theory*, Sage, London.

Turner, P., 2001, The occupational prestige of physiotherapy: perceptions of student physiotherapists in Australia, *Australian Journal of Physiotherapy*, 47(3), p. 191.

Williams, L., 2005, Jostling for position: A sociology of allied health, in J. Germov (ed.), *Second opinion*, Oxford University Press, Oxford, pp. 349–72.

2   Physical therapies before 1894

Introduction

In the summer of 1894, four British nurses and midwives decided to form a professional organisation to represent masseuses and establish a legitimate basis for
their practice. This organisation would lay the foundation stone for many other
physiotherapy societies around the world and create the conditions under which
many physiotherapists still practice today. In Chapter 3, I look at what the founders
actually did to convince the public and the medical profession that it was possible
to use physical therapies in a respectable way, but here I want to explore some of
the conditions and events that would make their actions possible.

Physical therapies are as old as recorded history and they are, in all possibility,
as instinctive to humans as migration is to birds. They involve many people and
practices and their evolution and development mirror many of the major events of
recorded history. A full account of massage, mobilisation and manipulation, remedial exercises, hydrotherapy and electrotherapy would require a book of its own,
and would not necessarily answer more specific questions of how physiotherapy
came to deploy and institutionalise these modalities for its own ends. In this chapter,
therefore, I attempt a more specific history of physical therapies; a history that is
less concerned with accounting for a succession of events leading to the formation
of the physiotherapy profession and more, with some of the critical discourses and
influences that made the profession possible.

I explore the important role physical therapies have played throughout recorded
history and their role in helping medicine establish its pre-eminence in the 18th
and 19th centuries. I look at the role the Industrial Revolution played in creating the
surplus and luxury necessary to allow people to enjoy massage and other therapies
as leisure pursuits. And I examine the role that gender has played in the history of
the physical therapies. This last question is particularly important because early
physiotherapy was almost exclusively female, yet all the practices and systems
they inherited came from a very masculine world of medicine. Unlike nursing and
midwifery, which were also female-dominated, physiotherapy adopted a very androcentric (male-centred) model of practice (see Chapter 3). How this might have
been achieved and why it might have been necessary are the questions at the heart
of this chapter. As with any analysis of the physical therapies though, we must
begin with the earliest accounts from recorded history.

Ancient physical therapies

The physical therapies, as systematically organised systems of treatment (as opposed to the reflex rubbing of one's skin or acts of comfort towards others), have their origins in ancient civilisations. Some of the greatest scholars of physical medicine have explored the long history of massage, manipulation, hydrotherapy and electrotherapy, and claim that they have their origins in the earliest recorded histories of humankind (Krusen 1942; Stewart 1925; Kleen 1918; Kamenetz 1960; Cutter 1934). Many of the words we now use today for physical therapies show how old these practices were and how much practices were hybridised as they crossed cultures. The word massage, for instance, may have its origins in Hebrew (*mashesh*), Arabic (*mass*), Sanskrit (*makch*) or Greek (*massein*), and words like shampooing – a popular term for massage in the 19th century – derives from the Hindu word *chamna*, meaning 'to press' (Kleen 1918, p. 4).

Physical therapies in China and India are considered by many to be the basis upon which later Egyptian, Greek and Roman practices developed (Calvert 2002), and although it is unclear to what extent practices were systematised, it is known that massage and exercise were regularly used as accompaniments to herbal and 'spiritual' forms of medicine as early as 2500 B.C. (Kleen 1918). Greek physicians provided the first systematic accounts of the widespread use of physical therapies, and so are credited with organising, if not necessarily 'inventing', many of the methods we now use today. Greek gymnasiums were places of learning, and students studied land- and water-based exercise, therapeutic gymnastics and massage as part of a general introduction to civil society. Young men from wealthy families studied the law, politics, history, the arts and medicine in schools that taught them debating, social etiquette, politics, ethics and aesthetics, as well as physical discipline, combat and bodily discipline.

Some trained as physicians, others as architects or politicians. Those specialising in medicine developed a range of skills including anatripsis (meaning *to rub up*). Hippocrates (460–377 B.C.), for example, 'mentions the utility of friction after sprains and reduced dislocations, recommends abdominal kneading for constipation, knew of chest-clapping, "terrain cures," etc'. (Kleen 1918, p. 2), and suggests that 'the physician must be acquainted with many things and assuredly with anatripsis . . . for rubbing can bind a joint that is loose and loosen a joint that is too hard' (Smith et al 2010, p. 44).

Roman medicine was heavily influenced by the work of Greek doctors, including Asclepiades[1], the 'father' of manipulative medicine, and Pedanius Dioscorides (40–90 A.D.), author of *De Materia Medica* (Krusen 1942, p. 10). Numerous references are made in their works to the use of natural elements in 'physical' medicine. These include possibly the first reference to 'electrotherapy', in which torpedo fish are used to treat headaches and gout (Krusen 1942, p. 10). But it was Galen (131–201 A.D.), who had the greatest influence on 'Western' medicine in the first millennium.

Galen of Pergamon (later Galen of Rome) provided the first systematic account of medicine, including the development of experimental physiology and the first accurate description of the bones and muscles. Galen's voluminous works contributed significantly to the celebration of Greco-Roman high culture in the centuries either side of the millennium. Romans made thermotherapy and heliotherapy central parts of daily life, and baths became highly sophisticated as 'Emperors vied with one another in erecting magnificent public baths, capable of accommodating thousands of persons daily' (Krusen 1942, p. 13).

With the rapid growth of the early Christian church and the subsequent decline of the ancient civilisations of Greece, Rome and Turkey after 300 A.D., physical therapies became the subject of moral scrutiny. Sensuality – in all its forms – was anathema to the early Christian faith. Grounded in a belief in original sin (in which Adam chose Eve over virginal fidelity to his Creator), the virtues of chastity, abstinence and purity of spirit, disciples began to purge any representations or practices that they felt breached Christian law. Bathing, massage and any other practices that involved touch and the celebrations of bodily form and function were considered sins of the flesh and were systematically eradicated. Books, including the hand-copied manuscripts of Galen, were burned for their profanity. Fortunately, it is thought that a few copies survived this purge and, over time, were taken to Persia and translated into Arabic and contributed heavily to an Arab Renaissance that lasted almost 1,000 years. At its high point, works by Avicenna (Ibn Sīnā, ابن سينا, c. 980–1037 A.D.) and other Arabic scholars developed Greco-Roman medicine, so that when European culture began to emerge from its long years of paganism and puritanism around 1500 A.D., the works of Galen and other ancient scholars were translated back into Latin and used as the basis for the European Renaissance.

Physical medicine from the Renaissance

The Renaissance was a period of profound change in European society. Loosely extending from the early 14th to 17th centuries, it represents a period in which people developed scientific principles to understand the natural world and challenge the power of religion and superstition. Natural philosophers (as scientists were originally called), artists and scholars like Leonardo da Vinci (1452–1519) and Michelangelo (1475–1564) observed and measured natural occurring phenomena, and they were followed by mathematicians, physicists and philosophers like Francis Bacon (1562–1626), Galileo Galilei (1564–1642), René Descartes (1596–1650), Immanuel Kant (1724–1804) and Isaac Newton (1642–1727), who developed subjects like anatomy, astronomy, geometry, chemistry and physics to instigate the European Enlightenment.

Many Enlightenment sciences explored 'man's' relationship to the natural world and one of its greatest philosophers – René Descartes – used the new sciences to propose a dangerously heretical idea that the body was separate from the mind. He argued that the body was based in the natural world and represented man's worldly suffering. It was profane and prone to corruption, whereas the mind was the seat of the soul, pure and God-like. Descartes also argued that because our dreams were so vivid and so real, we could never know when we were dreaming and when we were not. Consequently, we could never know for sure that objects we perceived around us (the chair we sit on, the cup we drink from etc.) were real, or part of our dream's imagining. The only thing we could say for sure was that we existed, in some form or another, because we were able to contemplate our own existence. Hence Descartes most famous aphorism – *cogito ergo sum*. I think, therefore I am.

Descartes suggested that because we cannot trust our senses, we should look for evidence of the real world using as much objectivity as was available to us. Experimentation, the independent validation of others and repeated measurements, for instance, were all preferable to individual opinion, faith or dogma. This approach can be seen in the work of people like Galileo, who showed that the Earth and the planets orbited around the Sun (heliocentrism), rather than the Earth being the centre of the universe (geocentrism). Such ideas suggested that the world followed natural laws and was not under the control of a supernatural force. The world could be studied, understood and even governed by humans – a view that may not be controversial to us now, but was dangerous enough to have Galileo put under house arrest for the last nine years of his life. The natural sciences only continued to develop over the next 200 years, however, and few areas grew more rapidly than the study of the human body (Sawday 1995; Bynum & Kalof 2010).

Enlightenment thinking largely saw the body and the mind as separate entities, and where the church kept its power over the person's soul, new sciences of anatomy, physiology and kinematics began to interrogate the inner workings of the body. Andreas Vesalius developed the study of anatomy, Zacharias Janssen produced the first functioning microscope, allowing Antonie van Leeuwenhoek to see red blood cells for the first time, Francis Bacon pioneered the experimental method and William Harvey discovered how the heart and circulatory systems worked. Robert Boyle refuted Aristotle's beliefs about natural elements, giving birth to modern chemistry, Isaac Newton discovered universal gravitation and described the world as a giant clock in which everything could be expressed mechanically. Edward Jenner invented the first vaccine for smallpox and Gabriel Fahrenheit produced the first thermometer. These inventions, and many others, marked a period of scientific ferment in Europe during the 17th and 18th centuries and many of the physical therapies drew on and amplified these discoveries.

Because of its name, electrotherapies are often thought of as relatively recent inventions, but this is not the case. In the late 1670s, for example, Isaac Newton began experimenting with the light spectrum, which led to discoveries by Römer (fixed speed of light), Huygens (light waves), Ebermaier (the effect of light on the human body), Herschel (infrared), Ritter (ultraviolet), Davy ('artificial' or 'carbon' light) and Gilbert (magnetism) (Krusen 1942, pp. 16–17; Colwell 1922). Krueger and Kratzenstein developed the first 'medical' electrotherapy devices around 1750, and Volta, Faraday and Tesla followed. With the discovery and commercialisation of electricity in the 19th century, a whole new branch of medical science emerged. People believed that electricity was akin to 'nervous energy' and that small galvanic and faradic batteries could replenish lost energy. This produced an enormous market in medical and commercial devices, and doctors used people's astonishment with electrical energy to promote their own practices (Morus 2006). Light therapies, too, became immensely popular, particularly for wealthy Victorians who escaped the city to holiday in spa resorts that offered plentiful fresh air and sunshine;

> Just as the sun is the principal of all life, so is it the source of all healing. It is the Sun, and uniquely the Sun, that sick people seek in winter on our coast. It is the Great Doctor, Doctor of the Faculty of the Sky, to whom the suffering come to demand a cure for their ills.
>
> (Orgeas 1889, p. 466, cited in Woloshyn 2013, p. 1)

Health spas, in general, saw a massive revival in the 19th century, particularly in Europe and North America. It should be remembered though that these were only really available to the leisure classes. The conditions of working class people did not provide the time or money to allow them to 'take the waters' or travel to the Alps for the air. This did not appear to slow the popular interest in mineral spas, hiking, or leisure tourism in general (Browne 1990; Porter 1990; Cowie et al 1997). Hydrotherapy had fallen out of favour during the Middle Ages, but was revived by Vincent Priessnitz who developed the idea of spa therapy in the early 19th century. Priessnitz's ideas quickly spread and doctors like Joel Shaw in America developed 'water cures' along European lines. Throughout much of the 19th century, spa therapies became some of the most popular remedies for overwrought, well-to-do people across Europe and North America and European spa centres promised a break from the hustle and bustle of new urban living and a chance to breathe fresh air, travel and regain one's vitality.

Exercise therapy, or gymnastics, occupied a difficult position in the consciousness of men and women in the 19th century. Those that worked in manual occupations toiled relentlessly and had no need for physical training, but new classes of sedentary workers grew to be a concern for health reformers. Unlike today, exercise in public was rare. There were no gymnasia that people could attend and swimming pools were for bathing only. While some physicians like Gustaf Zander pioneered the development of therapeutic exercise equipment, it would take until World War I before they came into widespread use (Hansson & Ottosson 2015). Sports, therefore, occupied the only significant outlet for vigorous physical activity, and men particularly took to football, horse-riding, tennis and other activities increasingly as the century wore on. Women's physical activity remained highly restricted, however; a point I will return to later in the chapter.

Mechanotherapy, including massage, bone-setting and other mobilisations had long been recognised as therapeutic techniques, including references by Hippocrates, Galen and later Johan de St. Amand (in the 13th century), Paré (in the 16th), Sydenham (17th) and Tissot in the 18th (Krusen 1942, p. 38). Eighteenth-century doctors like John Hunter, Percivall Pott, James Paget and Nicholas Andre gave rise to the orthopaedic medicine, studying the value of movement and mobilisation of the tissues after an injury, formalising the bone-setting that had been its crude forerunner (Paris 2000).

The most systematic development in the physical therapies during the 19th century, however, occurred in the field of therapeutic gymnastics, under the work of poet and fencing master, Pehr Henrik Ling (1776–1839) at the Royal Central Institute of Gymnastics (RCIG) in Stockholm, Sweden. Ling established forms of gymnastics to 'recreate some of the physical splendour that had previously distinguished the Swedish and Gothic people' (Ottosson 2011, p. 89), and this concern for individual and collective (masculine) degeneracy made Ling's system popular among romantic idealists, aesthetes, doctors and the military (Ottosson 2011). Ling's classes were grounded in natural sciences and were closely allied to anatomy, physiology and pathology, and strongly emphasised the Enlightenment belief that man was the agent of his own destiny (Eichberg 1995; Ottosson 2010; Russell 2013; Climent & Ballester 2003). Drawing on powerful Enlightenment discourses, advocates of Ling's system argued that the natural sciences were the 'true leveller that widens and cleanses the artery from which the truth of Gymnastics flood' (Branting's speeches 1842, vol. 6, GCI:s Enskilda arkiv, RA (National Archives), cited in Ottosson 2011, p. 91). Anders Ottosson has argued that the many of the systematic principles adopted by doctors, and later physical therapists, in the 20th century, drew on systems developed at the RCIG under Ling (Ottosson 2011). Significantly, medicine's adoption of orthopaedic medicine owes a great deal more to Ling's physical therapies than Cyriax, Mennell, Still, Palmer and others have acknowledged. Indeed, it was 'Physical Therapists "instructing medical physicians," [that laid the foundations stones of orthopaedic medicine] and not the other way around' (Ottosson 2011, p. 85).

All branches of the physical therapies blossomed in the latter years of the 19th century, with many doctors writing comprehensive treatise on the science and application of these approaches. Books by Douglas Graham (Graham 1884), John Harvey Kellogg (Kellogg 1895), William Murrell (Murrell 1886), Hartvig Nissen (Nissen 1899), Kurre Ostrom (Ostrom 1891), Mathias Roth (Roth 1852), Joseph Schreiber (Schreiber 1887), Thomas Stretch Dowse (Stretch Dowse 1887), A. Symons Eccles (Symons Eccles 1895), George Herbert Taylor (Smith 1860) and others all provided comprehensive evidence that the physical therapies had become mainstream medical modalities and had achieved an unprecedented public popularity. Physiotherapy was born into this environment and appeared just at the point when doctors were beginning to turn their attentions elsewhere.

Doctors had shown for some time a desire to hand over the more repetitive and technical aspects of the physical therapies to others. Morus argues some doctors, uncomfortable with new technology, sought to hand over the use of electrotherapy to nurses who would be trained to use 'the battery' and other devices: 'By making nurses into electricians, some electrotherapists hoped that a suitably skilled and trained workforce for medical electricity could be found without compromising doctors' own skills and status'. (Morus 2006, pp. 247–8).

There were clearly advantages in this for nurses looking to establish new professional careers, but there were risks too, and some of these will be explored later in the chapter. Before then, I want to reflect on what we know about the physical therapies in the centuries before the birth of the physiotherapy profession and consider how some of these discourses would have influenced the actions of the profession's founders at the end of the 19th century.

A particularly partial history

History is never without its biases and the stories we are told about our past are always inflected with the author's own interests and perspectives. So, we must always read accounts of past events as partial, incomplete and as only one of a number of possible portrayals. A critical reading of history is less about a search for the objective truth of past events and more about seeing what made the account we are given possible, what is said and not said and whose interests these particular narratives serve. To that end, we need to look at the histories of the physical therapies with a critical eye and try to look beyond the surface detail.

The first observation one might make of recorded history of the physical therapies is that it clearly draws heavily on Enlightenment beliefs that emphasise 'man's' conquest of nature. There are, for example, quite comprehensive accounts of the discovery and application of electrotherapy, actinotherapy and systematised forms of gymnastics, but much less on massage, indigenous healing practices and lay beliefs. All of these accounts focus on the processes by which we came to learn about the elemental forces of magnetism and electrical energy; how we developed tools to measure it, capture it and then generate it ourselves; how this was tested and, eventually, used therapeutically. Every step of the way conforms to a Western narrative of scientific discovery that was particularly powerful as a public discourse from the 18th century onwards. In this narrative, the might and primordial power of God's natural creation was tamed by science and commanded by man for the greater good of society. There is nothing to say that this account is wrong or a falsehood, but many might agree that it is unbalanced and in many ways self-serving. This is particularly important when we consider how these ideas influenced early physiotherapists because the profession was almost exclusively female in its early years and women's voices are completely absent from the story of the physical therapies before 1900.

It is entirely possible that counter-narratives of man's progress to enlightenment exist (and can be seen in the work of people like Rachel Maines, Elaine Showalter, Susan Rubin Suleiman and others (Maines 1999; Showalter 1985; Suleiman 1985)), but these remain marginal within the history of physiotherapy at the moment. Recent work in the critical history of the body has also pointed to a second observation that stems from an emphasis on the systematic command of bodies (Czachesz 2014; Metzler 2010; Bynum & Kalof 2010; Zweiniger-Bargielowska 2010; Gilbert 2005). Many of the accounts of remedial gymnastics and therapeutic exercise from the 18th and 19th centuries concern the disciplined and systematic application of particular regimes (Morus 2006, 1999). Those approaches that provide the best example of this kind of regimentation – including Ling's approach to Swedish Remedial Exercise – are promoted as the dominant narrative. Other modalities with less instrumental or biomechanistic foundations feature much less prominently. One of the arguments for this has been that the physical therapies played an important role in governing people's conduct and disciplining the way bodies were 'used'. Rhythmical gymnastics, turnverein, Muscular Christianity and other forms of physical culture, for example, played a hugely significant role in eugenically-inspired attempts to arrest racial decay during the late 19th and early 20th century (see Chapter 8) (Macdonald 2013; Zweiniger-Bargielowska 2006; Putney 2009; Vertinsky & Hargreaves 2006). The association between these approaches to movement and the Nazism of the 1930s and 1940s Germany reminds us that we cannot afford to read these accounts as politically or socially neutral.

What is also clear from accounts of the history of the physical therapies, is how prominent men are. Prior to 1900, there are no scientific accounts of the physical therapies written by women. Indeed, there are no accounts of *any* form of physical therapy in print from that time written by women. The history we read is, therefore, a gendered history; a history inflected through and largely serving men, in which masters of science have crafted a narrative of their achievements. This gives weight to the long-held argument that the history of science written by men often privileges the conquest of nature and man's ability to be free from bias in his judgement of objective truth. Given this, it is perhaps not surprising that the history of the physical therapies is most developed where men have been able to promote this narrative. How much this provides a partial picture of the physical therapies prior to 1900 is hard to say. If it is a distinctly one-sided account, it almost entirely excludes women's accounts of physical therapy practice from consideration and so must, ironically, be seen as distinctly biased.

One of the striking features of 19th century accounts of physical therapy, is how profoundly successful simple treatments like massage seemed to be. Lacking the scientific rigour of today's texts, doctors would often include case studies of patients who had benefitted from their treatments, and some of these make you wonder if the physical therapies acquired Lazarus-like power in the hands of a skilled manipulator. Arthur Symons Eccles (surgeon, and author of a number of texts on massage in the late 19th century, and certainly one of the most scientifically-informed practitioners of his day) illustrates this approach. In his book, *The Practice of Massage* (Symons Eccles 1895), the author tells of a 38-year-old woman, for instance, who presents with a three-year history of diarrhoea, including two years spent in bed. In the year before being seen by the surgeon (1889), she begins passing 'foetid' stools containing pus, blood and mucus (1895, p. 187). The patient was given a simple course of abdominal massage in October of 1890 and by December was reporting weight gain, the end to her diarrhoea and return to full health.

Rest and massage were also prescribed to a medical colleague who had been thrown from a dogcart in June 1889, and 'fell on to the back of his head, turning a somersault, so that the head was forcibly thrown forwards, the chin being pressed firmly against the breast-bone', rendering him unconscious for 20 minutes (1895, p. 294). Six weeks after recovering in bed from his head injury and broken ribs, the patient developed tingling and numbness in his fingers, giddiness, headaches, depression, loss of appetite and disturbed sleep. Symons Eccles reports that his neck movements were severely restricted, and any forwards flexion caused numbness in his hands. However, after a short course of massage, the symptoms completely cleared and by mid-November, the patient was restored to normal health.

Massage was used for a wide variety of conditions that would be treated with drugs and surgery today: skin diseases, muscle atrophy, early stage fractures (before fixation), constipation, anaemia, obesity, rickets, scoliosis, neuralgia, sciatica, chronic alcoholism, asthma and heart disease. In each case, extensive records account for the remarkable success of these therapies in the hands of a skilled operator[2].

For many doctors, the physical therapies not only provided a powerful demonstration of medicine's command over nature, but also showed that man was not *opposed* to nature, per se, but rather sought to harness it and work in harmony with it. Physicians like John Harvey Kellogg in America, for example, established entire systems of living based on a return to nature and a rigorous application of bodily discipline. Kellogg, along with many other social commentators of his day, was concerned that modern man had lost touch with nature; that inventions like the railways and the telegraph were isolating people in offices, forcing them to endure long hours of 'brain work'. Kellogg was convinced that this was injurious to people's health and set about turning the dilapidated Battle Creek Sanatorium into a world-leading health spa (Schwarz 2006). Kellogg favoured a highly regimented, systematised approach to life, including diet (Kellogg developed a now famous nutritious cereal that provided specific health benefits for his patients), rest, relaxation and vigorous exercise – often in groups, following principles similar to Ling's gymnastics (Hartelius 1896).

Kellogg tapped into powerful anti-progressive discourses that permeated Western society in the 19th century and that found their expression in the writings of people like Henry David Thoreau and romantic poets and painters. For some, science was a profanity and evidence of man's folly in the face of God's creation. For others, it was rampant technological progress that they feared. It is ironic then that many turned to medical science and the rational application of the physical therapies for the cure. Notwithstanding these concerns, man's seemingly insatiable will to power (Nietzsche 1973) only accelerated the pace of medical and social innovation in the years leading up to the 20th century, and central to this drive was the pervasive influence of the Industrial Revolution and the changes this brought about in attitudes towards 'man the machine' (Bizup 2003; Fracchia 2008; O'Neill 1986).

Industrial bodies

As much as anxiety surrounding the pace of life accompanied the rapid expansion of European and American civilisation in the 18th and 19th centuries, it did not slow down progress or stem the drive for greater individual and collective power among the developing economies of Europe and North America. Significantly for the physical therapies, many of the societal reforms were directed at the bodies of the state's citizens and treatment techniques advocated by doctors were used for a broader 'orthopaedics' of the population in the years following the Industrial Revolution.

The Industrial Revolution transformed civil society in the developing economies. Life in the 16th and 17th centuries was almost exclusively based around small agricultural settlements, where most people were engaged in the production of the necessities of life. The welfare of whole communities depended on an annual supply of food and this, in turn, was subject to the vagaries of the weather.

Food production also depended on the availability of labour and so the yearly cycle of sowing, cropping and harvesting dictated the community's prosperity in the year ahead. Because food production was so labour intensive and volumes produced relatively low, diseases of malnutrition were common, leading to premature death for many and high infant mortality rates prior to the advent of industrialised food production.

With the discovery of the seed drill (1701), the iron plough (1730), the threshing machine (1784) and other new agricultural technologies like crop rotation and selective breeding of animals, agriculture became a much more productive activity. The effect on rural communities was profound. Now, instead of needing 30 people to work the fields to feed a small village, enough food could be produced for 300 people with only a handful of workers needed to tend the agricultural machinery. This created surpluses that could be traded at nearby towns for new consumer goods and services. The availability of surplus food for less manual labour concentrated profits in the hands of those who owned the means of production generating a sudden and dramatic rise in wealth for landowners and employers. At the same time, the health of the population improved as food became more plentiful and calorific. Longevity increased as infants lived longer and death rates from community-acquired diseases fell. These benefits were offset somewhat, however, because people who had once been employed in their community's yearly agricultural cycle were now themselves surplus labour and many were subsequently driven off their land. Thus began the long exodus from the countryside that represented one of the great social revolutions of the Industrial Revolution.

Over the course of the 18th century, the populations in the great cities of Europe and North America expanded rapidly and became increasingly polarised. Those with capital developed civic society and pushed for cultural improvements in the arts, news, transportation, economic and political reform, while those who had fled the countryside in poverty often found themselves living in overcrowded, filthy, squalid conditions with few prospects and little hope of a happy, satisfying life. Not surprisingly, much of the 18th century saw social revolt as politically active and urban poor protested their appalling living conditions.

How, one might ask, does this relate to the history of the physical therapies? In the first instance, as well as social upheaval, the 17th and 18th centuries saw the birth of modern governments whose primary purpose was to ensure that the population *did not* revolt. Nation states increasingly came to realise that the traditional power of the sovereign was being eroded and that the threat of beheading and summary execution was insufficient as a way of managing whole populations (Foucault 1977). New approaches were required that centred on the needs of the population as a whole but also on the actions of individual citizens (a new word at the time, connoting someone with rights *and* responsibilities). Censuses and surveys, services and institutions, duties and freedoms were all 'technologies' developed by governments in this period to better manage the population and increase its health, wealth and happiness.

At the heart of the emergence of modern government lay a realisation that civic leaders could not, themselves, administer every corner of social life and that some control needed to be vested in the hands of trusted agents – people that agreed to promote the government's desires, in return for state patronage. Doctors, teachers, local councillors, the police and others all benefitted from a mutually agreeable relationship with the state where access to patients, subsidies and legal protections were offered in return for attention to people's needs (Rose & Miller 1992).

Initially, these focused on the causes of social unrest (poverty, illiteracy, sickness etc.) and medicine willingly took on the responsibility for the health and wellbeing of the population. Central to doctors' authority was their ability to define what constituted sickness and what constituted normality; how the body would be understood and the language with which that knowledge would be communicated (an exclusive language like Latin was particularly significant here); how the nascent health system would be organised and how services would be distributed; who was entitled to care and who was not (Armstrong 1998; Rose 1994). Although this sounds very clear cut, these transformations took many years to eventuate and they were not without their contests and challenges[3], but the effect was to consolidate power in the hands of the medical profession and give it a monopoly on how we would be conditioned to think about health for the next 200 years.

Many of the governmental reforms brought about by medicine in the name of the state were directed at the individual's body and had a distinctly 'moral' tinge to their function. Boys had rings lined with metal studs fitted to their penises to prevent them from masturbating, 'hysterical' women were locked away in asylums and experimented upon and epileptics had their skulls opened without anaesthetic to relieve their symptoms (Annandale 1998; Samson 1999). Slowly, though, like governments at large, doctors learnt to be more circumspect and humanistic in their approach to medicine and subtler technologies were deployed to engender health. Medical care moved from the home to the hospital as doctors learnt to use constant surveillance as a way to encourage compliance (Armstrong 1995). Epidemiological data began to be increasingly important in differentiating those who fell within and those who fell outside the range of normal seen across the population. And the growth of medical specialties consolidated knowledge and power in the hands of doctors such that only a lengthy and costly training could equip a person with a necessary licence to practice.

Naturally, this licence carried with it a cachet that elevated doctors to some of the most elite members of society (the trade-off for years of service to the state), which meant that until the 20th century and the birth of the welfare state, few could have afforded regular medical care. And while a few doctors undertook charity work and a number of hospitals operated under charitable status, they were often overcrowded, dirty and poorly staffed. Thus, good medical care was largely the province of the rich and 'well-to-do'. This returns us to one of the achievements of the Industrial Revolution – the creation of a wealthy professional class that physiotherapists would aspire to become part of in the early part of the 20th century.

Formal medical care prior to 1900 was largely delivered by a medical elite to a population of middle- and upper-class patrons who could afford the cost of care. Treatments, therefore, concentrated upon conditions that were common in these sections of the population and physical therapies were some of the most respected, accessible and benign remedies available (Armstrong 1995). Compared with the primitive and largely untested pharmacopoeia possessed by physicians or the barber surgery of the pre-anaesthetic, pre-antibiotic 19th century, physical therapies were popular and largely well regarded by the general public. Doctors insisted that to practice the physical therapies, one needed a detailed working knowledge of anatomy, physiology and kinesiology, and they couched their practices in uncommon language to give the public the sense that their years of study and high cost of care was grounded in a deep appreciation for science (e.g. effleurage, petrissage, actinotherapy, galvanism, mechanotherapy, balneotherapy etc.). Their regimes were firm and they insisted on them being strictly adhered to (Nissen 1899; Stretch Dowse 1887; Symons Eccles 1895). To deepen their social significance even further, doctors frequently connected the person's suffering to deeper concerns (for the pace of life, moral decay, poor habits, noxious environment etc.) so that the patient would see that the doctor had profound insights beyond the limits of their ailment (Lutz 1991).

Importantly, up to the end of the 19th century, there were few calls for doctors to provide physical therapies for the whole population. No welfare state existed, there were few large hospitals and formal rehabilitation services would not become commonplace until the early 20th century. So, medicine faced little competition and only looked to nurture other professional groups if it wanted to hand some of its techniques on to subordinates. Thus, doctors were the sole providers of orthodox physical therapy prior to the 20th century, essentially serving a population of patients who could afford their care. There was then a second tier of unregulated salesmen, healers, masseurs and bone setters who had less choice about the location of their work.

Things began to change as the 19th century drew to a close, however, with the discovery of germ theory and over the course of the next 50 years, medicine would transform itself into a modern, techno-science-based profession and would largely turn away from the time consuming and rather 'old-fashioned' physical therapies. Many of the approaches developed by medicine would remain and would be a powerful influence on the founders of massage professions around the world. In contrast to medicine, however, many of these founders would be women and the way they chose to absorb, challenge or reinvent the strategies deployed by doctors in the previous two centuries would have a powerful influence on physiotherapy for the next 100 years.

Women and the physical therapies

Medicine is often portrayed as having a very masculine history, with its grounding in Enlightenment science, its inventors and technology. By contrast, physiotherapy was a profession founded by women and has remained female-dominated for its entire history. So, when we consider how physiotherapy began, we must consider how its founders navigated this very androcentric (male-centred) world of medicine and established their own legitimacy. This is important because the discourses that influenced the founders of physiotherapy in England, America, Australia,

Canada and elsewhere were discourses that almost entirely *excluded* women (or only included them as willing accomplices or patients of the masterful doctor). How did the androcentric world of physical medicine influence their practice and the way they decided to establish the profession? How did they successfully occupy the space left by doctors who migrated away from physical therapies and towards surgery, microbiology and germ theory? How could they share in medicine's state patronage, while promoting new professional roles for women acting, sometimes, against societal conventions? And how were their actions comparable with nursing and midwifery – other female-dominated health professions that were also gaining a foothold in orthodox healthcare?

I want to approach these questions by examining the role that the treatment of neurasthenia played in the founding of the physiotherapy profession. There has been a great deal written about neurasthenia over the last 150 years yet, remarkably, nothing from the perspective of the therapists who were so instrumental in administering the treatment[4]. There are lengthy accounts from doctors, even biographies of some of the figures who gained fame from their work on the disorder, and we have many accounts from those patients who endured its ruthless treatment regime, but nothing from the therapists themselves. Some of the possible reasons for this will be explored next.

Neurasthenia was one of the most widely recognised conditions of the 19th century. It was closely related to hysteria and hypochondria and presented mainly in affluent working age women (although cases were also seen in men). Its symptoms bore remarkable similarities to those presenting in present-day conditions like anorexia, breathing pattern disorders, anxiety and depression, chronic fatigue and fibromyalgia, and included loss of appetite, widespread non-specific neuromuscular pain, headaches, light-headedness and a feeling of detachment, poor sleep and restlessness. Although the symptoms were debilitating, the condition was thought to be prevalent in women who had been overwhelmed by modern life and, unlike hysteria – which was characterised by women who were vain and self-serving – neurasthenia concentrated on the leisured classes of society who suffered from too much 'brain work' or social refinement. Neurasthenia carries with it a certain cachet, such that William Marrs, writing in his book *Confessions of a Neurasthenic*, argued that the best thing about neurasthenia was that it allowed one to 'move in neurasthenic circles' (Lutz 1991, p. 7). The causes for neurasthenia were as uncertain as its presentation. Some doctors – all men, we should remember – suggested that it was a function of women's reproduction. All humans, they argued, were like batteries and carried a certain capacity for activity. Women's energy reserves were primarily directed at reproduction. Menstruation, pregnancy, labour and childrearing placed heavy demands on the woman's body, resulting in only a limited capacity for other types of work. Mental work especially but also sexual activity of any kind (except passive intercourse) were prone to deplete the woman's limited resources, leaving her exhausted. Rest, food and freedom from mental stimulation were critical if the woman was to retain her health.

This argument about women's physical capacity fed closely into 18th and 19th century thoughts about electricity, which explains to some extent why electrotherapy became so popular in the Victorian era. It was also offered as a justification for restricting access to education for girls, because too much mental work might tax their limited nervous resources. Such ideas are easily dismissed as misogynistic today, but they cannot be ignored not least because they played such an important role in the formation of the physiotherapy profession.

There were strong suggestions of hereditary links to neurasthenia and it was thought that it did not appear in the lower classes or uncivilised races. Citing George Beard – the doctor who coined the name neurasthenia in his 1869 book *Neurasthenia, or Nervous Exhaustion* (Beard 1869) – Lutz points to the overtly racist beliefs surrounding the disorder:

> Neurasthenia struck brain-workers but no other kind of laborer. It attacked those, such as artists and connoisseurs with the most refined sensitivities. It affected the more "advanced" races, especially the Anglo-Saxon. It affected only those of the more "advanced" religious persuasions, proof of which was that "no catholic country is very nervous". Some people or peoples in other racial or social categories have been "moderately nervous," according to Beard, but only if they were at "stopping-places between the strength of the barbarian and the sensitiveness of the highly civilised".
>
> (Lutz 1991, p. 6)

Neurasthenia represented an idealised image of femininity. Pale, weak and dependent on the support of a paternalistic male figure, neurasthenic women captivated late 19th century society in Europe and America, where paintings captured the refined sensitivity of these virtuous, 'Gilded Age' women (Williams et al 2004). We now know that simple things like corsetry caused many of the symptoms experienced by neurasthenic women, and many of the psychological sequelae may well be explained by the mental and physical confinement of the time, but at the time women's 'nature' was thought to be a more likely cause.

There were no professional roles for educated middle- and upper-class women in the 19th century other than as a governess or a nurse and neither of these offered respectability or necessary income to support an independent life (even if society had allowed this). Thus, women of wealthy families had to 'marry money' if they were to retain their social status. Women who did find a wealthy partner often entered loveless marriages that involved a regimented daily routine of social customs and practices. These activities often centred around daily 'performances' in which the woman would dress for breakfast, then dress for a walk in the park, before performing some minor philanthropic work in the community. She would dress again for dinner and finally dress for bed. Each occasion warranted a different costume, but all (even sleeping in some instances) involved corsetry.

Social conventions maintained that girls as young as five began using 'stays' in their clothes to control their posture and develop the exaggerated and idealised womanly form (see Figure 2.1). Years of lacing had a serious effect on women's physiology. It increased intra-abdominal pressure causing uterine prolapse and hypoxia of the liver, spleen and other organs; it made it possible to eat only small

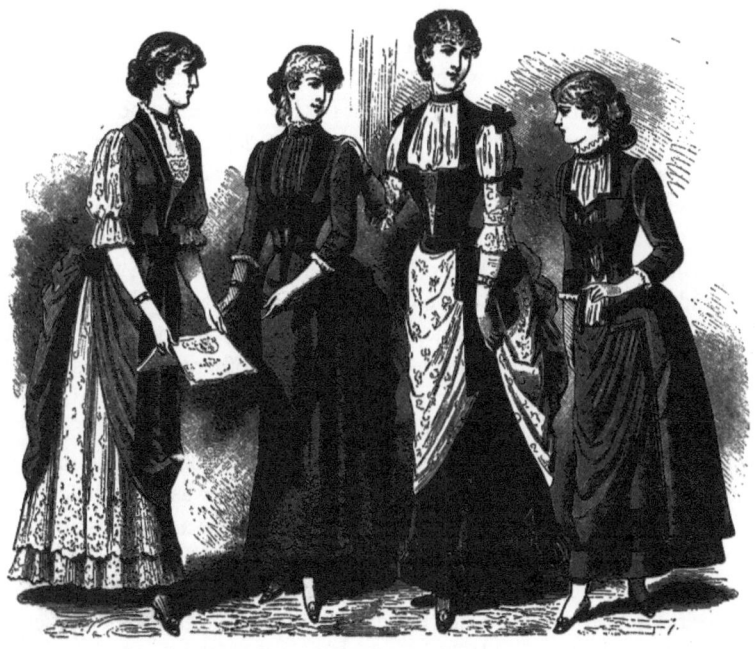

Figure 2.1 Popular fashions for 'young ladies' showing extreme corsetry circa 1883. Alan Bott (1932), *Our Mothers*, published by The Orion Publishing Group.

amounts of food and disrupted normal gastro-intestinal flow; it restricted venous return and diaphragm excursion, leading to the classical image of the swooning 'sofa wife'. Added to this, the life of an educated woman, forced into a marriage as one of the few options available to her, was unremittingly dull. There were few opportunities for meaningful work, there was little significant social engagement or opportunity to use whatever knowledge or skills she had been 'allowed' to develop. Such was the life of exactly the same class of woman who found the Society of Trained Masseuses and Physiotherapists.

If the conditions that led to neurasthenia were bad, the treatment that was proposed was possibly even worse. In an act of remarkable cruelty and unconcealed brutality, a treatment programme known as the 'Rest Cure' came to prominence and became not only the treatment of choice for sufferers of neurasthenia, but also an important influence on rehabilitation medicine in the early part of the 20th century.

The Rest Cure was devised by one of America's foremost neurologists, Silas Weir Mitchell. Weir Mitchell had achieved some notoriety for his work on peripheral nerve injuries during the American Civil War, but found his greatest success with an approach to the treatment of hysteria and neurasthenia that was exported to Britain, France, Germany, Holland and elsewhere (Gijswijt-Hofstra & Porter 2001; Bezio 2014; Poirier 1983; Lovering 1971). Weir Mitchell was clear that neurasthenic women suffered greatly from pandering family and friends and suggested that only if the patient was free of their interference would s/he be able to bend to the doctor's will and effect a cure. Thus, under the Rest Cure, women were removed from their families and housed in a nursing home or other residence for six to eight weeks, during which time they were prevented from engaging in *any* form of mental activity. Reading the news or letters from home was forbidden, as was taxing conversation or anything that might deplete the woman's mental resources. The patient was confined to bed for a large part of the treatment and was dressed, toileted and attended to for the entire period by a nurse. To re-establish the woman's vitality, a strict course of feeding was instituted, sometimes by force, and Weir Mitchell felt that the key to recovery lay in restoring the woman's bodily strength and tone (Mitchell 1884). To ensure that the woman regained her strength, a careful course of (passive) treatments was instituted – and here we come to the part played by the physical therapies. Massage, electrotherapy and passive movements were begun from day one, gradually increasing in their intensity each week until the woman regained her vitality.

The treatment was brutal and cruel, and Weir Mitchell made no attempt to hide that the woman needed to be treated like a child if she was to be healed. Thus, much of the approach was predicated on a desire to impose a strict discipline. This regimentation and infantilisation was personified in the 'cell' that the patient came to occupy during her confinement and became the focus for a great deal of bitter feminist critique over the last century (Schuster 2005; Bassuk 1985; Poirier 1983; Oppenheim 1991; Sicherman 1977). Central to many of these criticisms were the accounts of women patients themselves, including the celebrated work of suffragette Charlotte Perkins-Gilman, who was a patient of Weir Mitchell's and documented her experiences in a semi-autobiographical novel called *The Yellow Wallpaper* (Perkins-Gilman 1899). Perkins-Gilman's account was by no means isolated though, and many educated and well-known figures of the era were neurasthenics, including Virginia Woolf, Jane Addams and Florence Nightingale[5].

The highpoint in the popularity of neurasthenia as a diagnosis was the 1890s, after which time new diagnostic categories like neurosis and psychosis replaced it under the influence of the new field of psychiatry. But the term neurasthenia continued to be used well into the 1930s and approaches to it were used extensively during the First World War to diagnose shell shock.

There are many striking things about the history of neurasthenia, not least its embodiment of masculine attitudes towards women's bodies, medicine and healthcare in general. The extensive body of literature that has now built up around the disorder also reveals some other important issues, not least the dearth of research on the work of the therapists who administered the Rest Cure. As I mentioned earlier, there is extensive research from the medical perspective, and a large volume of commentary on the patient's experience, but nothing from the perspective of the women who administered the treatment itself. We know that a nurse was resident with the patient during the course of their confinement, but we also know that many doctors employed additional nurse-masseuses to perform the therapeutic work. In either case, the delicacy of the situation demanded that the practitioner possessed the right balance of skills, strength and tact to manage the complex psychological situation. The doctor needed to trust that the therapist would administer his treatment programme exactly as it had been prescribed, effectively acting as a surrogate in his absence as Gilbert Ballet explained in 1908;

> Whenever it is possible, the patient should be placed in a special establishment where there is a physician who will supervise the carrying out of the therapeutic measures of which the treatment is composed. A nurse should be told off [sic] to attend her. The choice of this nurse is not a matter of indifference; the success or failure of the treatment may depend on it. The nurse's functions are of the highest importance; she must not only be sufficiently trained to execute the physician's orders satisfactorily; she must also be well enough endowed in respect of intelligence and character to understand thoroughly the task she has undertaken, and to bring to it all the tact and firmness required. It must not be forgotten that this woman will be for weeks and for months the patient's only companion. She must be amiable and kindly enough not to inspire her charge with hatred or aversion, skillful enough to distract her by conversation and reading, and to help her to support patiently both the details of the treatment ordered and the weariness of a long isolation; and finally, firm and intelligent enough to have a certain ascendency over her, and to impose on her without harshness the discipline of the treatment. It is easy to see that it would be absurd to give to a woman of cultivated mind a nurse who was altogether illiterate and uneducated, or as we have occasionally seen done, a quiet young girl without experience or authority.
>
> (Ballet 1908, pp. 350–1)

Despite the popularity of physical therapies among the medical profession, it was recognised that some treatments were repetitive and uninteresting, and did not require the expertise of a doctor to perform them. Thus, a large number of unlicensed and differently qualified masseurs and masseuses operated in the larger cities across Europe (some of the finest having trained in Sweden under Ling's instruction). Many of these female practitioners were brought in by doctors to help manage the neurasthenic women.

Most masseuses had knowledge of 'the battery' (galvanism), which had become a popular treatment for a range of health and beauty concerns, and its use fed into the 19th century notion that machines that generated electricity could replace lost vitality in patients (hence its popularity as part of the Rest Cure). Alongside galvanism, masseuses were skilled in passive and active movements, general and localised massage and most were familiar working with doctors. They were, therefore, an ideal ally to the doctor.

The question remains, how these educated women, from similar social backgrounds to their patients, reconciled their role as surrogate doctors – with all its paternalistic overtones – when they imposed his will in the rooms of the neurasthenic patient?[6] Unlike nursing, which took to heart the idea of the noble, virtuous woman and was the bedrock of the suffragette movement, masseuses needed a closer affinity with more masculine notions of science and the body. And yet, many of the early masseuses were nurses and midwives exploring the possibility of new professional roles. Likely, a thorough training in medical science and the opportunity to work alongside doctors, and actually help people, was a far more seductive image than the life experienced by many of the women they often treated. But this, in itself required some significant costs and sacrifices. Masseuses would have walked a fine line between being seen as 'new' women[7], and functioning only as handmaidens to the medical profession. The question remains though, how members of the Society of Trained Masseuses in the UK managed to do this and establish physiotherapy as a profession is, in my view at least, a remarkable story that I pick up on in the next chapter. To conclude this chapter, though, I want to recap over some of the important tensions that I have explored so far.

Closing words

The story of the physical therapies before the 20th century is an important one because it points to the conditions that made physiotherapy possible. The founders of the profession were responding to important social issues when they formed their Society and so if we are to better understand what they did and why, we must interrogate some of their influences. In this chapter I have largely concentrated on four social discourses that have made physiotherapy historically and socially possible, and influenced it throughout its long history.

The first is the influence of Judeo-Christian beliefs about the sinfulness of sensuality that played so heavily upon Victorian attitudes towards touch. Physiotherapy in most organisationally countries developed with a strong European heritage where Christianity is still the predominant faith, and its influence can be seen throughout the entire history of the profession. The second is the role that Enlightenment ideas about science, knowledge and truth played in shaping ideas and beliefs about the gendered nature of physical therapy. The history of science in the West is a very 'male' history, littered with accounts of brilliant inventors and rational thinkers who sought to conquer nature and command the body. Physiotherapy, by contrast, has always been a female-dominated profession and so much of this chapter has focused on the tensions that must have been encountered by the founders of the profession as they sought to navigate the masculine world of Victorian medicine and find their point of difference.

One of the most fascinating questions that requires much greater consideration is how the founders of the profession balanced the need to be subservient to doctors with their own interests in developing new professional roles for women. Nurses and midwives had their own response (which met with a great deal of social opposition in some quarters)[8], which held strongly to feminist values, but it seems physiotherapists took a different path. It may be that physiotherapy was the first female-dominated profession to successfully embrace an androcentric model of practice and this may be a significant and underexplored aspect of women's labour history (Heap 1995; Parry 1995; Miles-Tapping 1989).

Clearly, this approach was highly successful. It met with the support of the medical profession and masseuses were able to establish the public's trust. It addressed many of the tensions surrounding the sensuality of touch and it provided women with new professional roles. But early masseuses also used their female patients (maybe to the point of exploitation) to gain professional recognition with the medical profession and the state. It would be interesting to read how the profession's founders grappled with this tension, but to date, no accounts of early masseuses have been found.

What we do know is that although female masseuses were common in the 19th century, physical therapy was, for a long time, doctor's work. We also know that before the welfare state was created, most people only received physical therapy if they could afford it. It was a product of luxury and surplus – the third discourse – that was made possible by the fourth, the Industrial Revolution. Medicine functioned as a therapeutic agent, but its success owes as much to its ability to respond to governmental priorities and become a trusted agent of the state. Medicine's orthodox status and its prosperity owes much to its willingness to manage the health of the population for the State and for this it was given immense power. Key among social discourses in the 18th and 19th century was the desire to translate the lessons of industrialisation into the lives of the populace, which blended beautifully with medicine's desire to see the body-as-machine. Thus, medicine operated in an intimate three-way relationship between industrial markets and the state to create a very powerful idea of what it meant to be productive, healthy, wealthy and wise.

If the founders of the physiotherapy profession were going to be successful, they would have had to find a way to assimilate many of these discourses into their practice, while also addressing some of the rising tensions around massage and touch. It would not be enough to simply be a good physical therapist. There were plenty of people who were good at all manner of physical therapies in the late 1900s. Indeed, the market for masseurs and masseuses was 'overstocked' by the time the Society of Trained Masseuses came into being (*The Morning* 1894). To be successful, the founders would have needed to have done much more than colonise a few trusted treatment methods. They would have only been successful if their actions dovetailed in with medicine's approach to the body, if they had been able to gain the trust of the medical profession and the public, if they had been able to attend to governmental priorities and prove the necessity of their work and if they had been able to do this while also pioneering new roles for women in a climate hostile to any form of therapy that involved sensuality and touch. In the next chapter, I explore how the founders of the Society of Trained Masseuses achieved this remarkable feat and put in place a template for the profession that would not only serve their needs, but also retain an enduring influence on the profession for the next 120 years.

Notes

1 Although exact dates are unknown, it is thought that Asklepiades lived from the 1st to 2nd centuries A.D.

2 Symons Eccles was almost certainly one of a number of doctors who employed masseurs to undertake some of his work. Many other doctors would have done so too, but their writings are incredibly vague on this point and, as far as I am aware, no first-hand accounts exist from masseurs prior to 1895 to verify their practices.

3 One of the principal challenges medicine faced was from the sham doctor or quack. Rather than seeing the quack as something doctors wanted to eliminate, however, we should consider how doctors used the popular image of the quack as a point of contrast. Doctors needed, and nurtured the idea of the quack as a tool to promote their own legitimacy (Fournier 2002).

4 There are some excellent resources for those interested in further study of neurasthenia, including (Loughran 2008; Schuster 2003; Sicherman 1977; Schuster 2005; Williams et al 2004; Haller Jr 1971; Gijswijt-Hofstra & Porter 2001).

5 Many notable men, including Marcel Proust, Charles Darwin, Theodore Roosevelt and William James, were also diagnosed as either neurasthenic or hypochondriacal, and here the diagnosis was used to promote a concern for the efete and somewhat feminising influence of culture on the more rugged ideals of 19th century manhood.

6 We know that the Rest Cure was important to the early Society of Trained Masseuses because some of the texts they used for training address the treatment directly. In M.A. Ellison and Margaret Palmer's books, written explicitly for Society members, large sections are given over to discussion of the 'Weir Mitchell treatment' (Palmer 1901, pp. 218–21; Ellison 1898, pp. 82–88). Other texts used by early registrants also give prominence to this approach (Creighton-Hale 1893, pp. 99–108; Symons Eccles 1895, pp. 254–341). Indeed, L.L. Despard was still discussing the Weir Mitchell treatment in her 1916 book written as a set text for members of the newly named Incorporated Society of Trained Masseuses (Despard 1916, pp. 287–8).

7 The idea of the 'new woman' began to emerge in the mid-1890s and was largely a derogatory term for a middle- and upper-class woman who defied gendered conventions around appearance, education, social intercourse, work and other spheres of social life. The term later became a clarion call for feminists and suffragetts (Nelson 2000).

8 In many countries, legal recognition of masseuses occurred before that of nurses and midwives.

References

Annandale, E., 1998, *The sociology of health and medicine: A critical introduction*. Polity Press, Cambridge, UK.

Armstrong, D., 1995, The rise of surveillance medicine, *Sociology of Health & Illness*, 17(3), pp. 393–404.

Armstrong, D., 1998, Decline of the hospital: Reconstructing institutional dangers, *Sociology of Health & Illness*, 20(4), p. 445.

Ballet, G., 1908, *Neurasthenia*, Henry Kimpton, London.

Bassuk, E.L., 1985, The rest cure: Repetition or resolution of Victorian women's conflicts? *Poetics Today*, 6(1/2), pp. 245–57.

Beard, G.M., 1869, Neurasthenia, or nervous exhaustion, *Boston Medical and Surgical Journal*, 80, pp. 217–21.

Bezio, L., 2014, S. Weir Mitchell, 1829–1914: Philadelphia's literary physician, *Journal of the History of Medicine and Allied Sciences*, 69(1), pp. 171–3.

Bizup, J., 2003, *Manufacturing culture: Vindications of early Victorian industry*, University of Virginia Press, Charlottesville, VA.

Browne, J., 1990, Spas and sensibilities: Darwin at Malvern, *Medical History Supplement* (10), pp. 102–13.

Bynum, W.F. & Kalof, L., 2010, *A cultural history of the human body in the Renaissance*, Berg, London.

Calvert, R.N., 2002, *The history of massage: An illustrated survey from around the world*, Inner Traditions/Bear & Company, Rochester, VT.

Climent, J.M. & Ballester, R., 2003, The link between technology and specialist practice in rehabilitation: The model of gymnastic technology in 19th century Spain, *Duynamis*, 23, pp. 269–306.

Colwell, H.A., 1922, *An essay on the history of electrotherapy and diagnosis*, Heinemann, London.

Cowie, L.W., Cowie, E.E. & Hembry, P.M., 1997, *British spas from 1815 to the present: A social history*, Fairleigh Dickinson University Press, NJ.

Creighton-Hale, A., 1893, *The art of massage*, The Scientific Press, London.

Cutter, I.S., 1934, History of physical therapy and its relation to medicine, in *Principles and practice of physical therapy*, W.F. Prior, Hagerstown, MD, pp. 1–115.

Czachesz, I., 2014, *The grotesque body in early Christian discourse: Hell, scatology and metamorphosis*, Routledge, Abingdon, Oxon.

Despard, L.L., 1916, *Textbook of massage and remedial gymnastics*, Oxford University Press, London.

Eichberg, H., 1995, Body culture and democratic nationalism: 'popular gymnastics' in nineteenth-century Denmark, *The International Journal of the History of Sport*, 12(2), pp. 108–24.

Ellison, M.A., 1898, *A manual for students of massage*, Bailliere, Tindall and Cox, London.

Foucault, M., 1977, *Discipline and punish: The birth of the prison*, Allen Lane, London.

Fournier, V., 2002, Amateurism, quackery and professional conduct, in M. Dent & S. Whitehead (eds.), *Managing professional identities: Knowledge, performativities and the 'new' professional*, Routledge, London, pp. 116–37.

Fracchia, J., 2008, The capitalist labour-process and the body in pain: The corporeal depths of Marx's concept of immiseration, *Historical Materialism*, 16(4), pp. 35–66.

Gilbert, P.K., 2005, *Disease, desire, and the body in Victorian women's popular novels*. Cambridge University Press, Cambridge.

Gijswijt-Hofstra, M. & Porter, R., 2001, *Cultures of neurasthenia: From beard to the First World War (Clio Medica 63)*, Rodopi Bv Editions, London.

Graham, D., 1884, *A practical treatise on massage*, William Wood & Co., New York.

Haller Jr, J.S., 1971, Neurasthenia: The medical profession and the 'new woman' of the late nineteenth century, *New York State Journal of Medicine*, 71, p. 474.

Hansson, N. & Ottosson, A., 2015, Nobel Prize for physical therapy?: Rise, fall, and revival of medico-mechanical institutes, *Physical Therapy*, 10.2522/ptj.20140284.

Hartelius, T.J., 1896, *Swedish movements or medical gymnastics*, Modern Medicine Publishing Company, Battle Creek, MI.

Heap, R., 1995, Physiotherapy's quest for professional status in Ontario, 1950–80, *Canadian Bulletin of Medical History/Bulletin Canadien d'Histoire de la Médecine*, 12(1), pp. 69–89.

Kamenetz, H.L., 1960, History of massage, in S. Licht (ed.), *Massage, manipulation and traction*, Elizabeth Licht, New Haven, CN, pp. 3–37.

Kellogg, J.H., 1895, *The art of massage: Its physiological effects and therapeutic application*, Modern Medicine Publishing Company, Battle Creek, MI.

Kleen, E.A., 1918, *Massage and medical gymnastics*, J. & A. Churchill, London.

Krusen, F.H., 1942, *Physical medicine: The employment of physical agents for diagnosis and therapy*, W.B. Saunders, Philadelphia, PA.

Loughran, T., 2008, Hysteria and neurasthenia in pre-1914 British medical discourse and in histories of shell-shock, *History of Psychiatry*, 19(1), pp. 25–46.

Lovering, J.P., 1971, *S. Weir Mitchell*, Ardent Media Inc, London.

Lutz, T., 1991, *American nervousness, 1903: An anecdotal history*, Cornell University Press, Ithaca, NY.

Macdonald, C., 2013, *Strong, beautiful and modern: National fitness in Britain, New Zealand, Australia and Canada, 1935–1960*, UBC Press, Vancouver, Canada.

Maines, R.P., 1999, *The technology of orgasm*, John Hopkins University Press, Baltimore, MD.

Metzler, I., 2010, *A cultural history of the human body in the Medieval age*, Berg, Oxford.

Miles-Tapping, C., 1989, Sponsorship and sacrifice in the historical development of Canadian physiotherapy, *Physiotherapy Canada*, 41(2), pp. 72–80.

Mitchell, S.W., 1884, *Fat and blood: An essay on the treatment of certain forms of neurasthenia and hysteria*, J. B. Lippincott and Co., Philadelphia, PA.

Morus, I.R., 1999, The measure of man: Technologizing the Victorian body, *History of Science*, 37(117), pp. 249–82.

Morus, I.R., 2006, Bodily disciplines and disciplined bodies: Instruments, skills and Victorian electrotherapeutics, *Social History of Medicine*, 19(2), pp. 241–59.

Murrell, W., 1886, *Massage as a mode of treatment*, H.K. Lewis, London.

Nelson, C.C., 2000, *A new woman reader: Fiction, articles and drama of the 1890s*, Broadview Press, Peterborough, Ontario.

Nietzsche, F., 1973, *Beyond good and evil: Prelude to a philosophy of the future*, Translated by R.J. Hollingdale, Penguin, London.

Nissen, H., 1899, *A manual of instruction for giving Swedish movement and massage treatment*, F.A. Davis, London.

O'Neill, J., 1986, The disciplinary society: From Weber to Foucault, *The British Journal of Sociology*, 37(1), p. 42.

Oppenheim, J., 1991, *'Shattered nerves': Doctors, patients, and depression in Victorian England*, Oxford University Press, Oxford.

Orgeas, J., 1889, *L'hiver à cannes, saint-raphael, grasse et antibes, guide descriptif, historique, scientifique, médical et pratique*, Chez tous les libraires, Paris.

Ostrom, K.W., 1891, *Massage and the original Swedish movements: Their application to various diseases of the body*, 2nd ed., P. Blakiston, Philadelphia, PA.

Ottosson, A., 2010, The first historical movements of kinesiology: Scientification in the borderline between physical culture and medicine around 1850, *International Journal of the History of Sport*, 27(11), pp. 1892–919.

Ottosson, A., 2011, The manipulated history of manipulations of spines and joints? Rethinking orthopaedic medicine through the 19th century discourse of European mechanical medicine, *Medicine Studies*, 3(2), pp. 83–116.

Palmer, M.D., 1901, *Lessons in massage*, 1st ed., Bailliere, Tindall and Cox, London.

Paris, S.V., 2000, A history of manipulative therapy through the ages and up to the current controversy in the United States, *Journal of Manual & Manipulative Therapy*, 8(2), pp. 66–77.

Parry, A., 1995, Ginger Rogers did everything Fred Astaire did backwards and in high heels, *Physiotherapy*, 81(6), pp. 310–19.

Perkins Gilman, C., 1899, *The yellow wallpaper*, Small & Maynard, Boston, MA.

Poirier, S., 1983, The Weir Mitchell rest cure: Doctor and patients, *Women's Studies: An Interdisciplinary Journal*, 10(1), pp. 15–40.

Porter, R., 1990, The medical history of waters and spas. Introduction, *Medical History, Supplement* (10), p. vii.

Putney, C., 2009, *Muscular Christianity: Manhood and sports in protestant America, 1880–1920*, Harvard University Press, Cambridge, MA.

Rose, N. & Miller, P., 1992, Political power beyond the state: Problematics of government. *The British Journal of Sociology*, 43(2), 173, doi:10.2307/591464.

Rose, N., 1994, Medicine, history and the present, in C. Jones & R. Porter (eds.), *Reassessing Foucault: Power, medicine and the body*, Routledge, London, pp. 48–72.

Roth, M., 1852, *Movements or exercises, according to Ling's system for the due development and strengthening of the human body in childhood and youth*, Groombridge & Sons, London.

Russell, K., 2013, The evolution of gymnastics, in D.J. Caine, K. Russell & L. Lim (eds.), *Gymnastics*, John Wiley, Chichester, pp. 1–14.

Samson, C., 1999, Biomedicine and the body, in *Health studies: A critical and cross cultural reader*, Blackwell, Oxford, pp. 3–21.

Sawday, J., 1995, *The body emblazoned: Dissection and the human body in Renaissance culture*, Routledge, London.

Schreiber, J., 1887, *A manual of treatment by massage and methodical muscle exercise*, Young J. Pentland, Edinburgh.

Schuster, D.G., 2003, Neurasthenia and a modernizing America, *JAMA: The Journal of the American Medical Association*, 290(17), pp. 2327–8.

Schuster, D.G., 2005, Personalizing illness and modernity: S. Weir Mitchell, literary women, and neurasthenia, 1870–1914, *Bulletin of the History of Medicine*, 79(4), pp. 695–722.

Schwarz, R.W., 2006, *John Harvey Kellogg, M.D.: Pioneering health reformer*, Review and Herald Pub. Association, Hagerstown, MD.

Showalter, E., 1985, *The Female Malady: Women, madness, and English culture 1830–1980*, Pantheon Books, New York.

Sicherman, B., 1977, The uses of a diagnosis: Doctors, patients, and neurasthenia, *Journal of the History of Medicine and Allied Sciences*, 32(1), pp. 33–54.

Smith, G.H., 1860, *An exposition of the Swedish movement-cure*, Fowler and Wells, New York.

Smith, J.M., Sullivan, J.S. & Baxter, D.G., 2010, Massage therapy: More than a modality, *New Zealand Journal of Physiotherapy*, 38(2), pp. 44–51.

Stewart, H.E., 1925, *Physiotherapy: Theory and clinical application*, Paul B. Hoeber, New York.

Stretch Dowse, T., 1887, *The modern treatment of disease by the system of massage*, Griffith, Farran, Okeden & Welsh, London.

Suleiman, S.R., 1985, *The female body in Western culture*, Harvard University Press, Cambridge, MA.

Symons Eccles, A., 1895, *The practice of massage: Its physiological effects and therapeutic uses*, McMillan, London.

The Morning, 1894, Massage scandals: Extraordinary charges, *The Morning*, 13 July 1894.

Vertinsky, P. & Hargreaves, J. (eds.), 2006, *Physical culture, power, and the body: Routledge critical studies in sport*, Routledge, London.

Williams, K., Ross, Z., Spies, K., Glesman, A., Perry, C. & Corn, W.M., 2004, *Women on the verge: The culture of neurasthenia in nineteenth-century America*, Stanford University, Stanford, CA.

Woloshyn, T., 2013, Le pays du soleil: The art of heliotherapy on the Cote d'Azur, *Social History of Medicine*, 26(1), pp. 74–93.

Zweiniger-Bargielowska, I., 2006, Building a British superman: Physical culture in interwar Britain, *Journal of Contemporary History*, 41(4), pp. 595–610.

Zweiniger-Bargielowska, I., 2010, *Managing the body: Beauty, health, and fitness in Britain, 1880–1939*, Oxford University Press, Oxford.

3 The quest for legitimacy (1894–1914)

Introduction

This chapter examines the very early history of a small organisation known as the Society of Trained Masseuses. Although relatively insignificant at the time, the Society would make an enormous contribution to the future face of healthcare, by offering a template for other professional massage organisations to follow and, in time, become the British Chartered Society of Physiotherapy (CSP) – one of the largest physiotherapy professional bodies in the world.

Possibly because the organisation was small; because it was dwarfed by the rapid expansion of medicine and nursing; or for other reasons that I will explore later in the book, the actions of the founders of the Society have previously gone largely un-noticed. The two histories that have been written about the Society speak matter-of-factly about the moment when physiotherapy as a profession was born. But as I shall show, the actions of the founders of the Society at the very moment of the profession's birth, played a vital role in defining the profession's future – a legacy that continues to have a powerful influence over the profession today.

Rather than being a purely historical account of the events themselves, this chapter will focus on what the founders did to secure the future for their profession. I will look at the reasons why the Society needed to be formed and how the actions of the four women that gave birth to the profession appear to have been a brilliant response to the tensions of the time. For their fledgling organisation to survive, the founders needed to prove that masseuses[1] could practice legitimately, safely and professionally, without any of the slurs that had become associated with massage in late Victorian England. Before I can analyse what the founders did, however, it is necessary to revisit the conditions that led them to act, beginning with the Massage Scandals of 1894.

The Massage Scandals

If we examine many of the physiotherapy systems that now operate around the world, and draw a line back in time to a point of common origin when we might say that physiotherapy as a profession was 'born', we would probably return to the summer of 1894 when a small group of British nurses and midwives met to form an organisation that they called the Society of Trained Masseuses. This would, in time, become the Chartered Society of Physiotherapy and spawn professional physiotherapy organisations around the world.

There have been two significant early histories of the Society. The first by Jane Wicksteed, written in 1948, which gives a rather breathless, romantic account of the events leading up to the formation of the STM; the other written by Dr Jean Barclay to commemorate the centenary of the CSP, is an altogether more academically robust text (Barclay 1994a, 1994b). What these books provide is the essential historical detail of the events surrounding the birth of physiotherapy, but what they do not explain is *why* certain choices were made, why certain strategies were employed and, most importantly, the effect those decisions have had on future generations of physiotherapists.

What is clear is that the decisions made by the founders of the STM in the first few months of the Society have had an enduring effect on the way physiotherapists think and practice, how they are trained, how they have come to define the limits of their scope of practice today. Most of the decisions that were made came in response to the Massage Scandals that erupted in London in the summer of 1894. But to locate the origins of these scandals it is necessary to identify its chief protagonist and this was Earnest Hart, eminent doctor and pioneering editor of the *British Medical Journal* (*BMJ*). Hart was one of the Journal's greatest editors. Famous for using his journal to promote social causes, he was a philanthropist, social reformer and strong advocate for Victorian moral values. His mantra was that 'a subject needing reform had to be kept before the public until the public demands reform' (Smith 1997) and the *BMJ* became the vehicle for realising his vision.

It is hard to imagine, given the size of the *BMJ* today, that at the time of Hart's appointment in 1866, the British Medical Association (BMA) had only 2,000 members and the Journal was a 20 page 'magazine'. By his death in 1898, the BMA had 17,000 members, and the Journal had been more than tripled in size. Hart's influence ranged from reform of the workhouses, to abolishing 'baby farming' (a practice of accepting custody of a child for payment) and to public works and sanitation. And for 25 years as Chairman of the BMA's Parliamentary Bills Committee, Hart was able to lobby the government of the day to instigate his social reforms.

In 1894, at the height of his influence, Hart's attention was drawn to the problem of massage parlours and the *BMJ* began publishing letters and occasional pieces on the problem hoping to bring about change, including one titled 'Immoral Massage Establishments' that beautifully summarised Hart's concerns:

> We have received communications suggesting that an association should be formed for those who have gone through a proper course of instruction in massage and obtained certificates of proficiency, and asking our assistance in the preparation of a list of good and satisfactory workers. The suggestion is, however, beset with difficulties. We understand that a good many 'massage shops,' the advertisements of which are frequently inserted in one or two of the

fashionable daily papers, are very little more than houses of accommodation . . .
Many of the girls have certificates, but they, as a rule, have spent their last
penny in getting instruction, and, little by little, drift into a mode of life which
is often most distasteful to them. The men are often not much better, and it has
become a fashionable fad for certain ladies of position to frequent the rooms of
a young and good-looking masseur . . . Certificates in 'massage' are given, even
by qualified medical men, after the most perfunctory course of instruction . . .
Our impression is that the legitimate massage market is overstocked, and that
no woman, unless she has a private connection, has the slightest chance of getting a living by massage alone – at all events in London. We are afraid that
nothing could be done in the way of registration unless the ground could previously be cleared of what is undoubtedly a great social scandal. It would be
difficult, at all events at first, to refuse a place on the list to any woman who has
a certificate from a legally qualified practitioner, and yet in many cases such
recognition would mean neither more nor less than a recognition of prostitution.

(*British Medical Journal* 1894a)

Stories of vice had been of particular interest to the Victorians and so it was no
surprise that these accounts drew public attention. Hart knew he had found a good
story and was keen to promote his brand of social reform through the *BMJ*. The
Journal launched its own investigation into massage practices which culminated
in the publication of a wonderfully titled booklet 'Astounding Revelations
Concerning Supposed Massage Houses or Pandemoniums of Vice, Frequented by
Both Sexes, Being a Complete Expose of the Ways of Professed Masseurs and
Masseuses' (*British Medical Journal* 1894c). This caught the attention of the local
and national media and, by the end of 1894, newspaper reports of the Massage
Scandals appeared in virtually every national and local newspaper across England.

The reports highlighted the resurgence of interest in massage as both a leisure
pursuit for the middle and upper classes and as a new career for women (*Reynold's
Weekly* 1894). They drew attention to the fact that the training of masseuses had
become shambolic, with a number of stories emphasising the poor working conditions experienced by masseuses (St. Paul's 1894; *British Medical Journal* 1894c).
A number of articles spoke of the scarcity of work that was driving down labour
costs and how this was exposing women to unscrupulous practices in which
the masseuse received no 'wages', but depended on the 'tips' of patrons – to which
they were expected to make themselves 'agreeable' (*Reynold's Weekly* 1894;
The People 1894).

Training in massage was most often provided by doctors or supposedly 'qualified'
masseuses, but there were clearly no standards governing the training and many
accounts came to light in the months following the *BMJ's* article that exposed a
trade in meaningless certificates and unreliable qualifications (*British Medical
Journal* 1894b,c). The women drawn into the brothels and bagnios of England's
large cities received no protection from the law because the authorities were
unable to distinguish legitimate massage from prostitution. As soon as the police
threatened to close down a suspicious practice, the proprietor claimed that it was

a massage parlour and the police were unable to take further action. This lack of differentiation between massage and prostitution caused a vexed response in the media, who openly reported their frustration – and that of 'the authorities' – that even the most well known brothels in London's West End were unable to be closed down (*The Star* 1894). The *BMJ* summed up the tone of the media reports thus;

> In these dens of infamy the worst passions of a man or a woman are excited by treatment they are pleased to call massage . . . We had thought that Christian England – especially the more aristocratic portion of it – could have given better illustration of her much-vaunted modesty for wicked France to peep at.
>
> (*British Medical Journal* 1894a)

In keeping with a growing interest in eugenics and the general question of the deteriorating 'quality' of the English race, reports emphasised that it was the 'aristocratic portion' of society that was frequenting the illicit massage parlours (*Reynold's Weekly* 1894) and, worse still, women were attending in considerable numbers as the fashion for massage reached its peak in the 1890s. The following quote captures the moral opprobrium that accompanied many reports within the popular press;

> . . . immorality is not . . . an offence against the law. If it were, indeed, the law would have its hands full, and we should find peer and peasant rubbing shoulders in the dock. In our opinion something far more dreadful than the existence of these immoral massage establishments is the thought that they are extensively patronised by persons who, in spite of rank and education, are a proof that man is, after all, the most disgusting of all the animals.
>
> (*Whitehall Review* 1894)

The lack of restrictions on the advertising of massage services, including where the adverts could appear and the nature of the claims made, meant that prospective patients would not know whether the person advertising themselves as 'Miss Nightingale' was a therapeutic masseuse or a prostitute. Legitimate masseurs and masseuses raised their voice in protest in the very same newspapers that published the advertisements of prostitutes. In a letter to the *St. James's Gazette*, for example, announcing the formation of the British Massage Association, T. Garner wrote, 'Unfortunately there are hundreds of most intelligent and useful men and women whose prospects have been well-nigh ruined by reported malpractice of unscrupulous persons' (Garner 1895).

Clearly, the normal processes of English law had been found wanting when it came to the prosecution of this social 'evil'. The *British Medical Journal* had appealed to the government to close the brothels down, regulate the advertising of masseuses and formulate a system of training to legitimise the profession (*British Medical Journal* 1894c) and, through its Parliamentary Bills Committee, even managed to reach as far as the Home Secretary. But ultimately Ernest Hart and the *BMJ* failed to bring about the change they sought. And so, over the course of 1895, the *BMJ's* interest, and that of the rest of the popular press, drifted away from the

Massage Scandals and found new avenues for its reforming spirit. But Hart need not have worried, because what followed would prove to be an even more effective mechanism for legitimising therapeutic massage than could have been provided through heavy-handed legislation and it would exemplify Margaret Meed's aphorism that 'A small group of thoughtful people [can] change the world. Indeed, it's the only thing that ever has'.

The birth of the STM

The problem facing the founders of the Society of Trained Masseuses was clear when they met in the summer of 1894. The massage market was overstocked with variously qualified practitioners with meaningless certificates and an entirely unregulated wage system that led to unscrupulous practices. There were no restrictions on advertising and no formal support for massage within the medical community. Women were openly massaging men and, worse still, men were massaging women. Massage had become indistinguishable from prostitution, and the brazen impudence with which the upper classes patronised brothels and bagnios of England's major cities only gave social reformers greater concern that the English race was in moral decline. The dire state of the massage market was particularly distressing and for the nurses and midwives who were beginning to develop new career paths and professional opportunities. Something clearly needed to be done.

We know that a combination of media reports and personal working circumstances led four London-based nurses and midwives to meet at the Midwives' Institute and Trained Nurses' Club in London in the summer of 1894. Of those four, Rosalind (later *Dame* Rosalind) Paget was a significant presence. Paget was a trained nurse and midwife and was a principal driving force in establishing legislation and registration for midwives in England. Paget came from a family of liberal reformers. Her uncle was William Rathbone, a famous Liverpool ship builder and Member of Parliament from 1868 to 1895. Her family were close friends with Florence Nightingale and her cousin was the suffragette Eleanor Rathbone. Paget was herself thought to be a strong advocate for women's suffrage[2].

Alongside Paget at the first meeting of the STM were Lucy Robinson, Annie Manley and Margaret Palmer who, together, convened the Society and organised its first formal meeting in December of 1894, at which a council of 12 members was elected and began the process of defining some rules of professional conduct for Society members. There is perhaps nothing striking in this, since many new organisations do something similar as their first formal act, but these rules provide a particularly good clue to the reasons why the Society formed and what it sought to achieve. According to an editorial in *Nursing Notes* – the rules

> protected our members from unpleasantness and [gave] the doctors a feeling of security that our rubbers [a colloquial name for masseuses] are not prescribing quacks, and the general public a feeling of trust that our members are masseuses of irreproachable character.
>
> (*Nursing Notes* 1900)

The rules stated that:

- No massage to be undertaken except under medical supervision
- No general massage for men to be undertaken but exceptions may be made for urgent and nursing cases at a doctor's special request
- No advertising in any but strictly medical papers
- No sale of drugs to patients allowed

(Society of Trained Masseuses 1895)

The rules were reproduced on the bottom of the certificates given to everyone who successfully completed the Society's membership examination, suggesting that these rules were significant in the founder's efforts to legitimise their practice. What can be seen in the rules is an eagerness to situate the Society's members in a subordinate relationship to doctors; to manage the problems associated in the public's mind when women massaged men; and to separate legitimate masseuses from those offering 'other' services.

The STM was not alone in trying to convince the medical profession and the public at large that it might be possible to form an organisation to legitimise massage, and many of the STM's competitor organisations also offered rules of conduct. In some cases, these rules were far more extensive and draconian. But by 1914, most of these rival organisations had disbanded. Organisations like the British Massage Association, the Incorporated Society of Trained Masseuses and Masseurs and the Harley Institute, all published rules of professional conduct between 1895 and 1898 as part of their quest for legitimacy (Barclay 1994b), but all, in time, would cease their operations and disappear.

Rules alone, therefore, cannot explain how the STM managed to survive and prosper. But the rules certainly give some clues to the way the founders set out to discipline the Society's members and thereby establish consistent standards that would give them the upper hand in the battle to establish a legitimate form of massage practice. Two important principles supplemented the rules set out previously and are of particular note here because they draw on critical principles established by the Society: the first is that STM members publish *only* in nursing and medical journals and the second is that the STM was a profession run by women, for women and that no men would be allowed to enter the Society.

Publishing only in the nursing and medical literature served two purposes; it showed the Society's intent to promote the profession within the medical community and it targeted the particular class of women who were now being attracted to nursing and midwifery – an aspect of the profession's identity that Rosalind Paget was most anxious to assert (Hannam 1997). The ability to influence nursing and midwifery practice was particularly enhanced by the fact that Ms Paget was the proprietor of the journal *Nursing Notes*, which subsequently carried reports of the Society's business and advertised the profession to nurses and midwives throughout Britain (Barclay 1994b).

Excluding men from the STM was a position the founders maintained until 1905, when men were finally allowed to sit the Society's examination. Men were only then allowed into the Society because the War Office approached the Society to examine Royal Army Medical Corps orderlies. Thornton explains that:

> This raised an interesting problem. The Society's rules clearly state that women must not give general massage to men or vice versa, nor were women allowed to examine men in practical massage. As men had been excluded from the Society, mainly because membership gave rights of access to the Nurses' Social Club, an exclusively female organisation, there were no male examiners. The problem was resolved by asking a son of one of the members, himself a trained masseur, to examine the practical component for the Society.
>
> (Thornton 1994, p. 12A)

Despite being allowed to sit the examination, men were still not formally allowed to register with the Society until 1920 (Parry 1995) and were thus prevented from receiving medical referrals – a vital component of the STM's pursuit of legitimacy. Finally, in 1920, the newly named Chartered Society of Massage and Medical Gymnastics (CSMMG) relented and allowed men to register, but only after the women of the now Incorporated STM had removed all competition and shown themselves to be *the* pre-eminent provider of legitimate massage treatment.

Anne Parry (1995) argues that the exclusion of men from the profession in its early years was motivated as much by the desire to protect the reputation of nurse- and midwife-masseuses during the Massage Scandals, as much as it was an attempt to create a new niche for women professionals (Parry 1995). While this may be the case, the actions of the founders were, in many ways, deeply ironic. Their belief was that massage between the sexes was dangerous, and that if contact between men and women was prevented, there would be less likelihood that Society members would be accused of acting inappropriately. The inevitable consequence of which was that a man living in one of Victorian England's large cities who wanted a massage *had* to take his chances with an unregulated practitioner or a prostitute. But the STM stuck to its strong ideological opposition to contact with men and actively promoted this view in its attempts to remove its competition.

The Harley Institute, for example, was accused of charging too little for treatments, giving false credentials, providing inadequate training, but 'worst of all, allowing young women to receive instruction from men and to work on male models (albeit from the Boy's Brigade)' (Barclay 1994b, p. 37). The Society engaged in a long, drawn out campaign against such practices, culminating in a petition sent to the London County Council asking for the Harley Institute's licence to practice to be revoked. Under the weight of the STM's campaign, the Harley Institute, like many before it, was closed down.

One important feature of any set of professional rules is that they rarely, if ever, address all the issues all of the time, thus approaches like those employed by the STM only ever served as a partial response to the breadth and depth of the issues raised by the Massage Scandals. Rules of professional conduct needed to be supplemented by other strategies that built on the moral foundations laid by the

Society and one of the Society's most powerful strategies was to seek the support of the medical community.

Courting medical patronage

The relationship the STM sought to establish with the medical profession took a number of forms. Firstly, the Society made it clear that a masseuse should not, in any way, overstep her authority by making her own diagnoses of patients' problems. This was strictly the domain of the physician, who had acquired newfound respectability towards the end of the nineteenth century with the discovery of germ theory. Masseuses were to treat only as directed by a doctor who, it was argued, knew more about the conditions requiring massage and the suitable modalities of treatment than the therapist. It should be remembered that before turning their interest towards germs, physicians had been very actively involved in physical medicine, but many willingly handed this work over to the masseuses when more modern forms of medicine appeared.

Secondly, the Society insisted that only patients referred by a recognised doctor were to be seen. This was not difficult to enforce in the hospitals and nursing homes where many of the early members were already working as nurses and midwives, but a growing number of masseuses were practising in private homes and so an additional level of regulation was needed. The STM, therefore, formed itself into a 'gate keeping' agency; taking referrals from doctors and passing them on to 'registered' and approved masseuses[3]. Through this mechanism, the STM was able not only to vet the referring doctor, but also to control the work of its registrants.

A third strategy employed by the founders was to seek medical patronage for their organisational endeavours. The STM went to quite considerable lengths to recruit medical support for their campaign to legitimise massage. The founders (probably using Rosalind Paget's social and political connections) worked assiduously to obtain medical signatories to the Society's principles and to promote them in the Society's advertising to the public. Signatories included Surgeon-General Sir Alfred Keogh, Robert Knox M.D., James Little M.D., Sir Frederick Treves and the retired Past President of the Royal College of Physicians, Sir Samuel Wilks[4].

Finally, if further recognition of medicine was needed, the founders made it clear that the knowledge that would form the basis for legitimate massage practice would be defined by biomedical, or more accurately, biomechanical, reasoning. Early texts used by Society members leant heavily on the writings of doctors who had specialised in physical medicine (Stretch Dowse 1887; Nissen 1889; Graham 1884; Ellison 1898; Creighton-Hale 1893; Bennett 1902). And so, the STM made it clear that it was a professional organisation prepared to work under doctors' instruction, that it accepted medicine's dominance and was eager to please the physicians. In doing so, it presented itself as an ideal solution to the vexed problem of who should take the practice of massage into the future.

Some authors have argued that the early founders of female-dominated professions like physiotherapy, hindered their professional progress by deferring so readily to medicine, which was dominated by men and a particularly strong masculine view of health and illness (Witz 1992). But this argument refers mainly to midwifery and nursing and ignores the evidence from the STM, which was remarkably successful in establishing a legitimate response to the Massage Scandals. Indeed, what professional histories have so far ignored is that physiotherapy may well be the first female-dominated profession to adopt an almost entirely androcentric (male-centred) view of the body. What is clear is that the STM benefitted greatly from the patronage of the medical community, it is possible that the STM would have gone the way of the Harley Institute and others who disappeared in part because of their inability to obtain medical cooperation and support.

What the founders did that was particularly insightful was to find a way to differentiate members of the Society from the medical profession (by not prescribing medications), while also fostering close connections with doctors (by deferring to the doctor in all things, by advertising only in medical and nursing publications and by adopting a medical view of health and illness). Taken together, these various strategies help explain why the STM survived while other massage organisations floundered. It may be, as Lynley Katavich argues, that the 'trade-off' for the profession was that it accepted a rather narrow view of the body (Katavich 1996), but in doing so, it made it possible for the Society to flourish.

The success of the Society in securing work for its members did not come about because the STM had merely developed some rules or gained the confidence of the medical profession, but rather because it was able to prove its allegiance and confirm its moral standing through an examination system that effectively functioned as a proving ground – a gateway – through which all prospective members should pass. Once the Society had established exclusive access to medical referrals, a masseuse had little choice but to submit to the STM's standards in order to find work. The establishment of an examination system was, therefore, another vital aspect of the Society's project to legitimise massage.

The creation of an examination system

More than all the other strategies, the creation of the Society's examination system was designed to govern the conduct of its members. Through this, the Society sought to give confidence to the public, the medical profession, the press and the government, and show that there could be a class of legitimate masseuses who could be distinguished from those with only the most basic training, or those engaging in licentious practice. On the surface, the examination system proved the competence of the applicant, but its primary function was much more sophisticated than this because it established the STM as the registering body and through this promoted the Society's values. The STM was very small at its inception and could not hope to deliver massage teaching throughout the country, but it could define standards of practice and restrict access to medical referrals for those who had bought into the Society's ideals. Through the examination system, the STM was able to establish itself, its massage ideals and demonstrate a strongly disciplined approach to professional conduct all at the same time.

An examination system was deemed necessary by members of the Society because; 'Massage is a scientific method of treating disease by means of systematic manipulations, and is very different from the ordinary shampooing or medical rubbing, which can be acquired without any definitive training' (Ellison 1898, p. 1). Mary Anne Ellison was one of its founding members of the Society and, alongside Margaret Palmer (Palmer 1901), published one of the first texts specifically for STM registrants. In these texts the authors were clear that training in the complexities of *legitimate* massage demanded testing and this testing needed to be sufficient to convince the medical profession particularly that the STM was graduating suitably qualified practitioners.

The significance of examinations to the STM's purpose was highlighted by Barclay, who states that while the first objective of the Society was to 'improve the status and training of masseuses', the second was to 'hold examinations and grant certificates' (Barclay 1994b, p. 31). The first council of the Society recognised that it had limited resources and was small in size, so decided against setting up a training school or defining a curriculum that would need to be policed around the country. Instead, it devised a registration examination that had to be passed by everyone who wanted to become a member of the STM. The effect of these changes was to establish a curriculum 'at a distance', since teachers would need to comply with this to be able to submit students for examination.

Students attempting to register with the STM sat a national examination – written, approved and delivered by the Society's Examination Committee. Training was offered by tutors dispersed around the country, many of whom were themselves STM members. Miss Manley, for example, was a leading massage teacher at Guys Hospital from 1888 to 1913, while Miss Palmer and Miss Despard were actively involved in training students in their own practices. Both of the latter would go on to develop texts for their students, which included information on the facets of practice necessary to be an effective masseuse (Despard 1916; Palmer 1901). But the STM would also examine students of tutors who were not STM members. These students stood little chance of succeeding unless they had studied for the STM's examination and so through this the Society was able to influence what quickly came to be the principal therapeutic massage curriculum that one studied if one wanted to find legitimate massage work.

To qualify for membership of the STM, students had to demonstrate theoretical and practical competence in massage, medical gymnastics and, later, medical electricity. These three domains were prefaced on the student's knowledge of anatomy and physiology, kinesiology, rudimentary pathology and elementary physics, including biomechanics. Importantly, however, the examinations also acted as a barometer of the students' attitudes towards their work and as a vehicle to reinforce the Society's own brand of professionalism and, unfortunately, practical performance did not always meet the required standard. In 1908, for instance, 18 students under the tutelage of Miss Manley were reported as performing 'useless massage; were painfully slow; knew few movements and had a casual attitude' (Barclay 1994b, p. 39; Barclay 1994a, p. 39). The following year the examiners criticised nurse candidates whose 'short petticoats, high heeled shoes, and transparent stockings, and an exceedingly obnoxious style of hairdressing' went 'extremely ill with a print dress, bonnet and veil' (Barclay 1994b, p. 42).

Every examination straddled the mutual concerns for the students' theoretical knowledge, practical proficiency and professional demeanour. The first written examination conducted by students in 1895, for example, included the following four questions:

1   How would you treat a case of constipation?
2   What symptoms occurring during massage of a sprain, strain or recent fracture would cause you to send for the doctor?
3   Give the position, origin and insertion and use of four leading muscles.
4   You receive a letter from a would-be patient asking if you can undertake a case. What would you do?

(Thornton 1994, p. 11A)

In the examination of June 1911, students were still asked to demonstrate 'How may the personal habits of the masseuse be responsible for success or failure in her profession?' (Incorporated Society of Trained Masseuses 1911), and in the November we of 1914, the first five questions concentrate on anatomical, clinical and practical issues, while the last question asked 'As a member of an honourable profession what do you consider to be your duties and obligations to that profession and to your fellow members?' (Incorporated Society of Trained Masseuses 1914).

It seems that the function of these 'professional' questions was to reassure the Society that the appropriate moral standards were being instilled in the students, with the students needing to demonstrate the right answer to these questions to register as a legitimate masseuse. Thus, the questions in the examination served to test a set of normalised moral values about the proper conduct of the masseuse. Importantly, these values were based not on either the masseuse's theoretical, practical or technical ability – these were tested elsewhere – they were explicitly directed at measuring the registrants against the STM's definition of legitimacy. They made the student subject to the gaze of the STM and, at the same time, reinforced the Society's status as the pre-eminent object of authority and expertise. They fused those practices that gave students pass grades with legitimacy and normalcy, and marginalised all practices that hinted at incompetence, licentiousness or a casual attitude to work.

Success in the examination, and subsequent registration with the Society carried some significant benefits for massueses – not least the access to patients referred by doctors. Thus, registration was an important corollary to examination and it seems that registrants were happy to accept the moral prescription of the Society in order that they should obtain gainful employment at a time when the massage market was overstocked with practitioners claiming to offer a skilled service.

The registration of members

The disciplinary strategies already mentioned were effective in their own right as tactics designed to regulate the conduct of the Society's members. They achieved particular significance for the Society, however, when they operated in concert; when one strategy triangulated with another to form an interconnected disciplinary network whose purpose was to define the registered practitioner.

Professional regulation of members is not, in itself, unusual in the history of the conduct of the established health professions, as Davies argues;

> Professional regulation, in essence, is a state-supported power to place names on a register. Nineteenth and early 20th century legislation in the UK gave the right to doctors, pharmacists, midwives, dentists, nurses and others to maintain registers, and to make decisions about entry and about removal. Legal restriction of title to those on the register separated sheep from goats and enabled regulators both to set standards for entry to practice and to remove those who failed to meet those standards.
>
> (Davies 2007, p. 234)

Davies' reference to 'sheep and goats' is interesting, because it is the same phrase used by the *BMJ* a century earlier to refer to the difference between legitimate masseuses and prostitutes. What Davies argues is that registration offers certain privileges to members of the professional group, but it also levies obligations upon them. For the STM, the privileges offered to members included the patronage of the medical profession, the advocacy of a legitimate professional body, a recognised examination system that provided a certificate that people trusted, standardised rates of pay and conditions of service and some degree of protection from the vagaries of the market. For their part, to gain membership of the Society, the student was required to pass a stringent examination, subscribe to the STM's rules, practice only in ways prescribed by the Society, register with the organisation and only take on patients that were offered to them through the Society's referral system.

For many, this arrangement was mutually advantageous. For instance, it allowed the Society to make public the claim that:

> We do not recommend any from our Institute unless they undertake only to attend cases under medical supervision. We never recommend masseuses to male patients for general massage. We have the name and directions of a few excellent masseurs [sic] whom we can recommend for such cases.
>
> (Young 1969, p. 271)

The appeal of these guarantees appears to have been a strong influence on the growth of the Society in its early years, since members were happy to endure work shortages and poor rates of pay in order to benefit from the legitimacy that the STM offered. Between 1894 and 1914, STM-registered masseuses worked independently as private practitioners and earned very poor wages. Unlike most of the founders – who as affluent single women were able to develop their interests in the Society largely as a philanthropic gesture (for which they received no financial reward) – most newly registered masseuses struggled to live on the wages prescribed by the STM (Barclay 1994a, p. 35–6). Securing periods of steady employment in the home of an affluent (e.g. neurasthenic) patient was a boon, but these opportunities were relatively rare, especially outside of the metropolis. In the overstocked massage market, masseuses often needed to compete by undercutting their rivals or by offering other points of difference. The main point of difference for STM members was the Society's guarantee of legitimacy, but this needed to be policed because some members' wages were so poor and they resorted to offering other services alongside those prescribed by the Society. Knowing this, the STM kept a close eye on its members and threatened to deregister anyone offering beauty, chiropody or nursing services as a way of supplementing their income.

The Society was repeatedly drawn into action against its own members, who offered services that drew on their massage skills to supplement their income. In 1908, for example, one member complained that she had earned only two shillings a week from massage (at a time when the massage examiners were charging 21 shillings an hour for their services). At other times the Society recorded instances where registrants traded with fashionable sounding pseudonyms like 'Sister Nightingale' to make their treatments more appealing (Barclay 1994b). Clearly, training in massage, exercise and electrotherapy was perfectly suited to this line of work. It was, however, deemed to be too close to an aesthetic of pleasure or luxury for the STM to countenance its practice.

To help police the profession and ensure noone brought the Society into disrepute, the STM appointed an Inspector (at significant cost to the personal wealth of the founders) whose job it was to visit each of the schools that prepared students for the registration examination and ensure that they were upholding the Society's standards. The Inspector's role was of critical importance and was only ever awarded to a masseuse of peerless principles and an unblemished professional career. Its first appointee, for example, was Miss Anne Gibson, 'a Nightingale protégée, who had recently retired as Matron of Birmingham's huge Poor Law Infirmary' (Barclay 1994b, p. 34). Not only was Miss Gibson an experienced nurse and masseuse, but also an early graduate of the STM and a therapist well-schooled in the Society's founding principles.

Where the Inspector focused on the quality of students and the various training institutions, the registered membership was reached through the publication *Nursing Notes* that, from June 1887 through to WWI, provided information for nurses, midwives and later, registered masseuses, as a supplementary magazine to the large circulation *Woman* magazine. Through *Nursing Notes*, the STM was able to broadcast not only the administrative functions of the Society, but also its aspirations, requirements and principles. In one example, Miss Wilson commented on the need for personal dignity as a vital quality in the 'making of the profession'; 'a masseuse with a fussy manner who was not sure where to put her cloak and bonnet made a nervous patient worse, and demeanour was important as servants recognized the standing of the doctor and the trained nurse but were unable "place the masseuse"' (*Nursing Notes* 1900). These opinion pieces reinforced the more authoritarian rules and guidance notes produced by the Society and sought to enhance the standards of practice that were built into the STM's examinations.

The environment the STM created for its practitioners acted like an 'enclosure' in which registered members operated. This enclosure gave members freedom to practice without fear of scandal, but it demanded a disciplined approach on the part of the individual member in the face of fierce competition from other masseuses, gender discrimination from the medical profession and the public at large, and subsistence wages. In this regard, the Society's members stood alongside other health professionals who were making their own strides towards legitimacy and respectability. Berghs and colleagues have argued that these kinds of professional discipline were the 'essence of moral training' in nursing, and that 'a nurse's character was more important than theoretical knowledge and more important than education' (Berghs et al 2006). The same emphasis on a masseuses' moral character holds true for the early massage profession. It is surely no coincidence that the motto carried on the badge of the Society from 1900 onwards was 'Digna sequens', or 'Follow worthy things'.

Closing words

In this chapter, I have examined some of the key events that led to the formation of the Society of Trained Masseuses and concentrated on the actions of the founders of the Society in disciplining the conduct of people who aspired to be legitimate masseuses. In some ways, a disciplined approach can be seen as a rather negative strategy because it is designed to constrain people's freedom. Today we are so used to the idea that freedom is a good thing that it can be hard to reconcile ourselves to the attitude of our forebears whose actions can, in hindsight, seem draconian. But discipline has another side – and one physiotherapy learnt from very early on – that it can be a very positive strategy in securing other people's trust.

The STM's actions in the first months of the Society were focused on creating a structure around massage practice that would convince people that it could be performed legitimately. Clearly, some things had to be sacrificed for this to occur and the masseuse's freedom to express in whatever way they chose was one of them, but this appears to have been willingly accepted by practitioners in order that they might find work. It is important to remember that the Society's early members were all educated single women who were striving to carve out meaningful and interesting career pathways. Many resolved to endure poor wages and long, hard working days in order to enjoy the benefits of the physical and mental challenge that legitimate massage offered. And many appear to have welcomed the opportunity to cross the threshold into an exclusive 'club' populated by other women of similar intention. For these women, then, the Society's rules were a contingent response to the Massage Scandals and a necessary step in demonstrating the superiority of their work.

There is a large body of historical analysis necessary to examine some of the tensions that the Society's early actions created, not least how it reinforced Victorian notions of gender roles and traditional 'heteronormative' notions of sexuality and morality, but there is no space here to examine these ideas further. One component of the early story of the STM that I will examine in much more detail is, in my view, the single most important dimension of the whole story of physiotherapy, and that is how the founders of the STM adopted a biomechanical view of the body as its founding principle and most valuable disciplinary strategy. I will tackle this question in Chapter 7. For now, I need to move beyond the early years of the physiotherapy profession to consider how the success of the founders put in place the necessary conditions for physiotherapy to become recognised as *the* orthodox provider of legitimate physical rehabilitation services, not only in England and the wider Commonwealth, but in most developed countries around the world.

Notes

1 The word 'masseuses' is the feminine derivitive of the word masseur. It is used in chapters that refer to the early history of the profession because only women could register with the STM in its early years – a point I will explore further later in the chapter.
2 Although, as Barclay reported in her history of the CSP, the founders of the STM were eager not to be seen to be too politically active – laying a further foundation stone in the profession's long held belief that physiotherapy was scientific and biomedical, not political. In the question of women's suffrage, for example,

> The Editor and Committee [of the JISTM] did their best to stick to professional and clinical matters and, although quietly pleased when the vote was granted to women over 30 in 1918, admitted that they had considered the question too 'political' to cover in the past.

> (Barclay 1994a, p. 54)

3 UK physiotherapists did not achieve formal registration until the passing of the Professions Supplementary to Medicine Act of 1960. Barclay argues that 'By establishing the machinery for state registration, the Act of [October] 1960 set basic standards for work in the National Health Service and conferred on physiotherapists and kindred groups a new professionalism' (Barclay 1994a, p. 190).
4 A sidenote worthy of consideration is that the STM was much more successful in gaining medical and regulatory support than midwives, who fought a long and at times bitter battle to gain recognition (see June Hannam's biography of Rosalind Paget (Hannam 1997) and (Donnison 1977)). The midwive's campaign was much more medically and socially divisive and it must have been a real relief for the founders of the STM to institute almost identical reforms for masseuses without the hours of endless lobbying.

References

Bennett, W., 1902, Address given to ISTM titled 'Some points relating to massage', Wellcome Institute Library, London, Ref. SA/CSP/P.1/3.

Barclay, J., 1994a, *In good hands: The history of the Chartered Society of Physiotherapy 1894–1994*, Butterworth Heinemann, Oxford.

Barclay, J., 1994b, The story behind 'In Good Hands', *Physiotherapy*, 80(12), pp. 857–60.

Berghs, M., Dierckx de Casterlé, B. & Gastmans, C., 2006, Nursing, obedience, and complicity with eugenics: A contextual interpretation of nursing morality at the turn of the twentieth century, *Journal of Medical Ethics*, 32(2), pp. 117–22.

British Medical Journal, 1894a, Immoral 'massage' establishments, *British Medical Journal*, 2, p. 88.

British Medical Journal, 1894b, Immoral massage, *British Medical Journal*, 2, p. 145.

British Medical Journal, 1894c, Astounding revelations concerning supposed massage houses or pandemoniums of vice, frequented by both sexes, being a complete expose of the ways of professed masseurs and masseuses, Wellcome Institute Library, London, Ref. SA/CSP/P.1/2.

Creighton-Hale, A., 1893, *The art of massage*, The Scientific Press, London.

Davies, C., 2007, The promise of 21st century professionalism: Regulatory reform and integrated care, *Journal of Interprofessional Care*, 21(3), pp. 233–9.

Despard, L.L., 1916, *Text-book of massage and remedial gymnastics*, Oxford University Press, London.

Donnison, C.J., 1977, *Midwives and medical men: A history of interprofessional rivalries and women's rights*, Heinemann Educational, London.

Ellison, M.A., 1898, *A manual for students of massage*, Bailliere, Tindall and Cox, London.

Garner, T., 1895, The massage question, *St. James's Gazette*, 23 December 1895.

Graham, D., 1884, *A practical treatise on massage*, William Wood & Co, New York.

Hannam, J., 1997, Rosalind Paget: The midwife, the women's movement and reform before 1914, in H. Marland & A.M. Rafferty (eds.), *Midwives, Society and Childbirth: debates and controversies in the early modern period*, Routledge, London, pp. 81–100.

Incorporated Society of Trained Masseuses, 1911, Massage examination paper, Wellcome Institute Library, London. Ref. SA/CSP/C.2/2/1/1.

Incorporated Society of Trained Masseuses, 1914, Massage examination paper, Wellcome Institute Library, London, Ref. SA/CSP/C.2/2/1/1.

Katavich, L., 1996, Physiotherapy in the new health system in New Zealand, *New Zealand Journal of Physiotherapy*, 24(2), pp. 11–13.

Nissen, H., 1889, *Swedish movement and massage treatment*, F.A. Davis, London.

Nursing Notes, 1900, Editorial, *Nursing Notes*, 25 (February).

Palmer, M.D., 1901, *Lessons in massage*, 1st ed., Bailliere, Tindall and Cox, London.

Parry, A., 1995, Ginger Rogers did everything Fred Astaire did backwards and in high heels, *Physiotherapy*, 81(6), pp. 310–19.

Reynold's Weekly, 1894, Massage and aristocracy, *Reynold's Weekly*, 22 July 1894.

Smith, R., 1997, Does the world need the *BMJ?*, *British Medical Journal*, 314, p. 1.

Society of Trained Masseuses, 1895, Minutes of Committee Meeting, Wellcome Institute Library, London, Ref. SA/CSP/C.2/2/1/1.

St. Paul's, 1894, The massage affair, *St. Paul's*, 4 August 1894.

Stretch Dowse, W., 1887, *The modern treatment of disease by the system of massage*, Griffiths, Farran, Okeden & Welsh, London.

The People, 1894, London massage houses: Police officer's remarkable statement (Special interview), *The People*, 15 July 1894.

The Star, 1894, Morals and massage: Mr. Asquith orders an inquiry in the system, *The Star*, 19 July 1894.

Thornton, E., 1994, 100 years of physiotherapy education, *Physiotherapy*, 80(A)(2), pp. 11A–19A.

Whitehall Review, 1894, Editorial: Immoral massage, 28 July 1894.

Witz, A., 1992, *Professions and patriarchy*, Routledge, London.

Young, P., 1969, A short history of the Chartered Society of Physiotherapy, *Physiotherapy*, 55(7), pp. 271–8.

4   The pursuit of orthodoxy (1914–1973)

Introduction

In the previous chapter, I argued that the actions of a small number of masseuses made the early physiotherapy profession possible. Drawing on a specific set of techniques, approaches and strategies, they brilliantly, if perhaps not always consciously, navigated the social and political tensions surrounding the physical therapies in the late 19th century. They created conditions that would legitimise their approach to touch, built close ties to medicine and created the foundations of a professional identity that would be exported to many other countries around the world and sustain the profession for much of the next century.

There are a number of critical lessons to be learnt from this period in the profession's history, but perhaps none more so than the way in which the founders were able to amplify the power of their actions by attaching social significance to otherwise practical measures. Massage, for example, was popular enough in the 1900s, but many people practiced as masseuses and masseurs. What the founders of the profession had to show was that their massage was different; that it was not just a massage, but that it was also a vehicle to say some bigger things about respectability, decency and the sensuality of touch. Adopting highly regimented Swedish remedial massage techniques, learning patho-anatomical language and only treating patients with a medical referral served to suggest that these masseuses were serious about the discipline of their discipline and determined to carve out a new professional identity.

In this chapter, I trace the broad period between the outbreak of World War I to the Oil Crisis of 1973. This 60-year time span was chosen because it represents what I see as a golden age in the history of the profession. The profession grew exponentially in countries that already had established physiotherapy identities going into WWI, and many new programmes emerged. War created the conditions necessary for the birth of the rehabilitation movement and the inter-war period deepened the collective sense of responsibility for many of the health problems that physiotherapists were asked to tackle. The Depression of the 1930s provided the political impetus to establish the Welfare State, and scientific advances after World War II changed the way that orthodox medicine was practiced and perceived. At each step along the way physiotherapy prospered. For each major social event of the period between 1914 and 1973, physiotherapy grew both in size and in social standing. Physiotherapists found that the challenges and uncertainties the profession had endured in the previous decades had only served to position it in the ideal place to take advantage of the economic, political and social changes affecting whole swathes of the population in developed countries. So, although the profession often struggled for recognition and members battled endlessly for better working conditions, by 1973 physiotherapy had established itself as the principal provider of physical rehabilitation services throughout the Western world. This chapter charts some of the sentinel events that made this possible and explores what must be considered the golden age of physiotherapy.

Serving the State

> An ever-present problem was the potential conflict between ambition and per-
> ceived needs and status of the profession and the true needs of the community
> it should serve.
>
> (Dyer 1994, p. 71A)

In the first half of the twentieth century, medical power and authority grew tremendously. The discovery of germs and later antibiotics, advances in surgery after the outbreak of WWI and the growing role medicine played in public health gave doctors a social standing such that the old saying that 'doctor knows best' began to be applied to the entire span of orthodox healthcare. Alternatives to medicine had always been available, but after WWI it became increasingly difficult to access healthcare that did not begin with a visit to the doctor. Medicine and surgery became increasingly technological and specialised, leading to the ironic situation in which 'general' practice became its own specialty. With the creation of each sub-discipline, the necessity to police professional boundaries became more and more important, and regulatory bodies and professional societies took on significant roles in setting standards and prosecuting marginal practices. New areas of practice were allowed to emerge – most notably with the formalisation of the 'psy' disciplines (psychology, psychotherapy and psychiatry) after 1900 (Rose 1997, 1999), particularly where doctors had decided they no longer wanted to focus as much on physical medicine.

Physiotherapy benefitted hugely from medicine's relatively rapid abandonment of the physical therapies in the latter decades of the 19th century. Prior to the discovery of germs, many doctors called themselves physical therapists. Indeed, it was not until 1947 that American doctors fully replaced the title of physical therapist with physiatrist, allowing American physiotherapists and physical therapy technicians to adopt it formally (Murphy 1995, p. 133). So, physiotherapy – alongside psychology, psychotherapy, radiography, occupational therapy and podiatry – emerged in a new space largely vacated by doctors, taking up new work as the occupational definitions of doctors and nurses became increasingly specific. Unlike professions like radiography though, physiotherapy did not emerge as a result of any specific new invention or discovery. Rather it became a gained its distinct professional identity through its ability to colonise a certain set of quite specific practices (massage, electrotherapy etc.). Thus, the act of 'constructing' the profession's identity became a significant, if not *the* significant professional project for the first half of the 20th century.

Physiotherapy's ability to engage with the agencies that would support its professionalisation project (most notably the State, the medical profession and the general public) became vital to the profession's prosperity. Physiotherapy's ability to 'serve the State' and respond to the changing economy of healthcare, was far more significant than any concern about the scientific merits of the therapies it drew on. To put this in starker terms, the adoption of particular modalities of treatment (Swedish remedial massage, as opposed to other forms of touch, for example) was much more to do with its ability to speak about the legitimacy and orthodoxy of the physiotherapists work than it was to do with any physiological or pathological benefits. The largely passive modalities used by physiotherapists were entirely uncontroversial and remained largely unchallenged until more active interventions began to be promoted in the 1920s and 1930s. Before then, their function was much more political than previous historians of physiotherapy have accounted for (see Part II).

The need to respond to the things that the State felt responsible for is arguably the single most important influence on physiotherapy in the first half of the 20th century. Young physiotherapists today who have grown up in an era of neoliberal economic reform may find it difficult to comprehend that, for much of the last century, public policy towards the health, wealth and happiness of the population was dominated by a belief in social insurance – the idea that the population as a whole should contribute to the welfare of society at large. The policy relied on a strong, healthy working-age population, paying relatively high taxes, to allow governments to organise social services and public infrastructure for all. Those in vulnerable positions (the elderly, children, disabled people, the unemployed etc.) would be given support, but everyone would benefit from free schooling, public services like libraries, free healthcare at the point of delivery, pensions and benefits, subsidised state housing and public services like transport, refuse collection and public administration. This welfarist model of social policy became the principal mode of government – in one form or another – in most developed countries after WWI and reached its zenith in the years between the end of WWII and the 1980s.

Central to this ethos was a belief that things like education, a home and security in retirement should be available to all (universalism); the importance of state intervention in people's lives (statism); equal opportunities and access (egalitarianism); state ownership of national assets (nationalism) and all made possible through the redistribution of wealth through taxation (Lovell & Cordeaux 1999) [1]. Critically, in the context of health and welfare, the State took much more responsibility for some of the problems faced by society. Prior to 1900, few countries had the necessary resources or political will to develop centralised social services, but with the advent of WWI, the economic Depression of the 1920s and 1930s, and the public health and welfare crises that followed, Western States realised that the welfare of the population was a political problem and that if a nation did not look after its people, they were likely to revolt. Industrialisation in the previous two centuries had created considerable prosperity. Infant mortality had declined and life expectancy increased, providing a large working-age population. Governments realised that this population could be leveraged to improve the living conditions of the population as a whole and tackle social problems like poverty, illiteracy and disability. But it also realised that these problems were largely caused by poor housing, overcrowding, poor sanitation, social inequity, poor workplace safety, unequal access to necessary services and war: things for which the State itself was responsible.

Consider many of the principal changes in physiotherapy in the years between 1914 and 1973, and they are almost entirely connected with societal problems that the State felt responsible for: disability caused by warfare leading to the development of the rehabilitation movement after WWI; polio, tuberculosis and influenza between the wars, caused by communicable diseases, giving birth to the neurological and cardiorespiratory physiotherapy sub-specialties; fractures, rheumatic diseases and innovations in orthopaedic surgery creating the need for musculoskeletal and manual therapists. So vast and so sudden was the recognition given to the physiotherapists' role in managing these problems that the profession was never able to supply enough therapists to meet the need.

Having proved its legitimacy with its disciplined approach to the massage scandals in the two decades before the First World War, physiotherapists found themselves ideally placed to respond to the State's call for help tackle the problems that had become an enormous economic burden. I will focus here on two of these responses to illustrate how physiotherapists' reaction to this call shaped the profession for much of the 20th century. The first example is the management of injured servicemen in World War I. The second is the treatment of infantile paralysis.

A noble cause

Much of the 19th century history of the physical therapies was dominated by modalities that were used largely by the wealthy and luxuried classes. Few factory workers, coal miners or seamstresses could afford massage when they were ill or injured, and hardly any had the leisure time to indulge in a week at a European spa or experience the disciplined paternalism of the Rest Cure. Much of this changed, however, after World War I as physiotherapy became available first to returned servicemen, then children afflicted with infantile paralysis and later anyone who entered the subsidised public health system. By 1950, physiotherapy had become such a recognised part of the orthodox healthcare system, and had grown in size to a sufficient degree, that physiotherapists operated across the full spectrum of physical health problems.

A significant reason for this shift lies in the adaptability of modalities like massage, electrotherapy, hydrotherapy and exercise. The ISTM's leaders and practitioners learnt quickly that the skills they had acquired in treating neurasthenic women and patients with weak constitutions before the war were perfectly suited to the treatment of injured servicemen. As Margaret Palmer illustrated in 1917:

> At the time of the founding of the Society massage was used as a luxury of the well-to-do, and regarded as a substitute for healthy exercise. Today it is serving an infinitely nobler end in soothing nervous wrecks, and is helping to save limbs shattered in many a grim battle fought for the country and for freedom.
>
> (Palmer 1917)

For this transformation to take place, however, some adjustments needed to be made by the profession, and some key early principles reasserted.

The first adjustment was needed because of the sheer volume of work created by the war. For example, in Great Britain, members of the Almeric Paget Massage Corps (APMC) – ISTM members who volunteered for war service – were embroiled with other health workers in a scramble to establish services and facilities to cope with the unprecedented toll that appeared within weeks of the outbreak of war in 1914. Of the 750,000 British servicemen killed and 1,500,000 injured during the war, 73,000 were injured in just the first four months (Barclay 1994, p. 63). Places like the London Command Depot in Shoreham, Sussex had 24 masseurs and masseuses treating 650 men daily and the 20 masseuses working at the Heaton Park Command Centre treated 4,000 soldiers in one year, returning half to full active service (Barclay 1994, p. 67). Clearly, no medical, surgical and therapeutic services existed to cope with the demand of that size and so many of the early structural arrangements were haphazard and uncoordinated.

With the intervention of Mrs Almeric Paget, a massage service was started and staffed by members of the ISTM. Masseuses were initially attached to orthopaedic facilities behind the front lines, with some working in convalescent centres at home. At the outbreak of war, there were only 1,000 members of the ISTM, but many of these answered the call for help. Their work, however, met with some considerable scepticism. Many of the doctors and military personnel saw little value in their work and expressed deep concerns about the intimate nature of massage delivered by young women to vulnerable young men. But massage services began and the masseuses quickly demonstrated their value. Olive Millard, in one of the only biographies written by a First World War masseuse, recalls working from 8 a.m. to 8 p.m. treating gunshot wounds, fractures, peripheral nerve injuries, frost bite and patients like Sir Eric V. Bowater, whose body had been crushed by falling earth. 'Fortunately', she explains, 'his head had escaped and weeks of the gentlest massage and progressive treatment brought good results' (Millard 1952, p. 57).

It is worth remembering that, until this point, the masseuses of the ISTM had been engaged in a small, cottage-like industry, largely tending to wrought nerves of society women (Olive Millard's book, for example, is subtitled *The Autobiography of a Society Masseuse*). Within a few months of the outbreak of war, massage became an intrinsic and overstretched part of the injured soldier's recovery.

Certainly, the insistence of the founders of the STM on the need for a strongly patho-anatomical basis to practice, and the close association made with the medical profession helped the masseuses immensely. As Olive Millard explains:

> The varied work that came 'under my thumb' was the most valuable experience imaginable. I had numerous cases of nerve suture following gun-shot wounds. Massage could not cure by itself but it kept alive fading nerveless muscles until the nerves recovered from their injury . . . The anatomy of every nerve and the action of each muscle were imprinted so firmly on our minds that they could never be forgotten.
>
> (Millard 1952, p. 66)

As the war dragged on, the work became more complex, and cases became more and more immutable. Ankylosis, gross muscle atrophy and paralysis were all common and the massage departments began to resemble production lines. At the Northern General Hospital in Leeds, injured servicemen occupied more than 3,500 beds and the massage department was staffed by 80 masseuses (see Figure 4.1). Each masseuse treated about 20 patients a day with 50 masseuses working together in the lecture hall that had been converted into a treatment department. Masseuses worked at small stations organised by particular injuries, with no partitions or privacy, and no variation; 'The monotony nearly drove me crazy but after a week of patiently attending one hundred ulnar injuries my menu was varied by one or two leg cases' (Millard 1952, p. 69).

This picture was repeated all over the Great Britain. At the Aberdeen Orthopaedic Annexe, for example, 550 returned servicemen were managed by three doctors, one

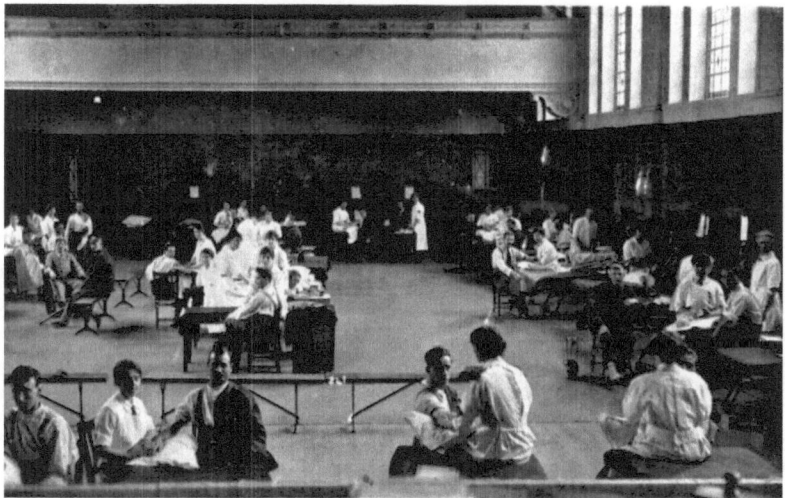

Figure 4.1 Massage room at the 2nd Northern General Hospital, Leeds, 1916. Olive Millard (1952) *Under My Thumb: The Autobiography of a Society Masseuse* published by Christopher Johnson Publishers Ltd.

nurse and 22 masseuses, in a department that the editor of the Journal argued 'could boast the latest massage, electrotherapy and exercise facilities' (*JISTM* 1919). Some of the older modalities like galvanism and faradism began to be used for muscle testing – perhaps physiotherapy's first recognised diagnostic role. And slowly, day-by-day, members of the CSMMG[2] established a foothold alongside the doctors and nurses, and some of the scepticism and suspicion directed at the masseuses from patients, other workers and the military establishment was allayed. In a reflective editorial from 1930, Margaret Palmer expressed this shift in mood: 'We were looked upon not with a little suspicion ... and could not relax efforts in educating the doctors. But we have arrived in every sense of the word' (Palmer 1930, p. 261).

By the end of WWI, membership of the ISTM had almost quadrupled, while the work of post-war was just beginning. In the United States, reconstruction aides – the forerunners of American physical therapists – began to be employed as the toll of the war began to be realised. The reconstruction aides, or RAs', role was created largely in isolation from members of the ISTM yet, like their Canadian and New Zealand colleagues, who formed their own massage associations in 1920 and 1921, respectively, their scopes of practice bore many similarities to those defined earlier by the profession in Britain (Anderson 1977; Cartwright 1924)[3]. This may be, in part, due to the work of the RA's chief instigator, Mary (or Mollie) McMillan. Born in Massachusetts in 1880, McMillan emigrated to Liverpool at the age of five and graduated from Liverpool University 1905. McMillan went on to complete a two-year course in physical culture and corrective exercises at the Liverpool Gymnasium College; 'one of several British institutions devoted to teaching Swedish Ling gymnastics' (Murphy 1995, p. 43), studying under Sir William Bennett – one of the patrons of the STM – and noted orthopaedic surgeon, Sir Robert Jones. At the outbreak of WWI, Jones asked for women to volunteer for a new Voluntary Aide Detachment (VAD). McMillan applied, but was turned down due to near exhaustion, at which point she returned to the United States to take up a post as Director of Massage and Medical Gymnastics at the Children's Hospital in Portland, Maine, from where she began to agitate for an organisation for physical therapists akin to the ISTM's model in Britain.

In August 1917, General William Gorgas authorised the establishment of the Division of Special Hospitals and Physical Reconstruction, which would create the necessary infrastructure and services to begin America's rehabilitation programme (Murphy 1995, p. 44). Men were initially treated at the nearest American Expeditionary Force (AEF) base hospital near the front line and, if possible, returned to the Front. Those with more extensive injuries were shipped back to America to be examined and distributed throughout the nation's 16 draft districts and associated hospital centres (Murphy 1995, p. 45). Mollie McMillan established the first American physical therapy training programme modelled on the ISTM's curriculum and, like Britain, the demand for RAs was enormous. In the 'two years following the Armistice, state-side reconstruction aides gave some 86,000 disabled soldiers more than 3 million treatments' (Murphy 1995, pp. 60–1).

One way of managing the complex and unrelenting workload was to move away from the masseuse's traditional approach of individual treatments. Wendy Murphy states that 'Because there were so many men in need of help, reconstruction aides often ran classes with a dozen or more men working simultaneously at a single task' (Murphy 1995, p. 63). Not only did this begin a new trend towards group exercise that would become a mainstay of physiotherapy throughout the next century (returning the profession to some of Lingian roots largely deviated from by the founders of the STM), but it would also necessitate the construction of larger, independent physiotherapy departments, including outpatient departments and gymnasia.

Following WWI, massage began to be increasingly seen as labour intensive and passive. Much more emphasis began to be placed on exercise as a modality for large groups and, as today, exercise was seen as a way to enhance the health and vigour of the population. Massage was seen as too indulgent, too 'caring' and likely to discourage men from taking responsibility for their own rehabilitation. Like many of his peers, R. Watson-Jones – orthopaedic surgeon to the Royal Air Force in WWII – was a passionate believer in the use of sport as a tool for recovery. RAF orthopaedic centres treated more than 35,000 injured servicemen between 1941 and 1944 (Anderson 2011, p. 109) in units that 'returned 85% of injured pilots to full flying duty' (Anderson 2011, p. 117). The culture in the RAF orthopaedic units was quite distinct from other treatment centres that followed traditional medical systems and structures. Here, rules were lax and the value of recovery through competition became an obsession. Men were grouped on arrival and competitions ran throughout the day to see who could do the most exercises, who could go faster or work harder. Central to this culture was sport and the use of Physical Training Instructors, or PTIs, as an alternative to orthodox health professionals.

Sporting and competitive exercise contrasted with the long periods 'wearisome convalescence' punctuated by massage, electricity, and 'monotonous machines', which 'too often leaves [the injured serviceman] discontented with hospital life' (Jones 1917, p. 514). Consequently, massage and electrotherapy treatments performed by masseuses, began to be focused on only the early, acute stage of injury, where wounds were suppurating or healing. But by WWII, masseuses had adapted to the competition and began to 'administer[ed] the various therapeutic agents there in use but also supervise the earlier stages of remedial exercise, with patients singly or in groups . . . exercising either freely or by means of gymnastic apparatus' (Stanton Woods 1943, p. 421).

Stanton Woods described the configuration of an ideal rehabilitation centre, staffed by one medical officer, one PTI and one masseuses for every 50 injured men, as including, 'A vast covered space' for physical rehabilitation, annexed to massage rooms which opens 'directly from the gymnasium or even be situated within it' (Stanton Woods 1943, pp. 435–6). Some of the earliest bespoke 'physiotherapy' departments were created in this image and many such departments persist today, even in smaller private clinics where exercise rooms are attached to individualised treatment spaces. Besides these structural changes, however, little practical development occurred in physiotherapy during and immediately after WWI.

Practice innovations and sexual tensions

> Most young women assisting in the field of allied health had very little expe-
> rience with men's bodies, but the First World War changed that. Massage
> created potentially awkward and complex physical and social interactions;
> patients and practitioners realised that it could be both painful and sensuous.
>
> (Carden-Coyne 2014, p. 290)

Evidence of real practice innovation is sparse in the years before physiotherapy
became a first contact profession (see Chapter 5). Physiotherapists used well-
known and established treatment techniques and followed medical prescriptions,
so there were few opportunities for the development of new assessment or treatment techniques. Perhaps the exception to this is the work of Olive Guthrie-Smith.
Guthrie-Smith stands out as being one of the few genuine practice innovators in
physiotherapy in the first half of the 20th century. Guthrie-Smith was Head Masseuse
at the London Command Depot in Shoreham, Sussex during WWI and later Principal of Swedish Institute and Director of Physical Exercise Department at
St. Mary's Hospital. She developed apparatus that could suspend limbs, or indeed
the whole body, in slings, and used gravity and various weighted springs as resistance. Once set up, the patient could relax the weightless limb or exercise with or
against gravity (see Figure 4.2). Following a tradition of exercise equipment used
by physical therapists going back to Zander's apparatus in the late 19th century, the
idea was to provide some way of objectively developing graduated free exercises
'permitting the patient to perform any degree or range of movement required'
(Krusen 1943, p. 457).

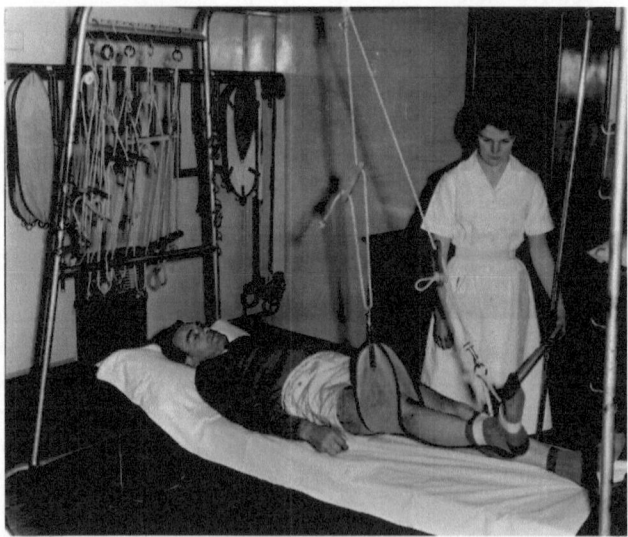

Figure 4.2 Senior student with patient on Guthrie-Smith suspension apparatus. Author's
personal collection.

Guthrie-Smith had become frustrated with the lack of specific exercise offered to the soldiers during her war service as a masseuse, believing that soldiers should be made to 'work hard and do [the work for] himself while [being] carefully kept under supervision, so that adjustments and suspensions may be corrected' (Lanckenau 1943, p. 615). The value of the equipment to physiotherapy was greater than just its role as an adjunct to massage and electrotherapy, though. Guthrie-Smith's apparatus could be stationed over the patient's bed so graduated exercise could begin while the patient was recumbent. Moreover, once set up, patients could exercise with only minimal supervision. Patients could begin exercise almost immediately, reducing the stagnation and potential atrophy of convalescence. They could even be taught how to walk while still in bed using 'ingenious methods of multiple joint work the patient while still recumbent' (Lanckenau 1943, p. 620). As Lackenau argued, 'The psychological effect of early active exercise in recumbency, graduated to active resistive exercise, is enormous' (Lanckenau 1943, p. 620). The apparatus became so familiar that some servicemen nicknamed the devices 'strafes' from the German *Gott strafe England* (God punish England) (Barclay 1994, p. 67).

The apparatus fitted perfectly into the ISTM's principal of treating the body-as-machine, effectively treating the body of the serviceman as one would treat a marionette or a puppet suspended on strings. It created a man-machine assemblage that could be assessed, controlled and measured, and repeated, accurate doses of treatment could be prescribed. It delineated the masseuse from the physical trainer because it required a much higher degree of patho-anatomical knowledge of the soldier's injury and its likely effects, while showing that labour intensive massage and electrotherapy were not the only modalities available to the masseuses. It reinforced and extended the Lingian heritage of remedial exercise based on fundamental and derived positions and it further delineated the masseuses from the doctors and nurses on the wards (Lanckenau 1943, p. 618). It taught masseuses about active, active-assisted and passive exercise – something that had only featured peripherally in their training and examination to date, and it replaced the need for an expensive and space-consuming hydrotherapy pool. It was, in short, an ideal therapeutic and 'political' apparatus and, not surprisingly, one that remained popular in physiotherapy departments for much of the remaining century.

Such apparatus also helped to manage the intimacy of touch that was necessary with so much massage practice. While it still required the female masseuse to touch the patient in some quite intimate ways (suspending the amputated thigh or wrapping the body in straps, for instance), it was essentially procedural and required much less of the sensual touch of massage. WWI brought massed ranks of young men and women into close physical contact for the first time and there were enormous concerns about the sexual tension that this might create, particularly around the use of massage as a therapy. The need to treat men created problems for the ISTM, which had built its reputation for legitimate massage by excluding men from training and treatment. With the advent of war, the profession's prosperity depended on the ability of its young women to demonstrate that they could work confidently and effectively on the bodies of young men. Ana Cardon-Coyne, Beth Linker and Joan McMeeken argue that masseuses navigated this tension by causing pain and, perhaps for the first time in any orthodox health profession, establishing dominant gendered positions over men. As Cardon-Coyne argues, 'Dispensing both pleasure and pain clearly affected relations between the sexes, as the therapist was given authority over a wounded man's body' (Carden-Coyne 2014, p. 291).

Traditional accounts of physiotherapy in the First World War tend to offer a relatively superficial narrative of the worthiness and nobility of the effort and energy brought by masseuses, but they often fail to examine some of the critically important gendered tensions that played a vital role in shaping the profession's identity. World War I presented some new challenges, however, because few masseuses had any experience of massaging 'tender stumps, buttocks, and groins [which] required sensitive arrangements, and could be embarrassing for both patient and therapist' (Carden-Coyne 2014, p. 288). There is no doubt that the masseuses were asked to perform treatments that were, at times, exquisitely painful. Despite what some orthopaedic surgeons like James Mennell argued, the kind of work required to break down adhesions and contracted wounds, stimulate moribund muscles and rehabilitate bodies weakened by disuse was arduous and painful. As Joan McMeeken explains, 'Gymnastics caused exhaustion, pain and muscle soreness, and electrotherapy was a constant source of pain, with some suggesting that modalities like faradisation were used to "shock" patients out of shell shock' (McMeeken 2015, p. 65).

Ana Cardon-Coyne describes the 'rough, uncaring handling of patients at the hands of doctors, nurses, and physiotherapists' as commonplace in the treatment of soldiers and recounts the way injured servicemen felt 'brutalised in the hands of strong women' (Carden-Coyne 2014, p. 286). Cardon-Coyne goes on to argue that 'men's fear of the masseuses was well documented' (Carden-Coyne 2014, p. 286), and that 'Patients often loathed the gymnasium where rehabilitation exercises were conducted . . . Indeed, some patients internalized and thus affirmed the medical and social perceptions of them as passive, weak, child-like and at women's mercy' (Carden-Coyne 2014, p. 287). Beth Linker has suggested the same, arguing that 'physiotherapists resembled drill sergeants more than bedside nurturers' (Linker 2005, p. 330).

But to view the masseuses' use of painful treatments as entirely negative would be to ignore the important role it played in defining the profession's burgeoning identity. Causing pain was, perhaps, a necessary evil given the pressure of work and the necessity to treat as many patients as vigorously as possible to manage the unrelenting workload. Beth Linker argues that the strength and physicality of the masseuses in WWI set them apart from the 'caring qualities embodied by nurses' (Mcmeeken 2015, p. 53) – 'an image taken one step further in Ana Carden-Coyne's depiction of British physiotherapists as brutal pain-inducing despots' (ibid). It would have functioned as a powerful placebo and it would have aligned physiotherapists, once again, with the medical interest in cure rather than the nursing focus on care. Unlike nurses, masseuses were women who could exercise control over men's bodies and were free, to a degree, to do whatever was necessary to return the men to the Front – a point not lost on military authorities and the medical profession. Their treatments tested the men's resolve to return to the Front and uncovered malingerers. It 'distanced' the female therapist from the male patient, but it also forced young men into a more subservient position, empowering the largely female workforce in a proto-suffrage response to male domination over women, giving the young masseuse a gendered power that they would never have known before. As Joan McMeeken argues:

> The [image] of a woman in an unusually dominant role indicates the professional control and power of the physiotherapist. Unlike nurses, physiotherapists were not generally depicted as soft and caring, however this harsher portrayal came to be associated with a service that was beneficial to the war effort in a different way, and it was from here that physiotherapy grew into its own.
>
> (McMeeken 2015, p. 67)

The potential for massage to be pleasurable was a significant concern for those charged with organising the wartime rehabilitation effort. The idea that injured men would return from the Front and be massaged back to health under the 'the loving lingering stroke[s]' (Carden-Coyne 2014, p. 290) of a young female masseuse was a cause of acute anxiety. As Anderson argues, 'the attraction for this type of treatment, apart from being able to lie down, was probably because many of the therapists were female' (Anderson 2011, p. 112). Massage Departments also needed to be large to cope with the numbers of casualties. This often meant that they were situated away from the main hospital. Men could therefore easily disappear in the Massage Department and military authorities could lose track of their whereabouts. Fortunately, the members of the ISTM knew all about how to separate effective and efficient massage from any kind of sensuality, having spent the last 20 years establishing systems to do just that. Deferring to medicine, using the examination system to reinforce its moral purpose, and treating the body-as-machine, allowed the masseuse to effectively depersonalise and desensualise the encounter. As Goodall-Copestake stated in 1917, the 'reasons for [the Society's] rules are obvious and only by adherence to them can certain dangers be avoided' (Goodall-Copestake 1917, p. 4). As Massage Departments became more common, their design, visibility and practical efficiency helped to emphasise the fact that the work undertaken was to be endured rather than enjoyed, with notable ISTM founders like Lucy Robinson writing reports of a 'big sergeant' saying to her that, 'If the Kaiser saw this he might say:—"The English Army is being tortured to make it go to the front"' (Robinson 1915).

The physical and metaphorical separation of the massage department, though, elevated the therapist to the status of specialist and created a new kind of hybrid authority: neither prescribing doctor nor caring nurse; a new kind of practitioner, and one that knew how to handle the trust that the authorities placed in them. WWI also broke the convention of the physiotherapist visiting the patient, in much the same way that doctors had asserted their authority in the 19th century by moving from bedside to hospital medicine (Armstrong 1995). This established a way of working for physiotherapists that would endure for the rest of the century and prepare the profession for the centralised secondary care model that developed under the Welfare State.

The war also made possible a shift in the public's attitude towards disabled people. Beth Linker has written about the changing attitudes towards men disabled in the American Civil War and how the cost of 'honouring' the largely indolent veterans of the Union nearly bankrupted America and brought about the concept of a rehabilitation movement (Linker 2011). Similarly, Wendy Murphy has argued that:

> Prior to the war, physical disability, particularly disability or deformity occurring as the result of birth defect or injury, was regarded by most Americans as irreversible. If those with disabilities could be made a little more comfortable, that was certainly to the good, but there was little expectation that medical intervention would make any real difference in the outcome. And the kind of extended care required to make even small improvements was not available to any but the very rich, which the disabled rarely were.
>
> (Murphy 1995, p. 40)

Taken together, the ruptures created by WWI, brought about a seismic shift in the structure and function of the physiotherapy profession, particularly in Britain. Prior to the war, the ISTM had around 1,000 members. At the end of the war, its membership had increased to nearly 4,000. The American reconstruction aide system only really began as the war ended and membership of the American Physiotherapy Association remained below 1,000 until 1940. But where war had provided the impetus for physiotherapists to prove that they were both legitimate *and* orthodox, the emergence of polio as a significant health problem after the war gave physical therapists a role that established its professional identity in the decades that followed.

Specialisation, differentiation and polio

In the years immediately after the Armistice, rehabilitation services began to be established across America. Progress was slow, however, and the RA's role was quite restricted; 'Diagnosing doctors filled out prescription forms on which were printed seven special types of functional treatment (abduction, adduction, flexion, extensions, pronation, supination, and circumduction) together with the parts of the body to which treatment was to be applied' (Murphy 1995, p. 48). Many of the same gendered concerns around touch also persisted for the American therapists, with student RAs being chaperoned in all of their dealings with their young, male patients (Murphy 1995, p. 48). Like their British masseuse sisters, much of the RA's work was tedious and formulaic. Facilities in the American field hospitals and back home at the newly commissioned rehabilitation centres were rudimentary and the women who served under the Army Medical Corps received poor salaries and none of the benefits of military service. Matters were made more complicated by the emergence of a range of communicable diseases almost immediately after WWI that stretched the already over-reaching rehabilitation services to their limit. Influenza added nearly three quarters of a million American casualties to the war wounded in 1919 and outbreaks of polio were recorded in every summer after 1916 until the 1960s.

After WWI, most masseuses re-entered private practice work at home. But with no well-established public role, and lacking the state support they had received during the war, numbers of RAs plummeted from 748 members working in 49 American hospitals to just 175 working in 11 facilities between 1919 and 1920 (Murphy 1995, p. 67). In isolated centres, however, American doctors and RAs began to apply their respective skills to conditions like polio. Therapists like Susan Roen – author of the influential *Techniques of Underwater Gymnastics* in 1937 in Boston – and Baltimore's Henry Kendall, began working with doctors on the application of traditional physical therapy techniques to paralysed children (Murphy 1995, pp. 94–5).

American physical therapies inadvertently received a boost to their popularity and significance when in August 1921, the 39-year-old future president, Franklin Delano Roosevelt, succumbed to polio while on holiday. Roosevelt was paralysed from the waist down but 'worked arduously for more than two years' after which time he 'succeeded only in gaining the use of a wheelchair' (Murphy 1995, p. 95). Roosevelt's experience of physical therapy was, however, entirely positive and he invested heavily in treatment facilities, especially at Warm Springs in Georgia, where physical therapists supervised all of the treatment. Two of the therapists who passed through the centre were Lucille Daniels and Catherine Worthington who would later co-author the highly acclaimed textbooks *Muscle Testing* (1946) and *Therapeutic Exercise* (1957).

Despite the privations of The Depression that nearly decimated training and private practice rehabilitation, the profession received a boost in 1932 when Roosevelt became President. In his 'first 100 days' Roosevelt initiated widespread welfare reforms. The 'New Deal' as it was called did not replace private benefaction, however, and centres like Warm Springs still relied on charity with the rehabilitation centre raising a million dollars each year after 1933 through charitable donations. Ironically, this was more money than the centre needed and so its manager, Basil O'Connor (who was also Roosevelt's old law partner), invested the money in the creation of a new organisation called the National Foundation for Infantile Paralysis (NFIP) in 1937, which would subsequently fund enormous expansion in physiotherapy programmes throughout the United States.

Alongside the support of the NFIP, Roosevelt's *Social Security Act* of 1935;

> provided the United States Public Health Service with the funds and the authority to build a system of state and local health departments . . . Before then children with polio wasted away at home, receiving only occasional visits from a doctor, waiting for a place in an orthopaedic hospital or convalescent home.
>
> (Murphy 1995, p. 99)

Although not all the money went directly into children's services, the demand for physical therapists to work in outpatient centres, convalescent homes, hospitals and schools grew exponentially. By 1939, and the outbreak of WWII, all 48 states had effective 'crippled children's' programmes treating the estimated 165,000 children affected by polio.

Before the arrival of Sister Kenny to America in 1940, there had only been one partially effective method of treatment characterised by bed rest and immobilisation (Murphy 1995, p. 123). When the belligerent, intolerant and stubborn Irish nurse Elizabeth Kenny arrived in America in 1940, after failing to convince the British medical establishment of the veracity of her approach during a year-long trial of her methods at Queen Mary's Hospital for Children in 1937 (Barclay 1994, p. 117), American doctors were equally challenged by her ability to promote herself and her cause. Kenny 'believed in aggressive physical therapy from the outset' (Murphy 1995, p. 123). She disliked splinting or bracing of any sort, arguing that orthodox practitioners were inadvertently worsening the paralysis and weakness when they used splinting and bed rest. Kenny preferred treating patients with 'round-the-clock hot "fomentations," or hot, wet packs applied to affected areas' (Murphy 1995, p. 123). Her approach was highly labour intensive, but she believed that it significantly reduced the muscle spasm that she believed caused muscle atrophy and the destruction of motor neurons.

Demonstration wards were set up at the Minneapolis General Hospital and the University of Minnesota Medical School and a staff of 20 physical therapists was 'loaned' for six months to implement Kenny's treatment regime. Results proved initially promising, which led to support from notable doctors (like Frank Krusen) and organisations, and a massive investment in new resources, including a purpose-built centre in Minneapolis. There were problems, however. Groups of three physical therapists were needed to continually rush boiling hot cloths from the steriliser to tubs near the patient. The cloths were then wrung through and applied in rapid succession to the patient's body. To treat a ward of 20 children with hot packs every two hours required 12–15 therapists (often students) to be in constant motion (Murphy 1995, p. 127).

A year after the trial, doubts began to emerge about the true efficacy of the treatment and severe shortages of physical therapy students meant that few regional centres could follow Minneapolis's lead. Claims that the Kenny Method succeeded in 90 percent of cases were cast into doubt, and centres in Boston, St. Louis and elsewhere began to renege (Visscher & Myers 1945). Slowly, practitioners returned to orthodox methods of treatment and persisted with more traditional, manageable treatment regimes. More than 25,000 cases of polio were treated by physiotherapists in the UK alone in this manner after WWII (Barclay 1994, p. 187).

If Kenny's methods ultimately proved no more effective than orthodox treatments – a question still being explored by scholars today (Rogers 2014) – they certainly succeeded in testing the orthodox medical establishment, and most especially the 50-year synergy between physiotherapists and doctors. Research into Kenny's methods forced the medical establishment to undertake some of the first large trials of physical therapies that had, until now, largely passed without challenge. Questions were raised both about the therapeutic benefits of heat, localised rest, active and passive movements, electrotherapy, and mobilisation, but also about the most beneficial ways to apply these modalities. Kenny's approach also challenged physiotherapists to think about their own profession.

Firstly, it drew physiotherapists together and emphasised their shared professional identity. Physiotherapists were considered by Kenny to be all alike; an assimilation that Kenny saw as negative, but proved hugely significant for the therapists themselves who, for perhaps the first time, began to share a collective professional identity. Kenny's challenge also made physiotherapists aware of the need for clinical differentiation. In previous decades, masseuses had used a relatively limited range of modalities in a quite undifferentiated way. It did not particularly matter, for example, if the patient was a polio victim, a child with cerebral palsy or war veteran with a peripheral nerve injury, they were all offered massage and electrotherapy. Because of Kenny's attention to the specific management of the patient with polio, physiotherapists began to realise that different groups of patients could be approached in radically different ways.

In hindsight, it is possible to recognise two significant effects of this. The first is the birth of specialisation in the profession – the gradual differentiation between the specialist and the novice practitioner – added to the growing distinctions that emerged between emerging branches of physiotherapy (orthopaedic, neurological, cardiorespiratory etc.) (Webb et al 2009). This, of course, would herald the development of special interest groups, that would mimic the growing medical organisation of the formal healthcare system. The second effect related to physiotherapists' growing sense of professional autonomy. While mirroring medicine's organisational structure, physiotherapy's increasing sense of specialisation pointed to a concern for its desire for self-determination[4]. This was especially seen in the structure of the profession's regulatory and professional bodies during the 1930s, 1940s and 1950s. Slowly, physiotherapists replaced doctors on their boards with a growing cohort of professional specialists and administrators.

The inexorable move from the 'general' to the 'specific' also implied a shift towards more applied knowledge, and a concurrent emphasis on the different ways that knowledge of the four main treatment modalities could be used. Cardiorespiratory physiotherapy is a case in point. Prior to Hester Angove's 1936 text on *Remedial Exercises for Certain Diseases of the Heart and Lung* (Angove 1936), patients with cardiorespiratory complaints were treated in much the same way as other patients. The sequelae of gas inhalation and empyema from gunshot wounds during WWI, followed by the use of artificial ventilation in cases of polio, taught physiotherapists that their basic treatment methods were highly adaptable and myriad different variations on some tried-and-tested techniques could be developed. (What is chest percussion, for example, if not a variation on basic tapotement?) This emphasis on applied knowledge also gave greater impetus to the study of biomechanics, ergonomics, exercise science and a range of other applied studies, and it pre-empted the profession's move to becoming a first contact profession in some countries by emphasising the importance of differential diagnosis and the study of pathology (Pagliarulo 2007). Some of the most popular and significant general physiotherapy textbooks of the 20th century were instigated with this impetus in mind. Nöel Tidy's books on massage and remedial exercise (currently in its 15th edition), Joan Cash's textbooks of medical and surgical conditions, neurology and orthopaedic disorders, and 'Clayton's Electrotherapy' series were all first published in the 1930s and 1940s following closely to the model of applied assessment and treatment differentiated by pathology.

It is worth remembering that physiotherapy was not a profession born from a new invention (like X-rays), so developments in physiotherapy have always been based on either the adaptation and refinement of 'old' knowledge, or a change in the practice context physiotherapists have found themselves in. The massage scandals, the World War, widespread economic disruption and epidemics presented such opportunities for professional differentiation and growth that, by the 1940s, physiotherapy was well on the way to established professional recognition and respectability where, once again, physiotherapy showed itself to benefit from accidents of history (French & Swain 2008, p. 45; Bourke 1996, p. 51), most especially the creation of the Welfare State.

Welfare State and the creation of a profession

Unlike World War I, which had such a profound impact on the structure and function of physiotherapy practice, World War II was less significant than the social reforms of the 1930s and 1940s that instigated what is now known as the Welfare State. Certainly, WWII was catastrophic on a human scale, but it was less profound for the physiotherapy profession. As Barclay argues,

> In the First World War orthopaedics had captured the public imagination and masseuses had shared in its glory, but the Second World War was not an 'orthopaedists' war' and newer specialisms like plastic surgery and the treatment of spinal injuries fired the public imagination.
>
> (Barclay 1994, pp. 125–6)

Proportionally fewer physiotherapists served in direct, front-line care in WWII than WWI; front-line surgical and medical services were much more advanced by 1939 and extensive rehabilitation services for amputees, fractures and other war injuries had been available in most regional centres for years. Indeed, if one looks at the journals and minutes of the professional bodies during the Second World War one would be hard pressed to know that a war was on. With a few obvious exceptions due to shortages of personnel and facilities, rationing and some re-allocation of services as a result of war damage, it appears that physiotherapy continued to function much as normal.

There were few practice innovations to speak of, with much of the change happening with the ongoing specialisation and differentiation seen in the inter-war years. Certainly, exercise became a more significant practice modality both because of its therapeutic efficiency, and because it was thought to focus more on the individual's own active recovery than massage, electrotherapy and other 'passive' modalities could. As one commentator argued, 'There can be no possible doubt that the danger of patients being buried alive in a workshop is even more grave than the former danger of patients being buried in the massage department' (Watson-Jones 1943, p. 406).

Anderson argues that:

> Although the medical profession considered remedial exercises and physiotherapy more important components of the rehabilitative process, sport was imbued with additional benefits that included the psychological. It was also felt that sport would re-create the sense of ordinary human association, particularly for those permanently disabled.
>
> (Anderson 2011, p. 82)

Physiotherapists were not immune to this shift, and felt equally as able as physical training instructors and others to promote and deliver active rehabilitation. As one editorial in the *British Physiotherapists' Journal* reported:

> We should be filled with the crusading spirit, gathering the population together in every empty hall in the winter and in parks and fields in summer, teaching them how to stand and breathe, how to walk, move and dance, how to develop a sense of rhythm, and how to march with elastic step towards 'physical literacy'.
>
> (*JCSMMG*, March 1936, p. 234 cited in Barclay, p. 100)

Notwithstanding these relatively minor shifts, a much greater shift was taking place in the structure and organisation of healthcare that would secure physiotherapy's professional future for the next half century. This shift can be understood in two relatively straightforward changes: the first is the creation of legislation that differentiated between orthodox and non-orthodox professions; the second is the access this legislation affords to patients within the public health system. These two features were pivotal structural elements of the Welfare State.

First explored at the turn of the century, the idea of *welfarism*, or social insurance, was a reaction to the liberalism of the late 19th century. Liberalism is a principal that espouses freedom, individual responsibility and the minimal intervention of the State in people's affairs. Many of the advances seen after the Industrial Revolution, and the political upheavals of the 18th and 19th centuries can be traced to an increasing concern for the 'rights of man' and a desire for people to be free from political and sovereign oppression. One of the consequences of liberal economic and political reforms, however, was a growing recognition that it did nothing to prevent exploitation or discrimination. Indeed, it relied upon a social gradient that amplified differences between the 'haves' and 'have-nots' leading George Orwell's to comment that clearly 'some animals are born more equal than others' (Orwell 1946). Realising that poverty, sickness, unemployment, delinquency, inadequate housing, pollution and infirmity were political as much as social issues, nation states began to take responsibility for the welfare of the population as a whole and enact legislation to centralise the organisation of some nationwide services. From the Danish and German pensions legislation of the 1890s, through the state home and hospital building projects in Commonwealth countries, to Roosevelt's 'New Deal' of the 1930s, a welfarist approach to government slowly replaced the laissez-faire liberalism of the previous century.

Returning to a point I made earlier, welfarism was as much about the state taking responsibility for social problems and this had a profound impact on healthcare because governments throughout the Western world enacted policies that organised the distribution and development of healthcare providers who could respond to the things the State felt responsible for. Physiotherapy, as a close partner to medicine, benefitted hugely from this. Although many physiotherapists express deep concern about the inroads chiropractors have made into physiotherapy territory since the 1950s, imagine how the history of the profession might have differed had chiropractors been chosen as the preferred provider of orthodox physical rehabilitation with the creation of the Welfare State in the 1930s and 1940s. Chiropractors would have been the ones benefitting from profession-specific legislation, enormous investment in training and research and privileged access to patients in the public health system. It is hard to imagine physiotherapy growing to a profession of nearly half-a-million registered practitioners or achieving the same social capital as it carries today, if it had been framed as the alternative or complementary therapeutic option. Welfare reforms, therefore, did infinitely more to advance the cause of physiotherapy than any practice innovation. Indeed, I would argue welfarism is a defining feature of physiotherapy's contemporary professional image and one that is significantly threatened by the growing importance of neoliberal economic, political and social reform. How did welfarism affect physiotherapy, though?

To begin with, it is important to realise that the 'State' part of the Welfare State was constituted by more than just central government. In effect, the Welfare State was a constellation of services and structures designed to coordinate and rationalise services. So, in America for instance, national institutions like the NFIP functioned as welfare providers to paralysed children, funding equipment, services and training for families and their support teams. As Wendy Murphy argues, 'acute and chronic poliomyelitis had been the principal engine driving the advancement of physical therapy', and the NFIP's funding provided the basis for exponential growth in the physical therapy profession in the 1940s and 1950s. After an annual grant of $10,000 to the American Physiotherapy Association the NFIP;

> set aside an additional $1,267,600 for the expansion of physical therapy on several fronts; funding allocations included scholarships to assist nearly 90 candidates in their undergraduate studies, a dozen exchange fellowships with Canadian physical therapists, still other fellowships to provide additional instructors in approved schools of physical therapy, and monies to underwrite various surveys and slide and film programs for distribution to schools and APA chapters.

(Murphy 1995, p. 129)

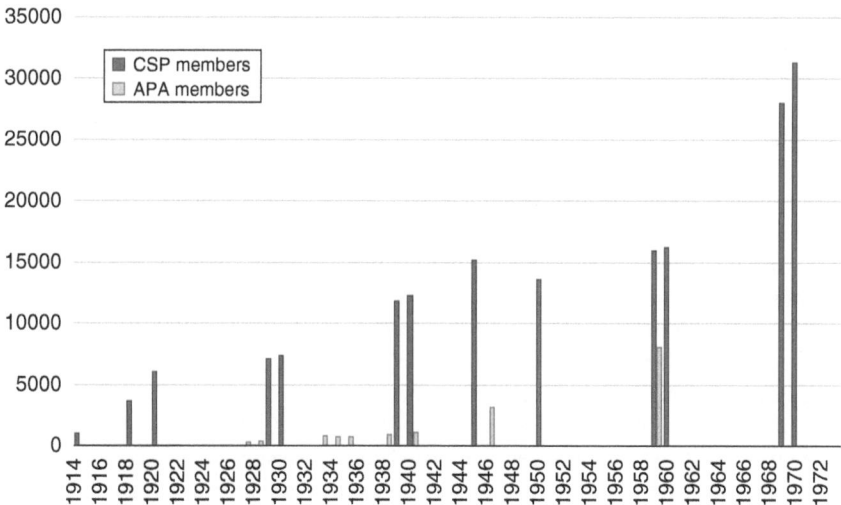

Figure 4.3 Chart showing growth in CSP and APA membership 1914–1974.

The NFIP provided a $5,000 grant to help the APA open its first national office in New York, which had become necessary because of the fourfold growth in professional memberships in the four years after the end of WWII (see Figure 4.3 and Murphy 1995, p. 113).

Although funding provided the means to grow and organise physiotherapy internationally, legislation was almost as influential in creating the necessary demand for work. Roosevelt's 1935 *Social Security Act*, was complemented by equally radical legislation in the UK in the 1940s. In all, six pieces of legislation were enacted that had a direct bearing on the care of ill and disabled people, including *Disabled Persons (Employment) Act*, The *National Health Service Act*, the *Education Act*, the *National Insurance Act*, The *National Insurance (Industrial Injuries) Act* and the *National Assistance Act* (Anderson 2011, p. 177). All of these acts became law between 1944 and 1948 and created both profession-specific roles and responsibilities for orthodox health providers like doctors, nurses and physiotherapists, but also connected together services and created care pathways for patients with acute illness and injury through to rehabilitation and workplace resettlement.

Welfare reforms brought about enormous investment in orthodox health services like hospitals, national general practice networks and health training institutes. It created the kinds of reductive models of secondary care that privilege the idea that patients move from the generalist to the specialist, who is centrally located and the head of a large team of professions 'allied' to medicine. Welfarism simplified the choices available to people, and cemented the belief that medicine offered the most trustworthy and affordable method of managing public health and wellbeing, and that professions that had the doctor's trust could, themselves, share in the reflected status carried by the medical profession. To understand how profoundly welfare reforms affected the nature of physiotherapy practice, we need only look at the effect of nationalised healthcare on private practice.

As large new physiotherapy departments opened up around Britain, like the London County Council (LCC) Hospital at Tooting in London, which carried out an unimaginable '482,452 massages and electrical treatments in 1933; 544,007 in 1934 and 623,253 in 1936' (*JCSMMG* 1937), private practice drifted into decline. Barclay argues that 'The coming of the National Health Service had reduced but not ruined private practice' (Barclay 1994, p. 207)[5], but that '[p]rivate practice declined after the introduction of the NHS and the [CSP's Appointments] Bureau reported that in 1953–1954 hospital appointments were up by 22% on the year before and private practice down by 37%' (Barclay 1994, p. 155). Prior to the NHS, '[p]rivate practitioners had been used to working (at 7s [shillings] and 6d [pence]) in small hospitals and clinics run by voluntary or municipal bodies and hoped to continue this service and extend it into the home', but the Minister of Health informed physiotherapists that under the new NHS, that 'physiotherapy should primarily be a hospital service carried out by properly supervised employees', and that 'only rarely would private individuals be asked to treat patients' (Barclay 1994, p. 154).

Australian physiotherapists, more used to independent private practice, shared the view of their medical colleagues, who 'worried that a National Health Scheme would see them controlled by bureaucrats and politicians' (Bentley & Dunstan 2006, p. 133). Australian physiotherapists, Bentley argues 'were chastened by the experience of their colleagues in Britain, where a similar health scheme had been introduced in 1948' (ibid), and that 'This had seen a significant fall off in patients attending private practitioners, whose fees were not subsidized, at the expense of those employed in hospitals, whose fees were' (ibid).

Under such competitive pressure, Australian private practitioners worked assiduously to secure their competitive advantage over other practitioners. Physiotherapy remained essentially a low-cost occupation, requiring little more than a room, a bed and a few pieces of basic electrotherapy equipment. As the 1950s passed into the 1960s, however, physiotherapists began to think of themselves as having commodities and consumables that might attract the interests of product manufacturers and marketing people. Partly born from a desire to see the profession develop a greater sense of autonomy through the production and dissemination of its own research, and partly from a desire to carve out a market advantage over nurses, doctors and complementary therapies, who were seen as a palpable threat to the economic and social capital now possessed by physiotherapy, technological advances emerged as a new frontier in physiotherapy's efforts to establish a unique professional identity.

Physiotherapy's white heat of technology

Harold Wilson's often quoted phrase that a 'new Britain' would need to be forged in the white heat of a new 'scientific revolution' (Francis 2013) perhaps pinpoints one of the most important discourses influencing physiotherapy in the long period of economic growth that followed World War II. Barclay describes the period from 1945 to 1960 as 'an era of reconstruction and redirection which gave birth to many features of today's Chartered Society' (Barclay 1994, p. 152). Physiotherapy had achieved professional credibility and a critical size significant enough for healthcare policy makers, politicians and professional leaders to explore its 'micro-economy'. Numbers of practitioners had increased to the point where physiotherapists represented their own market to advertisers and product manufacturers and, although physiotherapy remained largely a manual occupation, there was still money to be made in selling new treatment beds, exercise equipment and, increasingly, electrotherapy devices.

The volumes of work that physiotherapists now had to manage had increased to the point where their departments had become small communities, with some physiotherapy departments operating their own internal hierarchies. This may not have been the case outside of the large urban centres, but in many cities, it was possible for novice practitioners to have a path towards expertise laid out for them by senior colleagues with whom they worked and learned. One of the largest sections of the physiotherapy department was Out Patients, where patients would be brought daily for individual manual therapies or group exercises. Patients progressed through here with production line-like efficiency. The front of the building would teem with patients waiting for their next appointment. Patients recovering from wrist fractures would be sitting with one arm wrapped in towels, encasing a hand that had just been given a wax bath; others would be called by the physiotherapist at an allotted time to come to join the latest 'Early Knee', 'Shoulder' or 'Hands' exercise class; and many would be taken off to the large cubicled room for one-to-one treatment.

The sheer number of patients that passed through the department in any one day was staggering, and it would not be unusual for a busy department to be staffed by 20-or-more physiotherapists. At Alder Hey Special Military Surgical Hospital, for instance, 58 masseuses and five masseurs treated 1,540 men each day, giving 800 massages, 380 electrical, 190 gymnasium and 170 hydrotherapy treatments (Chuck, n.d.). One way in which the department could manage the workload was to put people into group exercise classes and this worked well where patients presented with relatively uniform problems and recovery trajectories (patients with colles fractures or post-hip/knee replacements, for example), but this did not work well with conditions that needed more individualised attention; problems like acute soft tissues injuries, burns and plastic surgery, nerve injuries and chronic pain. Here the patient often needed an individual assessment, and an individualised treatment plan. Massage, mobilisations and bespoke exercise programmes (using sling suspensions or proprioceptive neuromuscular facilitation techniques, for instance), were time consuming and labour intensive. Perhaps it is not surprising, therefore, that labour saving devices like short-wave diathermy and interferential became popular and increasingly used after the 1950s.

Adverts placed in professional journals after WWII show an increasing appetite for such devices, as physiotherapy became a viable new market for many companies. Companies like Enraf-Nonius, Rank Medical and Siemens fed into the need to provide specialised therapeutic input to idiosyncratic illnesses and injuries, and benefitted from the demand for the therapist to treat multiple patients in parallel. The new wave of ultrasound, interferential, short-wave and microwave devices was a boon to the private practitioner and the busy outpatients department alike, because a patient could be set up on their machine and monitored for the duration of their treatment, while other patients were being set up on their own devices. Of course, this naturally led to a long period in which departments became enormous equipment stores and treatment became a euphemism for 'plugging the patients into the wall'. In many countries, the funding mechanisms were such that private practitioners were often paid for each patient they saw, which served to encourage the more unscrupulous practitioners to treat multiple patients at the same time and bill funders in multiples.

Fortunately, these kinds of unscrupulous billing practices were isolated and short-lived, in part because of the rapid increase in quantitative research that accompanied the 'white heat' emanating from every physiotherapy room. The increasing affordability, portability and efficiency of electrotherapy modalities gave physiotherapists their own equivalent of the medical drug trial. For the first time, physiotherapists could manipulate variables; establish intervention, control and placebo groups; calibrate test measures and talk of standard deviations in ways that had, until now, been the preserve of their medical colleagues. Of course, electrotherapy devices had been prevalent before the 1950s, but physiotherapists had neither the critical mass, the necessary level of scientific scholarship nor the particular market to justify wide-ranging trials of the efficacy of their treatments. Now, all of these were in place. Physiotherapy programmes had also begun to move from vocational training institutes to universities, and the profession began to offer academic pathways for lecturers and researchers. Electrotherapy offered the perfect opportunity for clinical scientists to develop their skills and so after 1960 there was a rapid increase not only in the volume, but also quality and criticality of published research.

Consequently, physiotherapists began travelling to international conferences to present the findings of their studies and a secondary industry began to emerge, made up of experts who were abreast of a particular field and able to provide critical commentary on the state of research into a range of therapeutic strategies. Soon, almost all the fields of physiotherapy practice were being judged by similar standards and the 1960s saw a transformation in the way physiotherapy was evaluated and presented. Journals slowly replaced their pages on births, deaths and marriages with brisk scientific reports on recent clinical trials; opinion pieces by worthy medical men were replaced with evidence-informed reviews of best practiceand well-meaning social pieces reporting on people's visits to exotic overseas locations were replaced with adverts for the latest piece of therapeutic technology.

Conferences too were transformed. The abstracts for the World Confederation for Physical Therapy (WCPT) conferences of 1963, 1967 and 1970 show a remarkable growth in popularity of scientific studies. Having been formed in 1953, the WCPT's three- or four-yearly Congress became the international showcase for the emerging scientific community in physiotherapy. Invited speakers provided evidence of a growing culture of theoretical excellence emerging in the profession, and thousands of small projects were presented and international collaborations launched. WCPT fostered the scientific credibility of physiotherapy by promoting the idea that knowledge of physical therapies could be universal – in other words, if a treatment could be shown to be effective in a clinic in Wyoming, the treatment should work the same way in Warsaw or Winnipeg. What mattered was that the quality of the research itself met the standards developed in the medical sciences. Naturally, physiotherapists began to consider the critical quality of their research, and explore – perhaps in very crude and simple terms by today's standards – what would be *their* clinical trial methodologies, randomisation, control, dependent and independent variables.

By the early 1970s, physiotherapy had become a highly diverse, popular, well-resourced and nationally supported profession, with its own developing body of scientific literature, secure professional bodies, protective legislation in many places and a large, energetic group of therapists with a strong sense of their past identity, but an eagerness to grasp the transformative possibilities of future science-led practice. You can see this eagerness in the writings of some of the profession's leaders at the time. Returning to the quote at the opening of the chapter, Helen Hislop, in her 10th Mary McMillan memorial lecture to the APTA in 1975 quoted Pericles, arguing that physical therapists should 'Fix [their] eyes on the greatness of your profession . . . fall in love with her' and 'remember that her greatness was won by people with courage, with knowledge of their duty, and with a vision that all things are possible' (Hislop 1975, p. 1069).

Hislop, like many of her colleagues, felt confident enough with her profession's newfound standing to argue that 'Physical therapy is knowledge. Physical therapy is clinical science. Physical therapy is the reasoned application of science to warm and needing human beings. Or it is nothing' (Hislop 1975, p. 1070). Hislop was speaking as if the profession represented the confluence of a number of rivers that had begun as small streams many years ago and had now come together to form a mighty river. Little did she realise that the potential energy held within this massive body of water, would not overflow and spread across the landscape with as much potential energy as she had anticipated, but become progressively more and more frustrated in its flow and tamed by the events that unfolded after 1973. These are the events to which I now turn as I consider the critical moments in physiotherapy's more recent history – the history through which most of the readers of this book will have passed. Here I ask why it was that the mighty river that Helen Hislop and others envisaged in 1975 did not eventuate, and how the profession's abundant potential and kinetic energy of the previous three quarters of a century was dammed.

Notes

1 It would be wrong to imagine that universal welfare was ever anything other than an idea. Many authors have highlighted the discrepancies and inequalities that were perpetuated under the welfare state. Indeed, physiotherapists were pivotal in this process of differentiation and inequality – an issue I address in more detail in Chapter 8. (See also French, & Swain 2008; Borsay 2005; Oliver 2009.)

2 The STM become the Incorporated Society of Trained Masseuses (ISTM) in June 1900, the Chartered Society of Massage and Medical Gymnastics (CSMMG) in June 1920, and the CSP in November 1943.
3 It is worth noting that although Australian masseuses began professional organisation as early as 1906, they also followed the 'preferred English model' (McMeeken 2015, p. 54). As Joan McMeeken argues: 'The "English" model of training that emphasised exercise, massage and electrotherapy, underpinned by a course in biomedical sciences had by 1914 become the backbone of physiotherapy training in Australia' (McMeeken 2015, p. 56).
4 It is interesting to note that the CSP had a doctor as its Chair from its inception in 1895 until 1974.
5 Prior to the formation of the NHS, almost 19 million people in Britain relied on private medical insurance for healthcare. As a result of the Depression of the 1930s, few could afford physiotherapy. Added to this, the profession retained its historical ban on public advertising and continued to graduate 500 new practitioners each year. Not surprisingly, the profession grew very little before the creation of the NHS.

References

Anderson, E.M., 1977, *New Zealand society of physiotherapists: Golden Jubilee 1923–1973*, New Zealand Society of Physiotherapists, Wellington, New Zealand.

Anderson, J., 2011, *War, disability and rehabilitation in Britain: "Soul of a nation"*, Manchester University Press, Manchester.

Angove, H.S., 1936, *Remedial exercises for certain diseases of the heart and lung*, Faber & Faber, London.

Armstrong, D., 1995, The rise of surveillance medicine, *Sociology of Health & Illness*, 17(3), pp. 393–404.

Barclay, J., 1994, The story behind 'In Good Hands', *Physiotherapy*, 80(12), pp. 857–60.

Bentley, P. & Dunstan, D., 2006, *The path to professionalism: Physiotherapy in Australia to the 1980s*, Australian Physiotherapy Association, Melbourne, Australia.

Borsay, A., 2005, *Disability and social policy in Britain since 1750: A history of exclusion*, Palgrave Macmillan, Basingstoke.

Bourke, J., 1996, *Britain and the Great War*, Reaktion Books, London.

Carden-Coyne, A., 2014, *The politics of wounds: Military patients and medical power in the first World War*, Oxford University Press, New York.

Cartwright, E.M., 1924, History of the Canadian association of massage and remedial gymnastics, *Journal of the Canadian Association of Massage and Remedial Gymnastics*, (March), pp. 5–6.

Chuck, S., Massage and electrical treatments at Alder Hey Special Military Surgical Hospital, retrieved from www.scarletfinders.co.uk/180.html, accessed 7 April 2016.

Dyer, L.E. 1994, The profession and the government. *Physiotherapy*, 80, 70A–71A. doi:10.1016/S0031-9406(10)60990-X.

Francis, M., 2013, Harold Wilson's 'white heat of technology' speech 50 years on, *The Guardian*. Retrieved May 6, 2016, from https://www.theguardian.com/science/political-science/2013/sep/19/harold-wilson-white-heat-technology-speech.

French, S. & Swain, J., 2008, *Understanding disability: A guide for health professionals*, Elsevier/Churchill Livingstone, Edinburgh.

Goodall-Copestake, B.M., 1917, *The theory and practice of massage*, H.K. Lewis, London.

Hislop, H.J., 1975, The not-so-Impossible Dream, *Physical Therapy*, 55(10), pp. 1069–80.

JCSMMG, 1937, Editorial, *Journal of the Chartered Society of Masseuses and Medical Gymnasts*, (May), p. 280.

JISTM, 1919, Editorial, *Journal of the Incorporated Society of Trained Masseuses* (July), p. 11.

Jones, R., 1917, Notes on military orthopaedics (review), *British Medical Journal*.

Krusen, F.H., 1943, Rehabilitation of the chronically disabled with special reference to the use of physical measures, in W.B. Doherty & D.D. Runes (eds.), *Rehabilitation of the war injured, a symposium*, New York, Philosophical Library, pp. 454–63.

Lanckenau, N.I., 1943, Rehabilitation by modern methods of exercise, in W.B. Doherty & D.D. Runes (eds.), *Rehabilitation of the war injured, a symposium*, New York, Philo- sophical Library, pp. 614–21.

Linker, B., 2005, Strength and science: Gender, physiotherapy, and medicine in the United States, 1918–35, *Journal of Women's History*, 17(3), pp. 106–32.

Linker, B., 2011, *War's waste: Rehabilitation in World War I America*, University of Chicago Press, Chicago, IL.

Lovell, T. & Cordeaux, C., 1999, *Social policy for health and social care*, Hodder and Stoughton, London.

McMeeken, J., 2015, Australian physiotherapists in the First World War, *Health & History*, 17(2), pp. 52–75.

Millard, O., 1952, *Under my thumb*, Christopher Johnson, London.

Murphy, W., 1995, *Healing the generations: A history of physical therapy and the American Physical Therapy Association*, Greenwich Publishing, Lyme, CT.

Oliver, M., 2009, *Understanding disability: From theory to practice*, 2nd ed., Palgrave Macmillan, Basingstoke, UK.

Orwell, G., 1946, *Animal farm*, Harcourt, Brace and Company, New York.

Pagliarulo, M.A. 2007, *Introduction to physical therapy*, 3rd ed., Mosby, St. Louis, MO.

Palmer, M., 1930, Editorial, *Journal of the Chartered Society of Massage and Medical Gymnastics*, (April), p. 261.

Palmer, M.D., 1917, Editorial, *Journal of Incorporated Society of Therapeutic Masseuses*, (November), p. 110.

Robinson, L., 1915, Editorial, *Journal of Incorporated Society of Therapeutic Masseuses*, (July), pp. 10–11.

Rogers, N., 2014, *Polio wars: Sister Kenny and the golden age of American medicine*, Oxford University Press, New York.

Rose, N., 1997, *Inventing ourselves: Psychology, power and personhood*, Cambridge University Press, Cambridge, UK.

Rose, N., 1999, *Governing the soul: The shaping of the private self*, 2nd ed., Routledge, London.

Stanton Woods, R., 1943, Rehabilitation in the British emergency medical service, in W.B. Doherty & D.D. Runes (eds.), *Rehabilitation of the war injured, a symposium*, New York, Philosophical Library, pp. 416–23.

Visscher, M.B. & Myers, J.A., 1945, Editorial: Sister Kenny – Five years later, *Lancet (London, England)*, 65, pp. 309–10.

Watson-Jones, R., 1943, Rehabilitation in the royal air-force, in W.B. Doherty & D.D. Runes eds., *Rehabilitation of the war injured, a symposium*, New York, Philosophical Library, pp. 424–39.

Webb, G., Skinner, M., Jones, S., Vicenzino, B., Nall, C., & Baxter, D., 2009, Physiotherapy in the 21st century, In J. Higgs, M.S. Smith, G.W. Webb, M.S. Skinner & A.C. Croker (eds.), *Contexts of physiotherapy practice*, Churchill Livingstone, Sydney, Australia, pp. 4–19.

5 Physiotherapy under neoliberalism (1973–present)

Introduction

In this chapter, I focus on physiotherapy's most recent past, specifically the last half century in the history of the profession. As with the other chapters in this first section, my focus is on the conditions that made today's physiotherapy possible rather than a descriptive historical inventory of events. I am interested in the changes, innovations and fluctuations in physiotherapy practice for what these events tell us about the profession's past, present and future; so less about what physiotherapists have *done*, per se, and more about what that doing has made possible and impossible. This is an especially important point at the beginning of this chapter, because, unlike the other chapters, every reader will have lived through their own version of this period and may look to see how well their particular clinical interest is represented. A specialist in non-invasive ventilation, constraint-induced movement or positional release techniques, for example, may be dispirited that I have not traced the course of these particular practice developments. Readers may be disappointed that I use particular examples that do not derive from their own specialisation to make my argument and may feel that the situation is quite different in their jurisdiction. These are, undoubtedly, valid criticisms. But if readers approach this chapter having read the previous chapters, or can appreciate that my goal is not to present an encyclopaedic history of the profession, then I hope they will be able to see the possibilities for a different kind of historical analysis that this approach opens up.

The chapter centres around the economic and political changes that occurred following the 1973 oil crisis – an event that has triggered fundamental shifts in the ways people in the West have come to think about the meaning of health and illness, ageing, authority, bodies, healthcare, human potential, knowledge and expertise, the role and regulation of professionals in society, research, self-image, technology and myriad other fundamental features of modern life (Wietz 2013; Dutta 2015; Yong et al 2010; Yagi 2015). Since 1973, the entire philosophy, economic rationale and organisation of Western healthcare that had been developed in the previous half century began to be dismantled. Where the State had once taken responsibility for the health and welfare of the population, now it began to withdraw, placing more and more emphasis on transforming the bureaucracy of health and social care into a market ethos; applying business principles to healthcare decision making and shifting the responsibility for society's health, wealth and happiness away from the State and more towards local communities and the individual (Bjornsdottir 2002; Salmon, & Hall 2003; Roy 2008; Rose 1999).

Political and economic reforms coincided with social reforms, as people demanded more freedom to choose how they lived, what they ate, how they worked, where they holidayed and when they had children (Gabe et al 2015). Many people have benefitted from increased work flexibility, the breakdown of social hierarchies and access to lifestyle-enhancing technologies, greater wealth and longer lives. But they have also experienced economic austerity, instability, problems achieving a comfortable work/life balance, anxiety about personal security, the paradox of having unbounded social networking and increased social isolation, fear for the environment and for the future health and wellbeing of themselves and their families. Where once people many people felt they had a 'job for life' and a State that provided a safety net in times of hardship, people today are much more used to the idea of shifting patterns of work and the necessity to take greater care of themselves because, as Cohn argues, if we do not do it, no one else will (Cohn 2014).

Physiotherapists themselves have not been immune from the costs and benefits of the kinds of neoliberal economic reforms we have seen over the last 50 years, but the profession has been somewhat more passive and disengaged than active in steering a course through these new waters. The reasons for this are, in broad terms, the basis for this book and clearly my argument is that the profession's traditional affinity with the idea of the body-as-machine has played an important role. Physiotherapists have largely ignored the cultural and socio-political world, preferring to leave the planning and organisation of health and welfare to others (Nicholls & Gibson 2010). Because the profession largely benefitted from the major health reforms that led up to 1973, it has seen no real need to interfere. And since it has even benefitted from some of the economic, political and social reforms that have happened since 1973 (in expanding private practice, for example, which, in turn, allowed for the growth of musculoskeletal and sports physiotherapy; the developing a research culture and a university system of education; moving with developing health technologies in areas like neurological rehabilitation and intensive care), it has felt no significant pressure to explore reform. (This point will be discussed in more detail in Part III.)

While some changes in healthcare have benefitted physiotherapists, there are a number of other reforms that now seriously threaten the profession's ability to remain a trusted and valued profession into the future: people's diminishing access to orthodox healthcare; the growing personal cost of chronic illness; the growing disparity between what people want and need from their health professionals and what the professionals provide; technological reforms that eliminate the need for traditional approaches to care and the loss of expertise in an age of digital ubiquity (Higgs et al 1999; Hao, & Tan 1999; Nicholls & Larmer 2005; Sanders et al 2014; Dahl-Michelsen 2015). So, in this chapter, I explore the major changes taking place in physiotherapy over the last half century in order to better understand how the profession is responding to the changing economy of healthcare.

I begin by outlining some of the major health reforms that have occurred since 1973 before considering how physiotherapists have responded. I trace the history of specialisation and the effect that masters – and doctoral-entry degrees are having on practice – particularly in North America. I then contrast physiotherapy in 1973 with practice today and explore how research and publication have changed the way people engage with physiotherapy. A discussion of the search for greater professional autonomy and the development of post-qualification training follows, before I explore some of the boundary conflicts that have beset the profession over the last 50 years. I then spend a little time looking at some of the major practice developments in cardiorespiratory, musculoskeletal and neurological physiotherapy, and make the argument that despite the appearance that so much has changed in practice, little has changed in principle with the way physiotherapists think and work: that approaches to physiotherapy have remained remarkably consistent, despite all of the superficial changes and the profoundly different world in which physiotherapists now operate. I close the chapter by exploring some of the reasons for this stability. To begin with, however, I need to consider some of the background changes taking place in the broader economy of healthcare to put the changes in physiotherapy into context.

Healthcare reforms since 1973

In the previous chapter, I examined some of the major innovations brought about by the move towards the welfare state that dominated most country's healthcare systems in the 60 years between the outbreak of World War I and the 1973 oil crisis. I chose 1973 as the joint line between the two chapters because it was at this point that many governments began the economic and political transformations that explain so much about the drivers of healthcare reform that are so familiar to many people today. In the following section, I provided a short account of some of the key economic and political reforms that followed the 1973 oil crisis. In hindsight, this appears to mark the point when governments began to realise that the years of 'big government' were at an end and began, instead, to explore new political economies. These economies would have a profound effect on the structure and organisation of all healthcare systems and structures, practice and professions, including physiotherapy.

The events surrounding the 1973 oil crisis – or oil 'shock' as some have called it – are now well known, but essentially involved an embargo on crude oil production by the main Organization of the Petroleum Exporting Countries (OPEC). This had the effect of quadrupling the price of a barrel of oil between October 1973 and March 1974 (Slomp 1998). Almost overnight, countries that had previously depended on oil for their essential infrastructure (electricity, fuel for transportation and heating etc.) were threatened with massive new costs and national balance sheets were thrown into deficit. The result of this crisis, which played out over the next few decades, were many and varied but centred on large scale cuts in public expenditure, the privatisation of previously nationalised industries, the creation of new competitive markets, global efforts to find secure and reliable sources of oil leading to war and widespread environmental exploitation and a shift from state to greater personal responsibility for one's health, wealth and happiness.[1]

The high cost of oil resulted in rationing and cuts to public services that, in turn, led to industrial disputes and civic unrest. Governments realised that they could not sustain the cost of free education; subsidised public housing; welfare benefits for the unemployed, disabled and elderly and healthcare free at the point of delivery (Cribb et al 2014; Engdahl 1993; Brownsey & Langford 1990; Einhorn & Logue 2003; Merrill 2007; Belcher 2014; Wietz 2013). In UK, for example:

> . . . The oil crisis brought immediate pressures for cuts in public expenditure. From this date, the UK, in common with other Western economies, set about urgent re-assessment of its welfare-state commitments. This brought about a sudden end to the long period of incremental growth in NHS spending. Henceforth the NHS was forced to accustom itself to growth levels insufficient to meet the demands of demographic change or medical advance.
>
> (Webster 1998, p. 34)

By the 1980s, an entirely new political landscape had begun to emerge, led by neoliberal and free-market economic reformers like Prime Minister Margaret Thatcher in the UK and President Ronald Reagan in the United States, who argued that the central government planning that had been the basis for welfarism stifled economic growth and limited people's personal freedoms. Baxter and Nall (2009) stated that;

> Managing health care expenditure, which is rising steadily in response to . . . new demands, has become a major concern for most national and state governments, and has led to an increasing focus on such areas as managed care, clinical governance, evidence-based practice and cost effectiveness of clinical services.
>
> (Baxter & Nall 2009, p. 21)

Neoliberal economic reformers – so called because they offered a new economic basis for classical liberal beliefs in freedom and individual rights and responsibility – believed that 'the institutionalisation of the welfare state . . . had given rise to a revolution of rising expectations' (Scambler 2002, p. 63), and that these expectations had become unsustainable. The neoliberal solution was to aggressively promote the idea of 'small' government, less taxation and greater public ownership of state assets. People began to pay less in direct taxation and this was used as a lever to stimulate stagnating economies (see Table 5.1). Market competition allowed private providers to replace nationalised industries and states began to take less responsibility for being the commissioners, regulators and principal providers of education, healthcare and social welfare services (Bury 2008).

Governments that sought to implement such radical economic reforms faced enormous resistance, not least from people employed in previously nationalised industries that were being decimated. Miners, teachers, doctors and nurses all

Table 5.1 Ten key principles of neoliberalism, adapted from (Lovell & Cordeaux 1999)

	Theme	Explanation
1	Decentralisation	Minimal role for State in welfare provisions with centrally managed funds and services devolved to local communities
2	Privatisation	Private companies owning, organising and delivering services
3	Self-help	People helping themselves and each other in communities
4	Competition	Raising standards and efficiency through groups competing with each other
5	Freedom of choice	Reduction in State monopolies and expansion of competitive market to give people more choice
6	Enterprise	Encouraging innovation and creativity in services
7	Individualism	Responsibility for ones own needs, including self care
8	Managerialism	Business principles applied to State services
9	Deconstruction	Breaking apart previous State structures (Unions, bargaining, legislation, networks of services etc.)
10	Consumerism	Shift from language of patient to consumer/client, purchaser/provider split created, contracting for services

took prolonged and damaging industrial action, but this only served to harden governments' resolve and focused state attention on the traditional authority and power held by these groups. In healthcare, for example, the traditional approach 'in which knowledgeable and skilful doctors [made] decisions on behalf of patients' was increasingly undermined, and 'more patient centred models of care in which patients play[ed] an important role in decisions about their treatment' were encouraged (Rogers et al 1998, p. 1818). Added to this, the introduction of widespread managerial and administrative practices forced healthcare providers to account for the economic basis of their clinical decisions (Klein 2010). These measures led directly to evidence-based medicine and an explosion of interest in outcome measures, cost-benefit analyses and classification systems like the ICIDH and ICF (see Chapter 8). The old medical language of 'patients' was gradually replaced with new terms like 'client' and 'consumer' that carried a cachet of greater personal choice and responsibility and subtly undermined the power of the medical profession, which was increasingly portrayed as detached from the realities of healthcare decision making. Healthcare monopolies were dismantled and legislation relaxed to allow for competitive tendering for hospital services and the advertising of goods, products and healthcare consumables. And reductions in personal taxation gave people more money to spend on the kinds of 'body projects' that are now taken for granted but were once either unavailable or considered medically unnecessary (cosmetic surgery, green prescriptions, health supplements etc.).

Surprisingly quickly, people's beliefs about the meaning of health and wellbeing began to change. It was not that long ago that many people understood health and illness as essentially a binary state, as Susan Sontag explained in 1977:

> Everyone who is born holds dual citizenship, in the kingdom of the well and
> in the kingdom of the sick. Although we all prefer to use only the good passport,
> sooner or later each of us is obliged, at least for a spell, to identify ourselves
> as citizens of that other place.
>
> (Sontag 1977, p. 3)

Within two decades, the traditionally biomedical idea of health as a binary
state, in which people were healthy for most of the time but occasionally took on
a 'sick role' (Parsons 1951), necessitating the intervention of a wise doctor, was
largely supplanted by the more diffuse notion of 'optimal' health. Optimal health
refers to an aspirational but also unachievable goal, since no-one can ever be optimally healthy: there is always more that can be done. The logical consequence is
that we are all now engaged in 'body projects' and can never be satisfied. We can
always be in better shape, eat better food, exercise more often, manage our mental
health better, see our friends more often, tackle our dependencies and so on. Under
the ideal of optimal health, people are always deficient and eager to consume
goods and services that will fill the gap between where their health and wellbeing
is currently and where they believe (and are repeatedly told) it should be. The very
idea of 'health' has now become unbounded and has been uncoupled from the
traditional association with healthcare professionals. 'Health' now pervades every
aspect of our lives and no longer merely means the absence of sickness. It is, in
many ways, one of the archetypal success story of neoliberalism. But, of course,
it is not without its critics, for one of the other 'achievements' of the last half century is a growing public scepticism towards anyone who claims to know how to
make things better.

At the same time as the public was gaining an appetite for greater autonomy in
healthcare decision making, healthcare practices were being opening up to greater
public scrutiny, as attempts were made to improve the quality and consistency of
healthcare delivery, increase people's choice, reduce inherent risks and improve
information, consistency and the spirit of public service (Nettleton 2006, pp. 214–7).
Quality improvement models were introduced from private industry and new
management positions were created to monitor patient throughput, 'service-user'
experiences and bed occupancy rates. A much greater focus began to fall on individual citizen's rights and responsibilities, not least people's responsibility for
their own health and wellbeing. People were increasingly encouraged to fill the
gap left by a retreating State, by taking greater responsibility for their own health;
by remaining healthy and active; being informed about, and constantly implementing good health practices; going to the gym, reducing their weight, stopping
smoking, eating the right food, being mindful and managing their life stresses and
taking responsibility for their friends' and relatives' health and wellbeing. A tsunami
of public health information and the democratisation of healthcare knowledge
available through the Internet followed and the age of the health consumer was
born (Higgs 2012).

Of course, these reforms were far from uniform and people's experiences varied
widely. Most people in Western, developed economies, who had the disposable

income and the time to take advantage of the more appealing aspects of these reforms favoured them and voted, year after year, for further tax cuts, reductions in public services and greater freedom to spend their money on body projects of their own choosing. This group, which Barsky called the 'worried well' (Barsky 1988), benefitted most from the neoliberal economic reforms. Others, however, fared less well. Without the social safety net of a welfare state, increasing numbers of children, women, older adults, disabled people, people living in poverty and others were left without the necessary means to enjoy the newly created healthcare markets. With this population, the increasing requirement to take personal respon-sibility for one's health has become something of a burden and a source of a grow-ing blame culture, rather than an opportunity for self-actualisation and personal growth (O'Byrne & Holmes 2007; Petersen 1996; Harthorn & Oaks 2003). A new term – the precariat – has been coined by Standing and others to describe the 'many millions around the world without the anchor of stability' that was once available to all as a basic human right (Standing 2011, p. 1).

The growth in personal responsibility over the last half century has arrived in parallel with a much greater interest in people's individual opinions. It is common today for people to express their opinion on everything, from how much they liked their local restaurant, what they think about their local council, to whether they need new home and contents insurance. We now live in what Silverman and others have called an 'interview society' (Silverman 1997; Gubrium & Holstein 2002). At the same time, social research methods as a subject has become commonplace, following on from the civil rights disputes of the 1960s, much of it directed at emancipating the voice of previously marginalised people (Leininger 1985; Field & Morse 1985; Morse 1990; Webb 1984). Before 1960 it was rare for people to be polled, balloted, surveyed or otherwise asked their opinion. There were few televi-sion or radio programmes that focused on people's individual achievements and aptitudes, like the endless cooking, house renovation and singing competitions we see today. And although social media obviously existed, they were much more didactic and took little interest in how much individual ideas and opinions were 'liked' or re-posted.

The increased attention given to people's individual beliefs and opinions that accompanied many of the social changes that accompanied neoliberalism mirrored the growth of more individual, behavioural approaches to health and social care. Rather than focusing on social determinants of health like unemployment, poor quality housing, lack of educational opportunity, social isolation, environmental pollution, urban safety and institutional discrimination as reasons for the persistence of poor health in society, governments, policy-maker, health professionals and others have adopted approaches that focus on an individual's responsibility for her or his own health and wellbeing (Marmot et al 2008; Keleher & MacDougall 2011). Physiotherapists have been enthusiastic adopters of behaviourism and have shown a willingness to explore how individual healthcare consumers might be 'enabled' to act in their own interests. Concerted and multi-directional efforts to reduce the negative effects of smoking, obesity and inactivity have come to repre-sent the 'low hanging fruit' of health promotion, as health policy makers look at different ways to influence the health and wellbeing of the population (Archer et al 2013; Clark & Bassett 2015; Brunner et al 2015; O'Rourke 2012).

As a result of this behaviourism, it is becoming increasingly difficult to mobilise Western governments to act in concerted ways against social and environmental conditions that, overwhelming evidence suggests, play a significant role in determining people's sense of wellbeing, consumption of health services, time off work and incidence of all major comorbidities (Carson et al 2007; Graham 2009; Bartley 2004; Marmot & Wilkinson 1999; Wilkinson & Pickett 2010; Davidson 2014). Keleher and MacDougall go further, arguing that we are now concentrating too much on 'soft targets' like physical activity, nutrition and weight control 'that target individuals rather than environments and structural conditions that . . . are causal pathways for heart disease, diabetes and cancer' (Keleher & MacDougall 2009, p. 28).

The growth in people's sense of individual choice, personal responsibility and economic freedom has been accompanied by a slow deconstruction of the systems and structures that had been set up in the 20th century. People have more choices today than they did in 1950. Many also have more disposable income and a belief that it is their right to spend their money the way that they choose. Because of this, the immense, centralised, closed market that characterised national healthcare system has been devolved, allowing new opportunities to emerge. Healthcare consumers are now making many more independent decisions about which health practitioner to engage, which services to purchase and which health promoting measures to deploy. Health has become much more than just the institutional management of acute and chronic illness, and has bled into our overall sense of wellbeing. Interventions that were once only available to people who were ill – like reconstructive surgery, exercise-based rehabilitation and orthodontics – are now used as tools of body enhancement by people who have no underlying pathology.

Many people now no longer accept the traditional medically-mandated boundary on what constitutes a normal body or normal ability. Binary gender roles and (hetero)sexual expressions, typical lifespans and lifestyles, and even traditional distinctions between such fundamental states as being alive or dead, are all being challenged now. People live in an age of increasing uncertainty for the things that we once took for granted or trusted to others. Many people reading this will have been born after the 1973 oil crisis and will know little of the 'old world' that preceded the neoliberal reforms of the last 40 years. It will, therefore, be hard to imagine healthcare where there were few private providers and everything was filtered either through the general practitioner or the local hospital. People had very limited options for their healthcare beyond the orthodox providers mandated by the state, and there was very little growth and innovation in health technology. Having said that, neoliberalism has brought with it many problems that were directly addressed by the welfare state. Not least among these is the social gradient that now exists between those who can afford to exercise their greater freedom to choose and those who cannot. It seems relevant, therefore, to consider how these changes have manifested in physiotherapy thinking and practice over the last half century.

Physiotherapy since 1973

Specialisation and new doctors

There have been some remarkable advances in physiotherapy over the last 50 years: advances in specialisation, assessment and treatment, education, regulation and research have all figured strongly in the profession since 1973. At the same time, physiotherapists have remained remarkably consistent in their application of limited set of underlying modalities and have retained their strong affinity with biomedicine. If today's new graduates could return to 1973, they might be surprised at the limited post-graduate educational opportunities; the lack of research evidence; the repetitive nature of treatment and the limited equipment available to them; the public's deference towards the medical profession and the fact that their patients always came with a prescription from the doctor. Despite this, they would still recognise the physiotherapy being practiced and people's desire to regain lost function, cope with debilitating pain or rehabilitate from illness or injury. So, in many ways, much has changed in physiotherapy, but much has also stayed the same. Perhaps one of the areas that exemplifies this best is in the growth of specialisation.

The first specialised section of the American Physical Therapy Association (APTA) was formed in 1974 by physiotherapists interested in orthopaedics.[2] This coincided with the formation of the International Federation of Orthopaedic Manipulative Physical Therapists (IFOMPT). At the same time, there were 11 special interest groups (SIGs) in the CSP, including Associations of Blind Certified Masseurs (first formed in 1919), special interest groups for teachers and superintendents and for those in specific clinical areas (industry, obstetrics, manipulative, sports and paediatrics) (Owen 2014). Since 1974, the APTA has added a further 17 special-interest sections, in 'traditional' areas of practice, such as acute care, cardiovascular and pulmonary, education, neurology, paediatrics and private practice. But it also added some newer specialties, including wound management, hand rehabilitation, home health, oncology, research and women's health. The CSP has gone further, adding 35 new SIGs, some dealing with quite specific areas of clinical practice (cystic fibrosis and haemophilia, for example), while others are groups for practices that were once marginal to mainstream physiotherapy (bioenergy and cranio-sacral therapies) or were almost entirely operational (medico-legal and retirement). Owen suggests that:

> [T]he evolution of physiotherapy practice is organic and complex. Some [SIGs] and practices develop and multiply (e.g. manual therapies), others become discursively reconstructed over time (e.g. practice with older people), while others seem to disappear from view (e.g. cranio-sacral therapy, rheumatic care, teachers of physiotherapy).
>
> (Owen, 2014)

The growth of specialised areas of practice has come with a growing desire to recognise the extra experience, knowledge and skills of specialists. In line with this, the Australian College of Physiotherapy was inaugurated in 1971 to confer

Fellowships on elite practitioners and in 1981 began awarding Fellowships by Specialisation. Fellowships were awarded for 'high standards of clinical skill and scholarship' (Australian College of Physiotherapy, n.d.) and could be granted in eight areas: cardiorespiratory, continence and women's health, gerontology, musculoskeletal, neurology, occupational health, paediatrics and sports – an almost identical list to that now offered by the American Board of Physical Therapy Specialties and the Canadian Physiotherapy Association (CPA) Clinical Specialty Program, which were established in the early 1980s (American Board of Physical Therapy Specialties, 2015; Canadian Physiotherapy Association, 2016).

Board certification in America involves a very lengthy and extensive programme, from the completion of a relevant bachelor's programme and a subsequent doctoral entry-level degree in physical therapy; to evidence of at least 2,000 hours of clinical experience in the specialty field (ideally through a recognised post-professional clinical residency); evidence of continuing education, including further degrees and certificated courses; to the completion of the Board Certification Examination. Despite these demands, of the more than 80,000 APTA members currently practising, just under 15,000 are certified, despite the facts that the merits of such programmes remain largely untested (Rodeghero et al 2015), and that the similarities and qualities of different residency and fellowship programmes are, as yet, unknown (Furze et al 2016).[3] Of these, the most popular categories for certification are orthopaedics (59%), geriatrics (11%), neurology, paediatrics and sport (9% each) (Source: www.apta.org/Certification/, accessed 13 March 2016). Across American universities, there are now 219 post-doctoral residency and 42 fellowship programs designed to equip therapists with the 'advanced clinical knowledge, experience, and skills in a special area of practice and to assist consumers and the healthcare community in identifying these physical therapists' (Source: www.abpts.org/Certification/About/, accessed 3 March 2016, see also Johanson et al 2016). These programmes have developed in less than two decades, but still the 'increased demand for advanced specialised clinical knowledge and skills by graduating physical therapist students and practising practicing clinicians far exceeds the current supply of accredited residency and fellowship programs', and all signs indicate that 'the applicant pool will continue to grow at a rate far exceeding the number of slots offered by accredited programs' (Furze et al 2016, p. 950). Professional programmes in Australia, Canada and the UK have, to an extent, followed suit, developing new post-qualification pathways to match the growth in new practice designations (physiotherapy consultants, fellows, specialists etc.), and, in some cases, creating links with specialist practice areas beyond the traditional boundaries of physiotherapy (Wagstaff 2001; Kersten et al 2007; Gardiner & Wagstaff 2001).

One of the most significant changes in physiotherapy since 1973, however, has been the move to create a doctoral degree as the entry qualification for American physical therapists. Instigated by the APTA's Vision 2020 statement, the Association set an ambitious target that;

> By 2020, physical therapy will be provided by physical therapists who are doctors of physical therapy, recognized by consumers and other healthcare

professionals as the practitioners of choice to whom consumers have direct access for the diagnosis of, interventions for, and prevention of impairments, functional limitations, and disabilities related to movement, function, and health.

(American Physical Therapy Association 2000)

Good to its word, there are now doctoral-entry programmes in every accredited physical therapy training school in the United States, and data from the Commission on Accreditation in Physical Therapy Education (CAPTE) suggests that there are in excess of 30,000 students currently enrolled in 233 accredited programmes throughout the country (Source: www.capteonline.org/home.aspx, updated 6 September 2016). First introduced by the University of Southern California in 1992, the DPT programme serves a number of important functions (for an historical overview of the development of the DPT in America, see Plack & Wong 2002 and Pagliarulo 2007). Firstly, its proponents argue that it puts physical therapists on a par with other para-medical professions who also refer to themselves as doctors (chiropractors, dentists etc.). Secondly, it promises to elevate the status of the profession in the public's mind, by sharing in the reflected kudos associated with being an orthodox 'medical' professional. Thirdly, it recognises the breadth, depth and complexity of knowledge and skills required by physical therapists in today's workplace. Finally, it helps to promote the idea that physical therapists should become first contact professions. Despite the fact that direct access to physiotherapists has been a feature of a number of countries since 1976, many North American physical therapists work for patients whose third-party payer requires evidence of a medical referral before funding treatment (Bury & Stokes 2013a, 2013b; Ojha et al 2013). As the costs of specialised healthcare rise, however, some have argued that direct access to physical therapy could replace some of the services currently being offered by overstretched medical specialists; help to reduce waiting times; and improve the efficiency of healthcare generally (de Gruchy et al 2015; Burn & Beeson 2014; Ferguson & Cook 2011; Napier et al 2013; Durrell 1996). Thus, there is a great deal of impetus behind the move to doctoral-entry qualifications.

Other countries have sought to follow the American model, and a plethora of entry-level educational models now exist, from three- and four-year bachelor's degrees with and without honours, to graduate-entry masters and doctoral programmes that require prior relevant degree-level qualifications. In Australia, for example, there are currently 19 institutions offering 35 approved physiotherapy programmes, including ten four-year bachelors programmes, 14 four-year bachelors with honours, eight two-year graduate-entry masters degrees, two three-year extended masters degrees and one three-year doctor of physiotherapy programme, all leading to the same professional entry point for graduates (Source: www.ahpra. gov.au/Education/Approved-Programs-of-Study.aspx?ref=Physiotherapist, updated 6 September 2016).

Given the diversity of qualifications and educational experiences, it is perhaps surprising that all of these qualifications lead to the same outcome: graduates suitable for registration with their respective professional bodies and legally qualified to practice as physiotherapists. Perhaps unsurprisingly, some have argued that the advent of masters- and doctoral-entry qualification has changed little about the essential competencies required for novice practice, and that instead they represent 'degree inflation' and 'credential creep' (Kot & Hendel 2012; Bollag 2007). Others, however, have argued that a doctoral qualification is entirely appropriate for physical therapists in an increasingly competitive marketplace (Rothstein 1998; Moffatt 1994). Jules Rothstein, for instance, wrote in 1998 that;

> For too long we have attempted to overcome limitations inherent in undergraduate education by burdening students with unrealistic course loads; for too long we have expected employers to train our not-quite-ready- for-practice graduates for the complexities of practice in a relatively unforgiving world ... Today, practice requires a greater knowledge of measurement, clinical decision making, and patient management – and the ability to work in a variety of settings with patients and clients who have a range of conditions not previously seen. Programs claiming to educate practitioners for contemporary practice cannot do so within the confines of baccalaureate education. Neither can they do it in good conscience within the equally stifling confines of master's degree education.
>
> (Rothstein 1998, p. 358)

Nearly 20 years later, however, there are still few fundamental differences in the design and constitution of physical therapy programmes in North America, the UK, and Commonwealth countries, regardless of their level. Bachelors, masters and doctoral degrees place very similar emphases on particular biological sciences (anatomy, physiology, pathology), applied sciences (kinesiology, biomechanics, imaging), clinical sciences (neurology, orthopaedics, paediatrics), humanistic/behavioural studies (communication, psychology, ethics and law), clinical practice (assessment, diagnosis, treatment), professional practice (patient/clinic management, health promotion, research skills) and an extended internship/supervised clinical placement. There are some differences based on pre-requisites, with higher degrees demanding that some relevant learning has already been acquired in other degree programmes and there are different timelines to completion, with some masters and doctoral degrees dramatically foreshortening the time taken to graduation, but otherwise, much remains the same. This has raised doubts in some people's minds that the reason for moving to masters and doctoral entry was really anything to do with raising standards and providing better care for patients.

Degree 'inflation' – if that is what it is – may, in reality, be less about an actual improvement in the quality and consistency of graduate practice, and more about a contingent response to workplace tensions now being faced by physiotherapists. All physiotherapists, whether they work in private practice or in public healthcare, are experiencing increasing competition, horizontal and vertical encroachment and reduced State support, with the rising flood of competition from less well trained, cheaper and less heavily regulated practitioners, forcing orthodox practitioners like physiotherapists to 'higher ground'. Higher ground, in this context, represents higher entry qualifications (baccalaureate degrees before entering masters- or doctoral-entry programmes), specialisation, fellowships and extended scopes. Physiotherapists can do this because, in most jurisdictions, the profession remains highly regarded and popular among prospective students. But the move to further specialisation and elite status also leaves a number of problems in its wake, not least the potentially crippling cost of extended training (which naturally priv- ileges certain affluent sections of the community and marginalises others); the scientisation of professional practice, which emphasises the profession's technical rationalism (Schön 1987) at the expense of its humanistic, tactile and inter-subjective qualities and, most significantly, the expectation that new graduates with superior qualifications will be able to demand higher pay from their patients.

This latter point is of little importance when a large funder (insurer or State provider) conceals the unit cost of treatment, but it becomes a matter of huge significance when patients need to meet the full cost of care themselves. Premium salaries demanded by increasingly elite practitioners mean higher costs for treat- ment; this risks concentrating physiotherapy in areas of affluence and diminishing services for the very people who are now of biggest concern for health policy makers and funders. This may, in time, force practitioners to focus on acute, short- term, self-limiting treatment, because this is all that people can afford and those with longstanding, chronic, disabling and debilitating conditions (stroke, chronic pain, COPD, cerebral palsy etc.), will see physiotherapists less and less (Jones & O'Shaughnessy 2014). Long-term care and rehabilitation will then be left to lower paid, cheaper to train physical therapy, rehabilitation and healthcare assistants, kinesiologists, athletic trainers and others, who will be left to manage the most complex, intractable and costly cases. In time, acute care, short-term treatments will be provided by people who do not need a five- or six-year training and do not command elite social status, and physiotherapists may find themselves struggling to provide a service in a market that no longer exists.

We have seen over the last 40 years a growing recognition of the inevitability of some of these changes, with the increased use of physiotherapy and rehabilitation assistants, who are being asked to take on roles that physiotherapists used to be therapeutically accountable for (Ellis & Connell 2001; Stanmore & Waterman 2007; Schmidt 2013). We are also seeing the legislative blurring of regulatory boundaries so that other professionals can more easily move into the foothills physiotherapists once occupied (Norris 2001; Gieryn 1983; Huby et al 2014); the growing use of standardised care pathways and best practice guidelines that evac- uate the kinds of clinical decision making that once defined practice (Tsiachristas et al 2011; Pearson et al 2000; Sulch et al 2000) and the increasing emphasis being placed on interprofessional collaborative practice, such that once-distinct profes- sional boundaries are becoming more fluid and amorphous (Cameron 2011; Baxter, & Brumfitt 2008; Tsiachristas et al 2011). The significant point about all of these changes, however, is not that the fundamental basis of physiotherapy has itself changed, but rather that the contexts, locations, politics, power dynamics and relationships that physiotherapy was once based on have altered irrevocably. There is perhaps no better illustration of this than in the clinical world, where so much is now different and yet so much has remained the same.

Clinical practice since 1973

There have been so many changes to physiotherapy since 1973 that it would be impossible to describe the developments in even one specialty area, let alone physiotherapy as a whole. But even if it were possible, it would not be appropriate for the book, because my purpose is not to provide a catalogue of incremental changes in manual therapy, critical care physiotherapy or spinal cord injury rehabilitation. Rather, I want to make four inter-related arguments. That, superficially at least, the period since 1973 has seen some dramatic changes in physiotherapy but, at the same time, the core principles and practices established by the profession's founders more than a century ago have remained largely intact. I want to show that the reasons for this lie in enduring influence of the body-as-machine and that this has actually made the last half century about an emphasis on the role of *explanation* in shaping the profession rather than substantive change to the way physiotherapists think or practice. To begin with then, how has physiotherapy practice changed?

In 1973, physiotherapy was almost entirely subordinate to medicine. Practitioners could not treat patients without a medical referral, which meant that physiotherapists did little diagnostic work. Without the need for differential diagnosis, there was little need for assessment beyond the need to check for contraindications. Treatment was largely formulaic and was laid down in textbooks that provided 'recipes' for the management of different clinical conditions. Knowledge of pathology and, increasingly, physiology had become increasingly significant (Kelman 1972; Guyton 1971; Eyzaguirre & Fidone 1975), but primarily as a vehicle to understand the mechanisms of therapeutic effect, rather than for their critical or evaluative significance. Jennifer Lee's *Aids to Physiotherapy*, for example, provides three kinds of information necessary to practice physiotherapy: technical notes about the modality, uses and contraindications. Infra-red radiation (IRR), for example, is outlined in this way:

Technical notes

1   Non-luminous generator
2   Electromagnetic wavelength 4000–7700 Å
3   Shorter wavelengths produce greatest heating effect
4   Depth of penetration 1–10 mm
5   Heat produced by absorption of radiant energy
6   Dosage 20–30 min, daily
7   IRR obey optical laws

Used to

1   Relieve pain
2   Relax superficial muscle spasm
3   Increase superficial blood-supply

Contraindications

1   Loss of large area of thermal skin sensation
2   Some skin diseases
3   Vascular insufficiency
4   Haemorrhage
5   Some skin liniments (Lee 1978, p. 18)

Similarly, Joan Cash's widely read and highly influential textbooks on the treatment of medical and surgical, neurological and orthopaedic conditions follow a similar formula. Chapters are devoted to clinical conditions, bodily regions and treatment locations (i.e. physiotherapy in the community) (Cash 1974, 1975, 1976, 1977).[4] In P.J. Waddington's chapter introducing the reader to intensive care, the reader is told that the role of the physiotherapist is threefold: Chest care (loosening and removing secretions, ensuring adequate ventilation throughout the lungs); movement (free active exercise, maintaining full range of movement, positioning to maintain good posture); and general care (understanding the patient, his [sic] condition and the medical problem, while also appreciating the 'nursing programme and techniques' (Waddington & Cash 1975, p. 57). In all cases, the emphasis was on the accurate and professional application of appropriate treatment modalities and there was little emphasis placed on the differential diagnosis or evidence-based practice.

Prior to 1973, physiotherapy journals still relied heavily on the contributions of doctors to provide updates on the latest clinical approaches. Works published by physiotherapists often focused on personal and professional insights into clinical practice and only a handful of authors cited other literature in their reports. The monthly *Physiotherapy* journal of 1966, for example, featured 69 original articles. Of these, 32 were received from physicians or surgeons, with 22 submitted by physiotherapists. The year's contributions included ten articles on amputee surgery and rehabilitation, 12 on neurological rehabilitation, eight on orthopaedic disorders of the knee and seven on respiratory disease and treatment. There were articles on walking aids and adaptations, hand and upper limb rehabilitation and electrotherapy.

There were very few clinical trials offered, and those that were available appear quaint by today's rigorous standards. In the June 1967 edition of the *Australian Journal of Physiotherapy*, for example, a one-page report on 'The Value of Diaphragmatic Breathing in the Patient with Obstructive Airway Disease' was published (Wines et al 1967). This paper stood out in the journal, not only because it reported on an empirical research study, but that it was also produced entirely by physiotherapists. Today, however, its value lies less in its rigour than in its novelty and its function as a marker of a change to come. Here, for instance, is the entirety of the methods section;

> Thirty-eight patients were divided into two groups by random selection on admission. Both groups were treated with 15 breaths of 2% Alupert, four hourly, on a Bird's respirator, and with steroids. Group I also had diaphragmatic breathing exercises.
>
> (Wines et al 1967 p. 72)

In hindsight, it is clear that the infrastructure was not in place to allow for extensive, well-funded, rigorously conducted clinical trials. There were few physiotherapists trained in research methods, few sources of contestable research funding and there was little professional appreciation for the merits of scientific testing. Even if rigorously conducted studies had been published, few readers would have been able to interpret their findings or account for their veracity.[5] All of this began to change after 1973 and by 1980, Cecily Partridge was able to write that;

> Physiotherapy has developed over the years in a practical way but there have been few systematic attempts to evaluate its effectiveness. The present position where there is little scientific evidence for the effectiveness of most of the practice of physiotherapy is no longer acceptable.
>
> (Partridge 1980, p. 153)

Today, the publication of research findings is *the* principal function of physiotherapy journal. The September 2015 edition of *Physiotherapy*, for example, is almost entirely dominated by highly rigorous empirical research studies, including three systematic reviews:

- Identifying potential moderators for response to treatment in low back pain: A systematic review;
- Effectiveness of land-based physiotherapy exercise following hospital discharge following hip arthroplasty for osteoarthritis: an updated systematic review;
- Interactions of sex and aging on spatiotemporal metrics in non-pathological gait: a descriptive meta-analysis.

And five original articles:

- Does outpatient physical therapy with the aim of improving health-related physical fitness influence the level of physical activity in patients with long-term musculoskeletal conditions?
- Understanding the barriers and enablers to implementation of a self-managed exercise intervention: a qualitative study;
- Abdominal exercises affect inter-rectus distance in postpartum women: a two-dimensional ultrasound study;
- Investigation of the immediate pre-operative physical capacity of patients scheduled for elective abdominal surgery using the 6-minute walk test;
- Validity of linear encoder measurement of sit-to-stand performance power in older people.

Part of the change that took place after 1973 can be explained by physiotherapists' growing desire for professional autonomy. Having achieved a significant critical mass and a presence in the public health system, educators, practitioners and professional leaders began to look for ways to differentiate their work and distance themselves from the paternalistic medical control that had cast a long protective cloak over physiotherapy in the past (Ovretveit 1985; Magistro 1984). The search for greater autonomy became embodied in the transition from hospital-based 'training' to University-based education that gathered pace in the 1980s, alongside the move from practice based within the hospital to private practice in the community. University education opened up new opportunities for more diverse curricula, incorporating more behavioural, human and social sciences and training in research methods. A greater range of post-qualification courses began to be developed, including post-qualification certificates, diplomas, masters degrees and doctorates. Post-qualification courses were few and far between prior to 1973. The CSP arranged for just four in the second half of 1966: a management course for superintendents and senior physiotherapists, and clinical courses in ultrasound, proprioceptive neuromuscular facilitation and intensive care (which was planned to involve ten lectures, nine of which were given by doctors). Three further regional courses were organised: a post-natal course run in Leeds, a course on connective tissue massage in Middlesbrough and, tellingly, a course on manipulations by Geoff Maitland in Manchester. This latter course coincided with the reprint of the CSP Congress Lecture given by Maitland on 'Manipulation – Mobilisation' (Maitland 1966). Maitland's paper, along with works by Cyriax, Kaltenborn, Mennell, Paris and Stoddard and others (Kaltenborn 1965; Stoddard 1959; Paris 1965; Cyriax 1955, 1956; Maitland 1964; Bourdillon 1973; Sim 1971; Mennell 1952) prefigured one of the more significant shifts to take place in physiotherapy at the time.

In America, the challenge from chiropractic had always been greater and more persistent than elsewhere in the world, but the need to demonstrate that physiotherapists had both the right and the requisite skills to work in manipulation and mobilisation of the spine and peripheral joints, had become a growing source of tension in the 1960s (Huijbregts 2007; Coburn 1994; Villanueva-Russell 2005, 2011; Theberge 2008). Physiotherapists had worked for years to establish their pre-eminence as *the* orthodox providers of musculoskeletally-based physical rehabilitation, so the aggressive competition and horizontal encroachment that came from the chiropractic profession in America after 1960 came as a profound shock and its ripples were felt by practitioners around the world (Dew 2003; Committee of Inquiry into Chiropractic, Osteopathy, Homoeopathy and Naturopathy, 1977; Martin 1994; Turner 2001; Clarke et al 2004; Kelner et al 2004; Huijbregts 2007; Ottosson 2011). The reaction to this shock, indirectly brought about some dramatic changes to curricula, post-qualification development, the organisation of gatekeeping SIGs and academic scholarship within the physiotherapy profession that, ironically, opened the profession up to new approaches to practice that shifted the profession from its traditional focus on musculoskeletal medicine.

Shirley Sahrmann labelled the period before 1960 as the 'musculoskeletal' era in physiotherapy. She called the period between 1960 and 1980 the 'neurological' era, the 1980s the 'joint' era and the 1990s onwards the 'movement' era (Sahrmann 1999).[6] However these periods are classified, it is clear that the neurological rehabilitation became a more significant conceptual influence on the profession after 1973. With lessons learnt from treating infantile paralysis and polio in the middle of the century, solid foundations existed for neurodevelopmental, motor relearning and (proprioceptive) neuromuscular facilitation techniques to develop, and allowing pioneers like Berta and Karel Bobath, Herman Kabat, Margaret Knott, Dorothy Voss, Margaret Rood and Signe Brunnstrom to emerge (Carr & Shepherd 2000; Bobath 1965, 1975; Stockmeyer 1967; Knott & Voss 1956; Lettinga 2002; Shepherd 1974; Brunnstrom 1966, 1972; Perry 1967). At the same time, better surgical techniques, post-operative anaesthetics and ventilator support meant that more aggressive and invasive surgery had become possible, resulting in many more people surviving trauma and critical illness. There was a corresponding boom in cardiorespiratory physiotherapy, firstly in acute care and later in the management of long-term illnesses like COPD, where the need to reduce acute events became increasingly important. The work of Barbara Webber, Jennifer Pryor, Alex Hough, Julia Bott and Sally Singh became increasingly influential (Webber 1973, 1991; Hough 1991; Webber & Pryor 1993; Bott & Singh 1998). In manual therapy, the influence of James Cyriax (Cyriax 1956, 1982; Cyriax & Russell 1977), James Mennell (Mennell 1960, 1964), Freddy Kaltenborn (Kaltenborn 1970, 1976, 1980) and Alan Stoddard (Stoddard 1959) loomed large over the emerging practices of Geoff Maitland (Maitland 1973, 1977a, 1977b, 1978), Rob McKenzie (McKenzie 1980, 1981, 1983), Brian Mulligan (Mulligan 1989, 1995), Stanley Paris (Paris 1965) and others.

Because many manual therapists began to operate semi-autonomously, away from the large consultant-led teams seen in hospitals and large clinics, they, perhaps more than others, pushed for a greater focus on diagnostic clarity; stronger, physiotherapy-specific anatomical and biomechanical knowledge and pathological coherence. Mark Laslett has credited Cyriax and Mennell with establishing 'a direct connection between his diagnosis and treatment', and 'ruthlessly rejecting time-honoured and popular therapies such as heat and most forms of massage' (Laslett 1996, p. 3). Certainly, many traditional forms of 'passive' manual therapy fell into decline through the 1970s and 1980s, while others, especially electrotherapy, regained their popularity. Whereas actinotherapy (infra-red, ultraviolet and other forms of radiation) had become the target for an emerging critical research culture around efficacy and potential harm and subsequently fallen into terminal decline, electrotherapy devices experienced something of a resurgence (Clayton & Scott 1975). The growth of physiotherapy in private practice opened up a new market for manufacturers, who showed an increasing appetite for advertising their products through the profession's journals. Clinicians readily accepted the opportunities to offer the potent placebo effect of the new interferential, ultrasound, microwave and diathermy machines, and appreciated the fact that patients could be treated (and billed) for treatments that did not require direct hands-on management by the clinician.

By the 1990s, educational reforms and the slow deconstruction of traditional healthcare systems had created the conditions for rapid professional specialisation, including into areas like sports physiotherapy, occupational, mental, older adult and women's health. The focus of practice began to centre on diagnosis, the assessment of outcomes and treatment efficacy, and the development of innovative adaptations to traditional approaches to practice. Incentive spirometry, postural draining and chest percussion began to be replaced by the Active Cycle of Breathing Technique, Positive Expiratory Pressure devices and, later, non-invasive ventilation (Pryor & Prasad 2002), and physiotherapists became increasingly interested in exercise-based rehabilitation (Bott & Singh 1998). In musculoskeletal physiotherapy, muscle imbalance, segmental movement dysfunction, neural tension testing and positional release techniques became increasingly significant, alongside 'real time ultrasound, electrotherapy, clinical trials, management of chronic pain, pelvic floor and pregnancy' (Beeton 2008, p. 373). Growing tensions between advocates of neurodevelopmental, neurofacilitational and motor control techniques created a rich seam of research and practice debate in the 1990s and early 2000s. From this, new developments in treadmill, repetitive task and bilateral arm training emerged, alongside constraint-induced movement therapies, kinematics, robot-assisted therapy and Transcranial Magnetic Stimulation (TMS) (Reinkensmeyer & Dietz 2016).

In recent years, there has been a newfound interest in practices at the traditional margins of orthodox physiotherapy, including acupuncture, mind-body medicine and cognitive behavioural therapy, and there has been a resurgence of interest in areas like breathing performance, EMG biofeedback and ergonomics. Significantly, perhaps, physiotherapists have seen much greater interest in the synergistic connections between traditionally isolated clinical specialties. This has been evident in areas like postural control and muscle balance, trunk stabilisation, pain management, exercise-based rehabilitation and the adoption of bio-psycho-social models of practice. Physiotherapists with a traditional bias towards musculoskeletal medicine are now engaging in the neurological literature and vice versa. Cardiorespiratory physiotherapists and others are exploring behaviour change strategies and traditionally siloed practices are being pioneered in women's health, paediatrics, care of older adults and community care. The current 'bleeding edge'[7] of practice is perhaps not directly clinical at all, but relates more to the future possibilities of new prescribing rights (Foreman 2003; McIntosh et al 2016; Morris & Grimmer 2014), knowledge translation and the use of evidence-based practice guidelines (Condon et al 2016; Scurlock-Evans et al 2014), activity-based health promotion (Scott-Dempster et al 2015; Harding et al 2015; Bury & Moffat 2014) and the management of complex problems like pain and multiple comorbidities (Moseley 2007; Butler, & Moseley 2013; Thomas et al 2006; Clini & Ambrosino 2005; Vancampfort et al 2013; O'Sullivan et al 2015).

Notwithstanding the obvious insufficiencies of any attempt to summarise more than 45 years of physiotherapy practice in a few paragraphs, it is possible to argue a number of significant things about the development of physiotherapy since 1973. Firstly, despite all of the innovative ways physiotherapy has been described and delivered over the last half century, it still remains firmly anchored to the four foundational modalities that it began with in the late 19th century. Some form of touch-based therapy (massage or other), manual therapies, modalities of tissue mobilisation and neurofacilitation, land- or water-based exercise and electrotherapy still lie beneath every innovation in physiotherapy practice. The few exceptions to this rule (cognitive behavioural approaches, acupuncture, prescribing) remain largely fringe practices and are not widely recognised yet as physiotherapeutic.

Secondly, the reasons *for* physiotherapy have remained the same. People still want to regain lost strength and movement, return to 'normal' function, overcome acute illness or injury and manage their pain. Nothing has changed in this regard. The conditions physiotherapists are treating today are largely the same as they were treating 50 years ago: people recovering from amputations, arthritis, stroke, multiple sclerosis, Parkinson's disease, cerebral palsy, cardiovascular diseases, asthma, chronic bronchitis, emphysema, tuberculosis, post-surgical problems, polio, fractures and arthroplasties, peripheral nerve lesions and spinal cord injuries still make up the bulk of physiotherapists' clinical caseload. And while there is now growing concern for some new clinical problems such as falls, chronic pain and lifestyle diseases like diabetes and obesity, the approach from physiotherapists remains anchored to a broad set of medically-defined diseases and disorders.

Treatment 'packages' have also remained essentially the same, with Ann Moore and Gwen Jull recently describing the three common elements found in all 'multimodal' treatment packages as consisting of; a 'passive/active intervention, the prescription of exercise, and education and advice, the latter being pivotal in many cases to enhance and facilitate effective self-management in patients, thus reducing the need for treatment in the future' (Moore & Jull 2011, p. 307). Treatment locations (hospital wards, physiotherapy departments and private community-based clinics) continue to be the locations where most people come into contact with physiotherapy. And even the electrical modalities, which were once criticised for having little or no evidence of effect are now being revisited, with some now suggesting that 'the swing away from using EPAs [electrophysical agents] in the last 20 years has been as little evidence-based as their prior overuse in the 1970 and 80s' (Chipchase 2012, p. 265).

Perhaps a clinical example will illustrate how closely physiotherapy has kept to its historical roots. Today's physiotherapy treatment of patients with acute and chronic respiratory disease borrow directly from techniques practiced throughout the last century. Chest clapping and vibrations are tapotement techniques applied to the chest (Angove 1936); non-invasive ventilation derives directly from the care given to polio sufferers who survived in cuirasses (Hansson 1942; Neumann 2004; Wilson 2005; Ritchie Russell 1952); pulmonary rehabilitation is a virtual replica of the exercise-based treatments offered to injured soldiers after the First and Second World Wars (Lanckenau 1943; Wrynn 2014). Even the more recent interest in the management of airflow (ACBT, PEP, etc.) can be seen in early physiotherapy work with asthma patients in the 1960s (Thompson 1968; Thompson & Thompson 1968).

Respiratory physiotherapy today holds to the same reductive approach to the body that has persisted unchanged in orthodox medicine for over 150 years. The respiratory system is still seen as distinct from the neurological, urogenital and even the musculoskeletal system, despite the fact that half of the respiratory system is made up of muscles and bones. Respiratory physiotherapists are differentiated from other specialists. Physiotherapists still look to 'normal' lung function as the benchmark against which the effect of lung and thoracic disease is assessed, and their haptic techniques deployed are little changed from those used by masseurs and masseuses for generations. It is true that in recent years they have become more active as diagnosticians and this has necessitated the development of new assessment techniques and outcome measures, but even these are largely borrowed from longstanding medical practice (stethoscopes, lung function, exercise tests) and perpetuate over a century's concern to locate and address the specific aetiology.

My argument here, then, is that the ideas, principles, rules, systems and structures, cultural objects and subjectivities that constitute physiotherapy today, are, in the broadest possible sense, consistent with those established by the profession's founders more than a century ago. What is more, the changes that have been evident in the profession since its inception – and perhaps even more so since 1973 – are less to do with fundamental shifts in the theoretical and practice basis of physiotherapy and are, instead, more contingent responses to the changing economy of healthcare. I will explore this argument in much more detail over the subsequent chapters, but if we can accept this position for now, we can consider a series of questions that are important in understanding how physiotherapy has developed over the last few decades. For instance, if little has fundamentally changed in physiotherapy over the last 100 years, have physiotherapists simply been intransigent, lazy or indifferent to the profound economic and social reforms that have so radically altered healthcare over the last century? Has physiotherapy remained stable because of a lack of evidence for or against their efficacy or for other reasons that are perhaps less visible and less obvious? And thinking to the future, does it follow that the approach that has served the profession so well in the past, will necessarily serve the profession as well into the future?

Firstly, I do not believe that the evidence suggests physiotherapists have been either intransigent, lazy or indifferent. Far from it, physiotherapists have been some of the most passionate advocates for new approaches to healthcare practice and have retained the respect of the medical profession, the public and the State because of that willingness to engage (see, for example, the profession's adoption of physical rehabilitation, care for polio victims and entry into the welfare state). Secondly, it does not follow that physiotherapy has retained a strong affinity for its traditional approaches to assessment and treatment because of a lack of evidence. There are now more than 34,000 randomised trials, systematic reviews and clinical practice guidelines relevant to physiotherapy available for review in the Physiotherapy Evidence Database (www.pedro.org.au) and more are being added daily. As these trials become more sophisticated, physiotherapists are gaining a deeper understanding of the reasons why people consistently turn to physical therapies in times of need. And thirdly, perhaps this book and the people and ideas it draws on constitutes evidence of a growing interest in exploring other ways of conceiving physiotherapy into the future.

For the entire history of the profession, physiotherapists' approach to touch-based and manual therapies, land- or water-based exercise and electrotherapy has been prefigured by an approach governed by the idea of the body-as-machine. This approach served a number of important functions: it allowed physiotherapists to train students to see body parts, not people; it de-sensualised practice and allowed practitioners to touch people without fear of scandal and licentiousness; it aligned the profession's view of the body with medicine and facilitated a close working relationship with doctors; it gave physiotherapy the kudos that came with an expert vocabulary that elevated the practitioners above their rivals and the lay public; it opened the door to objective methods of assessment and research evaluation and it gave practitioners licence to do things to people's bodies (cause pain, perform suction, give electric shocks etc.) that would not be possible otherwise. Most importantly, it has defined the boundaries around physiotherapy, such that practitioners could perform their assessments and treatments in certain ways *because* they conformed with the idea of the body-as-machine; it allows physiotherapists to touch people, but only if there is a patho-physiological justification for doing so (it could not be purely for pleasure); it encourages practitioners to measure the effect of their treatments objectively, while discounting polluting variables like affect, culture, emotion or the social construction of meaning, which might otherwise complicate matters and it allows practitioners to specialise, but only by continuing along the pathway made possible by a reductive, deconstructed view of the body. Not surprisingly, perhaps, innovations that go beyond the boundaries set by the body-as-machine (qualitative research, embodied phenomenology, mind-body approaches, even population health, e.g. – see Moe 2009),[8] suffer at the margins of orthodox practice, struggling to identify how they can be considered consistent with the long history of orthodox physiotherapy.

The question remains therefore; how might it be possible to understand how physiotherapy has adapted over the last half century then, if the basis of its practice has remained ostensibly the same? When we look at some of the most fundamental changes affecting physiotherapy since 1973, I would argue that it is possible to see a pattern emerge: the growth of evidence-based practice and outcome measures; attention to the cost and benefit of physiotherapy; curriculum reform and the development of new pathways to practice; the flowering of research, book and journal publication; the more invested role being played by professional societies and regulatory boards and promotional campaigns and the recent widespread uptake of social media. It becomes clear that physiotherapists have become adept at analysing, auditing and testing their treatments, researching the efficacy of their interventions and explaining to people what they do.

Over the last half century, physiotherapists have learnt the necessity of explanation: explanation to themselves about the nature of their practice delivered through academic scholarship and publication; explanations to their funders through practice audits and evidence-based practice; explanations to their patients who demand more than just a technician to fix their problems and explanations to their professional colleagues and peers in interprofessional meetings. Physiotherapy over the last four decades or more has been dominated by a growing reflexivity in the profession, underpinning a desire to know better how the profession has arrived at this point in its professional history (Higgs et al 2001; Tyni-Lenne 1989; Noronen & Wikstrom-Grotell 1999; Jorgensen 2000; Carpenter 1996; Owen 2014; Kell & Owen 2008; Ottosson 2015; Terlouw 2007; Nicholls & Cheek 2006; Hiller & Vears 2016). Physiotherapists are increasingly asking whether their practices really work, how much do they cost and are the really better than those offered by competing professions. The profession, like many other health professions and organisations in society, has developed a zeal for explaining how and why physiotherapy works. As Gwyn Owen argues, much of the evidence-based literature that has emerged over the last three decades 'does not critique or resist the changing construct of the profession. Instead, it focuses on the opportunities created by the change to promote the acceptance of physiotherapy as a profession and a science' (Richardson 1999b p. 15, cited in Owen 2014).

The enthusiasm for showing how physiotherapy works is based on a strong belief in the efficacy of physiotherapy and a confidence that the profession will endure. Consider this recent statement from Natalie Beswetherick, Director of Practice and Development at the CSP;

> Wherever you work in the UK, it is clear that your government wants to reduce the cost of providing NHS services. While each country is adopting a different approach, the result is the same. Physiotherapy services in the NHS and beyond have to demonstrate they can provide a high quality cost effective service in order to compete with other providers.
>
> Why is this so important? The answer is if you don't, your service will no longer be bought. The NHS is being commercialised, particularly in England, where large private sector companies such as Virgin Care and Care UK are winning tenders and chiropractors and osteopaths are entering the market under the any qualified provider initiative.
>
> NHS physios are pitching against their colleagues in the private sector for the right to continue to offer their services from within the NHS. They don't want to see existing provision destroyed, or to see shortcuts made in care. And they want their patients to receive a good service whatever their financial means.
>
> For those of you who have your heads in the sand and those that are on a hamster wheel, too driven by the day to day pressures to see the bigger, strategic picture, now is the time to stop, wake up and find out what is happening in your geographical patch.
>
> What should you do next? Take action. Start with your website. Remember that in the electronic age this is your shop window. Get it updated with easily accessible information for all. And if you don't already have one, then get one – and soon.
>
> Next, if you have not done so already introduce a PROM (patient related outcome measure) and a PREM (patient related experience measure) for your service. Do not wait for the development of an outcome measure that is sensitive to a specific physiotherapy intervention – while you are waiting you may lose your service to multi-nationals.
>
> (Beswetherick 2012)

The need to spread the message about physiotherapy's value has become a priority. Significantly, the call is for physiotherapists to *demonstrate* 'they can provide a high quality cost effective service in order to compete' (ibid), and, this can be achieved 'If all [51,500] CSP members in the UK relentlessly tell everybody how effective physiotherapy is, then we'll be heard' (ibid). The zeal shown for reform is based on both a position of strength and weakness, however. It is a strength because the profession has engaged in conversations about its place in the world from a position of authority, power and high social standing. What is more, most physiotherapists believe passionately in their practice and are vocal advocates for the profession (which often makes it all the more bemusing when the evidence does not back up their enthusiasm). But there are weaknesses too, not least the fact that the profession's core philosophy allows for practitioners to focus very narrowly on the biomechanical body of the person in front of them, effectively dismissing the full breadth and depth of human life that makes up a person's sense of health and wellbeing.

This weakness becomes profoundly important when we consider that, if physiotherapy has remained largely the same over the last 50 years and advances in practice have remained within the rigid confines of the body-as-machine, then physiotherapists are very badly placed if all of the changes taking place in healthcare are economic, cultural, geographical, historical, philosophical and political. If physiotherapists cannot lift their eyes from the biomechanical body and contemplate, understand, embrace and actively engage in these 'other' ways of understanding health and illness then their explanations will increasingly fall on deaf ears. They will continue to research the efficacy of their treatments, but people will cease to purchase them, going instead to someone who is less of an expensive technical rationalist. They will continue advocating for a dispassionate and de-sensualised approach to practice – a model that works wonderfully for short, episodic bouts of acute care that do not require the therapist to know the patient's motives and experiences – but consumers will increasingly abandon physiotherapy in favour of practitioners who celebrate their individuality and turn it into a virtue. They will keep arguing that their work is better than their competitors, but funders will continue to look to diverse markets among disparate groups of healthcare providers and abandon the professional silos that took so long to establish.

Closing words

Most existing histories of physiotherapy suggest that the last half century has been marked by a progressive journey towards professional enlightenment, marked by advanced clinical practices, sophisticated educational provisions and well-developed methods of verification. Bentley and Dunstan's history of physiotherapy in Australia provides a good example of this approach; 'From massage therapists occupying a subordinate position in the medical hierarchy, the profession has organised itself into an active Association [sic] and developed a discrete body of knowledge on body mechanics and neurophysiological function' (Bentley & Dunstan 2006, pp. 217–8). 'Along the way', the authors argue 'the profession has established and redefined educational curricula, set professional standards, supported the pioneering of new areas of endeavour and therapeutic practice, and adopted a new name, 'physiotherapy', to indicate the growing breadth of its practice' (ibid). Physiotherapy 'has developed a collegiate spirit though a journal, college, and congresses. It has survived division, both within and between the states, and has established itself firmly enough that it can attain unity in its diversity' (ibid). Bentley and Dunstan conclude by arguing that 'Most important, it has nurtured and in return been supported by practitioners of skill and vision who have furthered the profession's standing until it has been able to take its rightful place in the pantheon of medical practice' (ibid).

Wanting to resist the urge to offer another celebratory account of the profession's history, I have taken a different route in thinking about physiotherapy since 1973, focusing instead on some of the competing discourses that have made today's profession possible. What is clear from this approach is that physiotherapy, in many respects, operates in many of the same ways that were established by the profession's founders more than a century ago. What has changed, however, is the economic, political and social context in which physiotherapy now operates and the greatest shift in the profession has been around its desire to explain itself better *to* itself and to others. Changes in education, policy, practice and research have not seen physiotherapists depart radically from the idea of the body-as-machine. On the contrary, the biomechanical view of the body has been enhanced. Physiotherapists have simply found more sophisticated and nuanced ways to explain the affinity.

In the following chapters, I explore in far more detail how the body-as-machine operates and makes certain ways of thinking and practising physiotherapy possible while denying others. Underpinning this critique is a belief that better explanations of physiotherapy's approach will no longer serve the profession in the way that it has done in the past and that a continued engagement with the idea of the body-as-machine as the core of physiotherapy thinking and practice could spell the end of the profession as we know it. The first chapter in the following section then turns, naturally perhaps, to the idea of the body and the role it has come to play in physiotherapy.

Notes

1 It should be pointed out that these changes were concentrated in European and North American countries and were felt more unevenly throughout the rest of the world. For instance, Norway gained enormous wealth with the discovery of North Sea oil almost immediately after 1973 and Japan's technology boom of the 1970s, 1980s and 1990s buffered it from many of the worst effects of the oil crisis. It should also be noted that the oil crisis, on its own, cannot account for all of these effects. The social reforms of the post-war era including the Vietnam War, people's growing awareness of historical civil rights abuses, feminism and the growing counter-cultural movements of the 1960s and 70s, television, space exploration, access to cheap consumer goods and so on, will all have played a signficant role in shaping the events that were to follow the tipping point that came with the 1973 oil crisis.
2 I have tried to retain different English and American spellings where it is contextually relevant to do so.

3 It is always interesting to consider how much emphasis physiotherapists place on evidence-based *clinical* decision making, but that the same principles rarely apply to evidence-based *policy* making which, arguably, affects people's working and practice lives just as much. Physiotherapists now expect every facet of their clinical practice to be tested and examined for its generalisability, reliability, sensitivity and validity, but do not expect the same to be applied to decisions about the very design and structure of their profession.

4 Faber and Faber did go on to publish a separate volume dealing specifically with orthopaedic and rheumatological conditions using Joan Cash's now well known name but under the editorship of Patricia Downie (Downie 1984). Prior to this, orthopaedic and rheumatological conditions had been dealt with in earlier editions of Cash's books on medical and surgical conditions.

5 The first dedicated 'Research Column' appeared in *Physiotherapy* in October 1979. It provided a summary of all reserach studied published by the journal since 1974. In five years there were only 37 studies reported – equivalent to just over seven per year, or less than one per edition of the journal.

6 Dale Larsen has offered a different categorisation, defining the period between 1880–1913 as the 'massage' era, 1914–1945 the 'peripheral neuromusculoskeletal dysfunction' era, 1946–1980 the 'neurological' era and 1981 to the present the 'movement' era (Pynt et al 2009, pp. 36–8), while Gwyn Owen has suggested that we can divide the period since the 1980s into periods dominated by 'functionalism' (1980s), epistemic arguments (1980s and 1990s), uncertainty (1990s) and latterly 'evidence-based practice' (1990s to the present) (Owen 2014).

7 The term 'bleeding edge' derives from business and refers to a radical new practice that breaks convention and attempts something bold. Often with high failure rates, these practices pave the way for other more stable ventures to follow (Kleinke 1998).

8 By comparison with general medical practice, nursing, dentistry and other health professions, physiotherapy has no history and no working concept of population health. Where doctors offered mass public health services, dental nurses monitored entire populations of children's teeth, innoculated them against communicable diseases and checked on the development of newborn babies, physiotherapists have had no such approach. I would argue that the principal reason for this is because they have always focused on the biomechanical body in front of them. The body-as-machine, once again, looms large here.

References

American Board of Physical Therapy Specialties, 2015, Specialist certification, Retrieved July 31, 2015, from www.abpts.org/Certification/.

American Physical Therapy Association, 2000, *Vision 2020*, Retrieved August 10, 2015, from www.apta.org/Vision2020/.

Angove, H.S., 1936, *Remedial exercises for certain diseases of the heart and lung*, Faber & Faber, London.

Archer, K.R., Motzny, N., Abraham, C.M., Yaffe, D., Seebach, C.L., Devin, C.J., Spengler, D.M., McGirt, M.J., Aaronson, O.S., Cheng, J.S. & Wegener, S.T., 2013, Cognitive-behavioral-based physical therapy to improve surgical spine outcomes: A case series, *Physical Therapy*, 93(8), pp. 1130–9.

Australian College of Physiotherapy, n.d., Retrieved July 31, 2015, from https://www.physiotherapy.asn.au/APAWCM/Careers/Career_Paths/APA_ACP/APAWCM/Careers/Career_Paths/ACP.aspx.

Barsky, A.J., 1988, *Worried sick: Our troubled quest for wellness*, Little Brown, Boston, MA.

Bartley, M., 2004, *Health inequality: An introduction to theories, concepts, and methods*, Polity Press, Cambridge, UK.

Baxter, S.K. & Brumfitt, S.M., 2008, Professional differences in interprofessional working, *Journal of Interprofessional Care*, 22(3), pp. 239–51.

Baxter, D. & Nall, C., 2009, Current trends in physiotherapy practice. In J. Higgs, M.S. Smith, G.W. Webb, M.S. Skinner & A.C. Croker (eds.), *Contexts of physiotherapy practice*, Churchill Livingstone, Sydney, Australia, pp. 20–32.

Beeton, K., 2008, Masterclass editorial, *Manual Therapy*, 13(5), pp. 373–4.

Belcher, H., 2014, Power, politics, and healthcare, in J. Germov (ed.), *Second opinion: An introduction to health sociology*, Oxford University Press, Melbourne, Australia, pp. 359–87.

Bentley, P. & Dunstan, D., 2006, *The path to professionalism: Physiotherapy in Australia to the 1980s*, Australian Physiotherapy Association, Melbourne, Australia.

Beswetherick, N., 2012, Director of practice and development at the CSP, 4 April, *Frontline Magazine*, Retrieved July 8, 2015, from http://tinyurl.com/ow7j44.

Bjornsdottir, K., 2002, From the state to the family: Reconfiguring the responsibility for long-term nursing care at home, *Nursing Inquiry*, 9(1), pp. 3–11.

Bobath, B., 1965, *Abnormal postural reflex activity caused by brain lesion*, William Heinemann Medical Books, Oxford.

Bobath, B., 1975, *Adult hemiplegia: Evaluation and treatment*, William Heinemann Medical Books, London.

Bollag, 2007, Credential creep, *The Chronicle of Higher Education*, 53(42), p. A10.

Bott, J. & Singh, S., 1998, Pulmonary rehabilitation, in J. Pryor & B. Webber (eds.), *Physiotherapy for respiratory and cardiac problems*, Churchill Livingstone, London, pp. 371–86.

Bourdillon, J.F., 1973, *Spinal manipulation*, 2nd ed., William Heinemann Medical Books, London.

Brownsey, K.L. & Langford, J.W., 1990, Economic policy-making in the Asia-Pacific region, in *Economic policy-making in the Asia-Pacific region*, Institute for Research on Public Policy/Institut de recherches politiques, Halifax, NS.

Brunner, E., Herdt, A.D., Minguet, P., Baldew, S.-S. & Probst, M., 2015, Can cognitive behavioural therapy based strategies be integrated into physiotherapy for the prevention of chronic low back pain?: A systematic review, *Disability and Rehabilitation*, doi:10.3109/09638288.2012.683848.

Brunnstrom, S., 1966, Motor testing procedures in hemiplegia: Based on sequential recovery stages, *Physical Therapy*, 46(4), pp. 357–75.

Brunnstrom, S., 1972, *Clinical kinesiology*, F.A. Davis, Philadelphia, PA.

Burn, D. & Beeson, E., 2014, Orthopaedic triage: Cost effectiveness, diagnostic/surgical and management rates, *Clinical Governance: An International Journal*, 19(2), pp. 126–36.

Bury, M., 2008, New dimensions of healthcare organisation, in D. Wainwright (ed.), *A sociology of health*, Sage, London, pp. 151–72.

Bury, T.J. & Stokes, E.K., 2013a, Direct access and patient/client self-referral to physiotherapy: A review of contemporary practice within the European Union, *Physiotherapy*, 99(4), pp. 285–91.

Bury, T.J. & Stokes, E.K., 2013b, A global view of direct access and patient self-referral to physical therapy: Implications for the profession, *Physical Therapy*, 93(4), pp. 449–59.

Bury, T.J. & Moffat, M., 2014, Physiotherapists have a vital part to play in combatting the burden of noncommunicable diseases, *Physiotherapy*, 100(2), pp. 94–6.

Butler, D.S. & Moseley, G.L., 2013, *Explain pain, Revised and updated*, 2nd ed., Noigroup Publications, Adelaide, Australia.

Cameron, A., 2011, Impermeable boundaries? Developments in professional and interprofessional practice, *Journal of Interprofessional Care*, 25(1), pp. 53–8.

Canadian Physiotherapy Association, 2016, Clinical specialty program, Retrieved July 21, 2016, from https://physiotherapy.ca/clinical-specialist-program.

Carpenter, C., 1996, The evolving culture of physiotherapy: Barbara Edwardson lectureship 1995, *Physiotherapy Canada*, 48(1), pp. 11–15.

Carr, J.H. & Shepherd, R., 2000, *Movement science: Foundations for physical therapy in rehabilitation*, 2nd ed., Aspen Publishers, Gaithersburg, MD.

Carson, B., Dunbar, T., Chenhall, R.D. & Bailie, R., 2007, *Social determinants of indigenous health*, Allen & Unwin, London.

Cash, J., 1974, *Neurology for physiotherapists*, Faber & Faber, London.

Cash, J., 1975, *Chest, heart and vascular disorders for physiotherapists*, Faber and Faber, London.

Cash, J., 1976, *A textbook of medical conditions for physiotherapists*, 5th ed., Faber and Faber, London.

Cash, J., 1977, *Cash's textbook of physiotherapy in some surgical conditions*, 5th ed., Faber and Faber, London.

Chipchase, L., 2012, Is there a future for electrophysical agents in musculoskeletal physiotherapy?, *Manual Therapy*, 17(4), pp. 265–6.

Clark, H. & Bassett, S., 2015, An application of the health action process approach to physiotherapy rehabilitation adherence, *Physiotherapy Theory and Practice*, 30(8), 527–33.

Clarke, D.B., Doel, M.A. & Segrott, J., 2004, No alternative?: The regulation and professionalization of complementary and alternative medicine in the United Kingdom, *Health & Place*, 10(4), pp. 329–38.

Clayton, E.B. & Scott, P.M., 1975, *Clayton's electrotherapy and actinotherapy: Including the physics of movement and hydrotherapy*, Bailliere Tindall Ltd, London.

Clini, E. & Ambrosino, N., 2005, Early physiotherapy in the respiratory intensive care unit, *Respiratory Medicine*, 99(9), pp. 1096–104.

Coburn, D., 1994, Professionalization and proletarianization: Medicine, nursing and chiropractic in historical perspective, *Labour/Le Travail*, 34, pp. 139–62.

Cohn, S., 2014, From health behaviours to health practices: An introduction, *Sociology of Health & Illness*, 36(2), pp. 157–62.

Committee of Inquiry into Chiropractic, Osteopathy, Homoeopathy and Naturopathy, 1977, *Report of the Committee of Inquiry into Chiropractic, Osteopathy, Homoeopathy and Naturopathy*, Australian Government Publishing Service, Canberra, Australia.

Condon, C., McGrane, N., Mockler, D. & Stokes, E., 2016, Ability of physiotherapists to undertake evidence-based practice steps: A scoping review, *Physiotherapy*, 102(1), pp. 10–19.

Cribb, J., Disney, R. & Sibieta, L., 2014, *The public sector workforce: Past, present and future*, Institute for Fiscal Studies, London.

Cyriax, J., 1955, *Textbook of orthopaedic medicine: Treatment by manipulation and massage*, Cassell, London.

Cyriax, J., 1956, *Disc lesions*, Cassell, London.

Cyriax, J., 1982, *Textbooks of orthopaedic medicine: Diagnosis of soft tissue lesions*, 8th ed., Bailliere Tindall, London.

Cyriax, J. & Russell, G., 1977, *Textbook of orthopaedic medicine: Treatment by manipulation massage and injection*, Bailliere Tindall, London.

Dahl-Michelsen, T., 2015, Curing and caring competences in the skills training of physiotherapy students, *Physiotherapy Theory and Practice*, 31(1), pp. 8–16.

Davidson, A., 2014, *Social determinants of health: A comparative approach*, Oxford University Press, Oxford.

Dew, K., 2003, *Borderland practices: Regulating alternative therapies in New Zealand*, University of Otago Press, Dunedin, New Zealand.

Downie, P.A., 1984, *Cash's textbook of orthopaedics and rheumatology for physiotherapists*, Faber and Faber, London.

Durrell, S., 1996, Expanding the scope of physiotherapy: Clinical physiotherapy specialists in consultants' clinics, *Manual Therapy*, 1(4), pp. 210–13.

Dutta, M.J., 2015, *Neoliberal health organizing: Communication, meaning, and politics*, Left Coast Press, Walnut Creek, CA.

Einhorn, E.S. & Logue, J., 2003, *Modern welfare states: Scandinavian politics and policy in the global age*, Praeger, Westport, CN.

Ellis, B. & Connell, N.A.D., 2001, Factors determining the current use of physiotherapy assistants: Views on their future role in the South and West UK region, *Physiotherapy*, 87(2), pp. 73–82.

Engdahl, W., 1993, *A century of war: Anglo-American oil politics and the new world order*, Dr. Böttinger; Concord, MA.

Eyzaguirre, C. & Fidone, S.I., 1975, *Physiology of the nervous system*, 2nd ed., Year Book Medical Publishers, Chicago, IL.

Ferguson, S. & Cook, F., 2011, Is a primary care orthopaedic interface service sustainable in a continually changing political and healthcare environment?, *Clinical Governance: An International Journal*, 16(2), pp. 137–47.

Field, P.A. & Morse, J.M., 1985, *Nursing research: The application of qualitative approaches*, Chapman & Hall, London.

Foreman, K., 2003, To prescribe or not to prescribe?: That is the question?, *Physical Therapy in Sport*, 4(2), p. 57.

Furze, J.A., Tichenor, C.J., Fisher, B.E., Jensen, G.M. & Rapport, M.J., 2016, Physical therapy residency and fellowship education: Reflections on the past, present, and future, *Physical Therapy*, 96(7), pp. 949–60.

Gabe, J., Harley, K. & Calnan, M., 2015, Healthcare choice: Discourses, perceptions, experiences and practices, *Current Sociology*, 63(5), pp. 623–35.

Gardiner, J. & Wagstaff, S., 2001, Extended scope physiotherapy – The way towards consultant physiotherapists?, *Physiotherapy*, 87(1), pp. 1–3.

Gieryn, T.F., 1983, Boundary-work and the demarcation of science from non-science: Strains and interests in professional ideologies of scientists, *American Sociological Review*, 48(6), p. 781.

Graham, H., 2009, *Understanding health inequalities*, McGraw-Hill, Maidenhead, UK.

de Gruchy, A., Granger, C. & Gorelik, A., 2015, Physical therapists as primary practitioners in the emergency department: Six-month prospective practice analysis, *Physical Therapy*, 95(9), pp. 1207–16.

Gubrium, J.F. & Holstein, J.A., 2002, *Handbook of interview research, Context & methods*, Sage, Thousand Oaks, CA.

Guyton, A.C., 1971, *Basic human physiology: Normal function and mechanisms of disease*, W.B. Saunders Company, Philadelphia, PA.

Hansson, K.G., 1942, Present status of physical therapy in anterior poliomyelitis, *Journal of the American Physical Therapy Association*, 22, p. 3.

Hao, P.Y. & Tan, C., 1999, The future of the physiotherapist: Boom, doom or gloom? *Physiotherapy Singapore*, 2(4), p. 148.

Harding, P.A., Holland, A.E., Hinman, R.S. & Delany, C., 2015, Physical activity perceptions and beliefs following total hip and knee arthroplasty: A qualitative study, *Physiotherapy Theory and Practice*, 31(2), pp. 107–13.

Harthorn, B.H. & Oaks, L., 2003, *Risk, culture, and health inequality: Shifting perceptions of danger and blame*, Praeger, Westport, CT.

Higgs, P., 2012, Consuming bodies: Zygmunt Bauman on the difference between fitness and health, in G. Scambler (ed.), *Contemporary Theorists for Medical Sociology: Critical Studies in Health and Society*, Routledge, Abingdon, Oxon, pp. 20–32.

Higgs, J., Hunt, A., Higgs, C. & Neubauer, D., 1999, Physiotherapy education in the changing international healthcare and educational contexts, *Advances in Physiotherapy*, 1(1), pp. 17–26.

Higgs, J., Refshauge, K. & Ellis, E., 2001, Portrait of the physiotherapy profession, *Journal of Interprofessional Care*, 15(1), 79–89.

Hiller, A.J., & Vears, D.F., 2016, Reflexivity and the clinician-researcher: Managing participant misconceptions. *Qualitative Research Journal*, 16(1), 13–25.

Hough, A., 1991, *Physiotherapy in respiratory care: An evidence-based approach to respiratory and cardiac management*, 1st ed., Nelson Thornes, Cheltenham, UK.

Huby, G., Harris, F.M., Powell, A.E., Kielman, T., Sheikh, A., Williams, S. & Pinnock, H., 2014, Beyond professional boundaries: Relationships and resources in health services' modernisation in England and Wales, *Sociology of Health & Illness*, 36(3), pp. 400–15.

Huijbregts, P.A., 2007, Chiropractic legal challenges to the physical therapy scope of practice: Anybody else taking the ethical high ground?, *Journal of Manual and Manipulative Therapy*, 15(2), pp. 69–80.

Johanson, M.A., Miller, M.B., Coe, J.B. & Campo, M., 2016, Orthopaedic physical therapy: Update to the description of specialty practice, *The Journal of Orthopaedic and Sports Physical Therapy*, 46(1), pp. 9–18.

Jones, L.E. & O'Shaughnessy, D.F., 2014, The pain and movement reasoning model: Introduction to a simple tool for integrated pain assessment. *Manual Therapy*, 19(3), pp. 270–6.

Jorgensen, P., 2000, Concepts of body and health in physiotherapy: The meaning of the social/cultural aspects of life, *Physiotherapy Theory and Practice*, 16(2), pp. 105–15.

Kaltenborn, F., 1965, *Frigjoring av ryggraden*, Olaf Norlis Bokhandel, Oslo, Norway.

Kaltenborn, F., 1970, *Mobilisation of the spinal column*, New Zealand University Press, Wellington, New Zealand.

Kaltenborn, F., 1976, *Manual therapy for the extremity joints*, 2nd ed., Olaf Norlis Bokhandel, Oslo, Norway.

Kaltenborn, F., 1980, *Mobilization of the extremity joints: Examination and basic treatment techniques*, 3rd ed., Olaf Norlis Bokhandel Universitetsgaten, Oslo, Norway.

Keleher, H. & MacDougall, C., 2009, *Understanding health: A determinants approach*, 2nd ed., Oxford University Press, Australia.

Keleher, H. & MacDougall, C., 2011, *Understanding health: A determinants approach*, 3rd ed., Oxford University Press, Australia.

Kell, C. & Owen, G., 2008, Physiotherapy as a profession: Where are we now? *International Journal of Therapy and Rehabilitation*, 15(4), pp. 158–67.

Kelman, G.R., 1972, *Physiology: A clinical approach*, Churchill Livingstone, Edinburgh, London.

Kelner, M., Wellman, B., Boon, H. & Welsh, S., 2004, Responses of established healthcare to the professionalization of complementary and alternative medicine in Ontario, *Social Science & Medicine (1982)*, 59(5), pp. 915–30.

Kersten, P., McPherson, K., Lattimer, V., George, S., Breton, A. & Ellis, B., 2007, Physiotherapy extended scope of practice – who is doing what and why?, *Physiotherapy*, 93(4), pp. 235–42.

Klein, R., 2010, *The new politics of the NHS*, 6th ed., Radcliffe Medical Press, London.

Kleinke, J.D., 1998, *Bleeding edge: the business of health care in the new century*, Jones and Bartlett, Boston, MA.

Knott, M. & Voss, D.E., 1956, *Proprioceptive neuromuscular facilitation: Patterns and techniques*, Hoeber-Harper, New York.

Kot, F.C. & Hendel, D.D., 2012, Emergence and growth of professional doctorates in the United States, United Kingdom, Canada and Australia: A comparative analysis, *Studies in Higher Education*, 37(3), pp. 345–64.

Lanckenau, N.I., 1943, Rehabilitation by modern methods of exercise, in W.B. Doherty & D.D. Runes (eds.), *Rehabilitation of the war injured, a symposium*, Philosophical Library, New York, pp. 614–21.

Laslett, M., 1996, *Mechanical diagnosis and therapy: The upper limb*, Self published, Auckland, New Zealand.

Lee, J., 1978, *Aids to physiotherapy*, Churchill Livingstone, Edinburgh.

Leininger, M., 1985, *Qualitative research methods in nursing*, Grune and Stratton, New York.

Lettinga, A.T., 2002, Diversity in neurological physiotherapy: A content analysis of the Brunnstrom/Bobath controversy, *Advances in Physiotherapy*, 4(1), pp. 23–36.

Lovell, T. & Cordeaux, C. (1999). *Social policy for health and social care*, Hodder and Stoughton, London.

Magistro, C.M., 1984, The clinician's role in the 21st century, *Clinical Management in Physical Therapy*, 4(6), pp. 10–13.

Maitland, G.D., 1964, *Vertebral manipulation*, Butterworth, London.

Maitland, G.D., 1966, Manipulation – Mobilisation, *Physiotherapy*, 52(11), pp. 382–5.

Maitland, G.D., 1973, *Vertebral manipulation*, 3rd ed., Butterworth, London.

Maitland, G.D., 1977a, *Peripheral manipulation*, 2nd ed., Butterworth, London.

Maitland, G.D., 1977b, *The vertebral column: Examination and recording guide*, 6th ed., Virgo Press, Adelaide, Australia.

Maitland, G.D., 1978, *Musculo-skeletal examination and recording guide*, Virgo Press, Adelaide, Australia.

Marmot, M., Friel, S., Bell, R., Houweling, T.A. & Taylor, S., 2008, Closing the gap in a generation: Health equity through action on the social determinants of health, *The Lancet*, 372(9650), pp. 1661–9.

Marmot, M.G. & Wilkinson, R.G., 1999, *Social determinants of health*, Oxford University Press, Oxford.

Martin, S.C., 1994, 'The only truly scientific method of healing': Chiropractic and American science, 1895–1990, *Isis: An International Review Devoted to the History of Science and its Cultural Influences*, 85(2), pp. 207–27.

McIntosh, T., Stewart, D., Forbes-McKay, K., McCaig, D. & Cunningham, S., 2016, Influences on prescribing decision-making among non-medical prescribers in the United Kingdom: Systematic review, *Family Practice*, doi: 10.1093/fampra/cmw085.

McKenzie, R., 1980, *Treat your own back*, Price Milburn, Wellington, New Zealand.

McKenzie, R., 1983, *Treat you own neck*, Spinal Publications, Waikanae, New Zealand.

McKenzie, R.A., 1981, *The lumbar spine: Mechanical diagnosis and therapy*, Spinal Publications, Waikanae, New Zealand.

Mennell, J., 1952, *The science and art of joint manipulation: The spinal column*, J. & A. Churchill, London.

Mennell, J.M., 1960, *Back pain: Diagnosis and treatment using manipulative techniques*, Little, Brown and Company, Boston, MA.

Mennell, J.M., 1964, *Joint pain: Diagnosis and treatment using manipulative techniques*, Little, Brown and Company, Boston, MA.

Merrill, K.R., 2007, *The oil crisis of 1973–1974: A brief history with documents*, Bedford/ St. Martin's, Boston, MA.

Moe, S., 2009, Another dance – about embodied knowledge. In E. Falk & H.-J.W. Weihe (eds.), *Living crafts: Preserving, passing on and developing our common intangible heritage: International and national ambitions.* Lillehammer; Stavanger: Norwegian Crafts Development (NHU); Hertervig Akademisk, pp. 101–6.

Moffatt, M., 1994, APTA presidential address: Will the legacy of our past provide us with a legacy for the future?, *Physical Therapy*, 74, pp. 1063–6.

Moore, A. & Jull, G., 2011, Musculoskeletal therapy and global challenges, *Manual Therapy*, 16(4), p. 307.

Morris, J.H. & Grimmer, K., 2014, Non-medical prescribing by physiotherapists: Issues reported in the current evidence, *Manual Therapy*, 19(1), pp. 82–6.

Morse, J.M. (ed.), 1990, *Qualitative nursing research: A contemporary dialogue*, Sage, London.

Moseley, G.L., 2007, *Painful yarns: Metaphors & stories to help understand the biology of pain*, Dancing Giraffe Press, Canberra, Australia.

Mulligan, B., 1989, *Manual therapy: "NAGS", "SNAGS", "PRP's" etc.*, Plain View Services, Wellington, New Zealand.

Mulligan, B.R., 1995, *Manual therapy*, 3rd ed., Plane View Services, Wellington, New Zealand.

Napier, C., McCormack, R.G., Hunt, M.A. & Brooks-Hill, A., 2013, A physiotherapy triage service for orthopaedic surgery: An effective strategy for reducing wait times, *Physiotherapy Canada*, 65(4), pp. 358–63.

Nettleton, S., 2006, *The sociology of health and illness*, 2nd ed., Polity, Cambridge.

Neumann, D.A., 2004, Historical perspective: Polio: Its impact on the people of the United States and the emerging profession of physical therapy, *Journal of Orthopaedic & Sports Physical Therapy*, 34(8), pp. 479–92.

Nicholls, D.A. & Cheek, J., 2006, Physiotherapy and the shadow of prostitution: The Society of Trained Masseuses and the massage scandals of 1894, *Social Science & Medicine (1982)*, 62(9), pp. 2336–48.

Nicholls, D.A. & Gibson, B.E., 2010, The body and physiotherapy, *Physiotherapy Theory and Practice*, 26(8), pp. 497–509.

Nicholls, D.A. & Larmer, P., 2005, Possible futures for physiotherapy: An exploration of the New Zealand context, *New Zealand Journal of Physiotherapy*, 33(2), pp. 55–60.

Noronen, L. & Wikstrom-Grotell, C., 1999, Towards a paradigm-oriented approach in physiotherapy, *Physiotherapy Theory and Practice*, 15(3), pp. 175–84.

Norris, P., 2001, How 'we' are different from 'them': Occupational boundary maintenance in the treatment of musculo-skeletal problems, *Sociology, Health & Illness*, 23(1), pp. 24–43.

O'Byrne, P. & Holmes, D., 2007, The micro-fascism of Plato's good citizen: Producing (dis)order through the construction of risk, *Nursing Philosophy*, 8(2), pp. 92–101.

Ojha, H.A., Snyder, R.S. & Davenport, T.E., 2013, Direct access compared with referred physical therapy episodes of care: A systematic review, *Physical Therapy*, 94(1), pp. 1–17.

O'Rourke, B., 2012, The role of the expert patient in compliance and concordance, in M. Davies & D.F. Kermani (eds.), *Patient compliance: Sweetening the pill*, Gower Publishing, UK, pp. 197–210.

O'Sullivan, K., Dankaerts, W., O'Sullivan, L., & O'Sullivan, P.B. (2015). Cognitive functional therapy for disabling nonspecific chronic low back pain: Multiple case-cohort study. *Physical Therapy*, 95(11), pp. 1478–88.

Ottosson, A., 2011, The manipulated history of manipulations of spines and joints? Rethinking orthopaedic medicine through the 19th century discourse of European mechanical medicine, *Medicine Studies*, 3(2), pp. 83–116.

Ottosson, A., 2015, One history or many herstories?: Gender politics and the history of physiotherapy's origins in the nineteenth and early twentieth century, *Women's History Review*, doi: 10.1080/09612025.2015.1071581.

Ovretveit, J., 1985, Medical dominance and the development of professional autonomy in physiotherapy, *Sociology of Health & Illness*, 7(1), pp. 76–93.

Owen, G., 2014, Becoming a practice profession: A genealogy of physiotherapy's moving/touching practice, doctoral thesis, University of Cardiff, Cardiff.

Pagliarulo, M.A., 2007, *Introduction to physical therapy*, 3rd ed., Mosby, St. Louis, MO.

Paris, S.V., 1965, *The spinal lesion*, Pegasus Press, Christchurch, New Zealand.

Parsons, T., 1951, *The social system*, Free Press, New York.

Partridge, C.J., 1980, The effectiveness of physiotherapy: A classification for evaluation, *Physiotherapy*, 66(5), pp. 153–5.

Pearson, S., Moraw, I. & Maddern, G.J., 2000, Clinical pathway management of total knee arthroplasty: A retrospective comparative study, *ANZ Journal of Surgery*, 70(5), pp. 351–4.

Perry, C.E., 1967, Principles and techniques of the Brunnstrom approach to the treatment of hemiplegia, *American Journal of Physical Medicine*, 46(1), pp. 789–815.

Petersen, A., 1996, Risk and the regulated self: The discourse of health promotion as politics of uncertainty, *Australian and New Zealand Journal of Sociology*, 32(1), pp. 44–57.

Plack, M.M. & Wong, C.K., 2002, The evolution of the doctorate of physical therapy: Moving beyond the controversy, *Journal of Physical Therapy Education*, 16(1), pp. 48–59.

Pryor, J.A. & Prasad, S.A., 2002, *Physiotherapy for respiratory and cardiac problems: Adult and paediatrics*, 3rd ed., Churchill Livingstone, Edinburgh.

Pynt, J., Larsen, D., Nicholls, D. & Higgs, J., 2009, Historical phases in physiotherapy, in J. Higgs, M. Smith, G. Webb, M. Skinner & A. Croker (eds.), *Contexts of physiotherapy practice*, Churchill Livingstone, Chatswood, NSW, Australia, pp. 33–43.

Reinkensmeyer, D.J. & Dietz, V., 2016, *Neurorehabilitation technology*, Springer, New York.

Ritchie Russell, W., 1952, *Poliomyelitis*, Edward Arnold, London.

Rodeghero, J., Wang, Y.-C., Flynn, T., Cleland, J.A., Wainner, R.S. & Whitman, J.M., 2015, The impact of physical therapy residency or fellowship education on clinical outcomes for patients with musculoskeletal conditions, *Journal of Orthopaedic & Sports Physical Therapy*, 45(2), pp. 86–96.

Rogers, A., Entwistle, V. & Pencheon, D., 1998, Managing demand: A patient led NHS: Managing demand at the interface between lay and primary care, *BMJ: British Medical Journal*, 316(7147), p. 1816.

Rose, N., 1999, *Powers of freedom: Reframing political thought*, Cambridge University Press, Cambridge, UK.

Rothstein, J.M., 1998, Education at the crossroads: For today's practice, the DPT, *Physical Therapy*, 78(4), pp. 358–60.

Roy, S.C., 2008, 'Taking charge of your health': Discourses of responsibility in English-Canadian women's magazines, *Sociology of Health & Illness*, 30(3), pp. 463–77.

Salmon, P. & Hall, G.M., 2003, Patient empowerment and control: A psychological discourse in the service of medicine, *Social Science & Medicine (1982)*, 57(10), pp. 1969–80.

Sanders, T., Ong, B.N., Sowden, G. & Foster, N., 2014, Implementing change in physiotherapy: Professions, contexts and interventions, *Journal of Health Organization and Management*, 28(1), pp. 96–114.

Sahrmann, S., 1999, Diagnosis and treatment of movement impairment syndrome [Lecture notes], authors personal copy.

Scambler, G., 2002, *Health and social change: A critical theory*, Open University Press, Buckingham, UK.

Schmidt, D., 2013, Supervising allied health assistants: A concerning skill gap in allied health professionals, *Journal of Allied Health*, 42(4), pp. 243–6.

Schön, D.A., 1987, *Educating the reflective practitioner: Toward a new design for teaching and learning in the professions*, Jossey Bass, San Francisco, CA.

Scott-Dempster, C., Toye, F., Truman, J. & Barker, K., 2015, Physiotherapists' experiences of activity pacing with people with chronic musculoskeletal pain: An interpretative phenomenological analysis, *Physiotherapy Theory and Practice*, 30(5), pp. 319–28.

Scurlock-Evans, L., Upton, P. & Upton, D., 2014, Evidence-based practice in physiotherapy: A systematic review of barriers, enablers and interventions, *Physiotherapy*, 100(3), pp. 208–19.

Shepherd, R.B., 1974, *Physiotherapy in paediatrics*, William Heinemann Medical Books, London.

Silverman, D., 1997, *Qualitative research: Theory, methods and practice*, Sage, London.

Sim, I.B., 1971, *Mobilization and manipulation of the spine: Basic techniques*, N.Z. Society of Physiotherapists (Inc.), Wellington, New Zealand.

Slomp, H., 1998, *Between bargaining and politics: An introduction to European labor relations*, Praeger, Westport, CT.

Sontag, S., 1977, *Illness as metaphor*, Penguin, London.

Standing, G., 2011, *The precariat the new dangerous class*, Bloomsbury Academic, London; New York.

Stanmore, E. & Waterman, H., 2007, Crossing professional and organizational boundaries: The implementation of generic rehabilitation assistants within three organizations in the northwest of England, *Disability and Rehabilitation*, 29(9), pp. 751–9.

Stockmeyer, S.A., 1967, An interpretation of the approach of Rood to the treatment of neuromuscular dysfunction, *American Journal of Physical Medicine*, 46(1), pp. 900–61.

Stoddard, A., 1959, *Manual of osteopathic technique*, Hutchinson Medical Publications, London.

Sulch, D., Perez, I., Melbourn, A. & Kalra, L., 2000, Randomized controlled trial of integrated (managed) care pathway for stroke rehabilitation, *Stroke: A Journal of Cerebral Circulation*, 31(8), pp. 1929–34.

Terlouw, T.J., 2007, Roots of physical medicine, physical therapy, and mechanotherapy in the Netherlands in the 19 century: A disputed area within the healthcare domain, *Journal of Manual and Manipulative Therapy*, 15(2), pp. E23–41.

Theberge, N., 2008, The integration of chiropractors into healthcare teams: A case study from sport medicine, *Sociology of Health & Illness*, 30(1), pp. 19–34.

Thomas, M., Dat Vuong, K. & Jankovic, J., 2006, Long-term prognosis of patients with psychogenic movement disorders, *Parkinsonism & Related Disorders*, 12(6), pp. 382–7.

Thompson, B., 1968, *Asthma and your child*, 3rd ed., Pegasus Press, Christchurch, New Zealand.

Thompson, B. & Thompson, H.T., 1968, Forced expiratory exercises in asthma and their effects on FEV_1, *New Zealand Journal of Physiotherapy*, 3(15), pp. 19–21.

Tsiachristas, A., Hipple-Walters, B., Lemmens, K.M., Nieboer, A.P. & Rutten-van Mölken, M.P., 2011, Towards integrated care for chronic conditions: Dutch policy developments to overcome the (financial) barriers, *Health Policy*, 101(2), pp. 122–32.

Turner, P., 2001, The occupational prestige of physiotherapy: Perceptions of student physiotherapists in Australia, *Australian Journal of Physiotherapy*, 47, pp. 191–7.

Tyni-Lenne, R., 1989, To identify the physiotherapy paradigm: A challenge for the future, *Physiotherapy Theory & Practice*, 5(4), pp. 169–70.

Vancampfort, D., Vanderlinden, J., De Hert, M., Adámkova, M., Skjaerven, L. H., Catalán-Matamoros, D., Lundvik-Gyllensten, A., Gómez-Conesa, A., Ijntema, R. & Probst, M., 2013, A systematic review on physical therapy interventions for patients with binge eating disorder, *Disability and Rehabilitation*, 35(26), pp. 2191–6.

Villanueva-Russell, Y., 2005, Evidence-based medicine and its implications for the profession of chiropractic, *Social Science & Medicine (1982)*, 60, pp. 545–61.

Villanueva-Russell, Y., 2011, Caught in the crosshairs: Identity and cultural authority within chiropractic, *Social Science & Medicine (1982)*, 72(11), pp. 1826–37.

Waddington, P.J. & Cash, J., 1975, Intensive care – 1, in *Chest, heart and vascular disorders for physiotherapists*, Faber and Faber, London, pp. 53–86.

Wagstaff, S., 2001, Extended scope physiotherapy, *Physiotherapy*, 87(1), pp. 2–3.

Webb, C., 1984, Feminist methodology in nursing research, *Journal of Advanced Nursing*, 9(3), pp. 249–56.

Webber, B. & Pryor, J., 1993, *Physiotherapy for respiratory and cardiac problems*, Churchill Livingstone, London.

Webber, B.A., 1973, *The Brompton Hospital guide to chest physiotherapy*, 1st ed., Blackwell Scientific Publications, London.

Webber, B.A., 1991, Evaluation and inflation in respiratory care, *Physiotherapy*, 77(12), pp. 801–4.

Webster, C., 1998, The politics of general practice, in I. Loudon, J. Horder & C. Webster (eds.), *General practice under the National Health Service 1948–1997*, Clarendon Press, London, pp. 20–44.

Wietz, R., 2013, *The sociology of health, illness, and healthcare*, 6th ed., Wadsworth, Boston, MA.

Wilkinson, R.G. & Pickett, K., 2010, *The spirit level: Why equality is better for everyone*, Penguin Books, London; New York.

Wilson, D.J., 2005, Braces, wheelchairs, and iron lungs: The paralyzed body and the machinery of rehabilitation in the polio epidemics, *Journal of Medical Humanities*, 26(2–3), pp. 173–90.

Wines, B., Nicol, L., Nicolson, R., Court, D. & Korsch, H., 1967, The value of diaphragmatic breathing in the patient with obstructive airway disease, *Australian Journal of Physiotherapy*, XIII(2), p. 72.

Wrynn, A., 2014, On the margins: Therapeutic massage, physical education and physical therapy defining a profession, *The International Journal of the History of Sport*, 31(15), 1882–95.

Yagi, E., 2015, *Health and healthcare at the crossroads of business and society*, ESSEC Publishing, Cergy-Pontoise Cedex, France.

Yong, P. L., Saunders, R. S. & Olsen, L. A., 2010, *The healthcare imperative: Lowering costs and improving outcomes: Workshop series summary* (p. 852), National Academies Press, Washington, DC.

Part II

6   The body

Introduction

Ask a physiotherapist what the body means to them and they are likely to look at you as if you had asked them a trick question. The body is so obvious to physiotherapists, so commonplace that to attempt to define it seem odd. The body is what physiotherapists work on. It is the object of their gaze and the defining feature of their work. The body is to the physiotherapist what the tree is to the carpenter or the cloth is to the tailor. Physiotherapists are artisans of the body. And yet the physiotherapists' view of the body is quite limited; concerned largely with the body-as-machine (the idea that the body can be understood biomechanically, as a series of intersecting parts that can be repaired or replaced when they malfunction). Other bodies, and other ways of understanding bodied, are for other people.

In this chapter, I make three arguments that are fundamental to this whole book: (1) that there are important historical reasons for the profession's adoption of the idea of the body-as-machine, (2) that the reasons to anchor the profession to these ideas belong in the nineteenth century and (3) that the profession's fidelity to these nineteenth century ideas is hampering the profession's ability to adapt to the needs of 21st century healthcare. How physiotherapists approach the body in the future is therefore a vital question for this book, but it is also an important question for the profession at large, because if physiotherapists cannot understand how the body has changed – and how they must change with it – they will almost certainly see the end of physiotherapy as a profession.

I begin the chapter by locating 'the body' in contemporary physiotherapy with a historical sketch of what the body has meant to physiotherapy in the past and how this was significant, before explaining a little about the idea of the body-as-machine and the problems this is causing the profession today. I will then outline some of the 'other' ways that historians, philosophers and sociologists have defined the body over the last century and how this has informed our understanding of what it means to be healthy or sick. An analysis of the radically transformed body that is now emerging in the 21st century follows and I examine two important fields of research around the lived body and the social body, and look at some of the research being conducted by physiotherapists in these fields. Clearly, this cannot be an exhaustive account, but I hope it provides enough material to encourage readers to recognise the strengths of the biomechanical body and then to consider how they might move beyond it.

The biomechanical body hiding in physiotherapy

One does not have to look far to find evidence of what the body means to physiotherapy. Look at the title of the articles in any physiotherapy journal or the index of one of the general guides to the profession and you will see lots of interest in the structure and function of the body; lots of evidence of anatomy, biomechanics, kinesiology, pathology and physiology; lots of attention to how the body's dysfunction can be measured, diagnosed and restored. And while you will also increasingly find evidence of physiotherapists looking beyond the confines of the biomedical body, by far the strongest influence on the academic writing about the profession is the idea of the body-as-machine.

To illustrate my point, at the time of writing this chapter, I looked at the contents of a major international physiotherapy journal to see what I might find out about physiotherapists' current interest in the body. There were eight original pieces of research published in the edition in addition to three systematic reviews. The reviews were of musculoskeletal triage, the clinical utility of cervical range of motion and the value of physiotherapy before knee replacement. The eight original articles included studies of normative data on hand grip-strength, movement and pain patterns in adhesive capsulitis and inter-rectus distance in postpartum women. These were the papers that specifically addressed issues of 'the body'. The other papers concerned more general health and organisational issues, including physical activity, fear of falling and clinical education.

The kinds of research being undertaken by the profession, like the subject headings in the indexes of physiotherapy texts, can tell you a lot about how the profession views fundamentally important ideas like 'the body' in its day-to-day practice. And two things are particularly striking here: firstly, how important the physical body is to physiotherapy and secondly, how unaware and unquestioning the profession is of this fact. While physiotherapists have had a long history of writing about the body, they have almost no history in writing about what the body is and what it means to them. Authors rarely explain that their studies are limited to a particularly biomechanical view of the body. It is merely assumed that the reader is 'on the same page' and has an implicit understanding that the body being spoken about in this study of hamstring stretching is the biomechanical body. No justification for this limited view is provided and, in reality, none is needed. By the time you have arrived at reading a physiotherapy journal article, you will have almost certainly experienced at least some of the physiotherapy curriculum. And this will have equipped you with all the 'fundamentals' of physiotherapy: the anatomy, kinesiology, pathology and physiology that you will need to begin along the journey towards a thorough biomechanical understanding of how the body fails and how to fix it.

And yet, at least in my experience, a lot of mature practitioners know that the body is so much more than that which you find in the scientific literature. In fact,

I would venture to suggest that you cannot become an expert practitioner unless you quickly realise that treating a patient's body as a machine is largely inadequate for the real world of practice. Unfortunately, lacking the necessary guidance from their own profession, many practitioners struggle to define *how* to move beyond their training. Their work demands a broader, more nuanced view of what health is and so it can feel sometimes as if one is actually moving away from one's scope to move beyond the body-as-machine. What is lacking, of course, is an acknowledgement that physiotherapy involves far more than just this narrow view of the body and efforts are now being made to do this. But we should not imagine for a moment that this task is easy. To be overt about the profession's historically limited view of the body and to open the door to a new more holistic view carries significant risks – risks that should be considered carefully before proceeding.

The body in Western culture

The body has been the subject of philosophy for as long as humans have thought about what they are, what distinguishes them from other animals and how they function as individuals and socially. Aristotle believed that it was our ability to speak and engage in discussion and debate that set him apart from animals and evidence suggests that most ancient cultures in Africa, Asia and South America had already developed specific practices that distinguished the body of the individual from the body of the group or tribe. The distinction between individuality and the social world was a concern for the early Christian church that saw the need to discipline the body through piety, but it was Rene Descartes' distinction between body and the mind (known as Cartesian Dualism) in the first half of the 17th century that marks a turning point in the scientific history of the body.

Descartes argued that we could not trust our senses and only knew that *we* existed because we could contemplate the very idea of our existence ('I think therefore I am'). He argued that to know anything about the world, we must suspend personal judgements and measure naturally-occurring phenomena as objectively as possible, thus providing a philosophical focus for modern-day science. He also argued that it might be possible to view the body as separate from the mind. The mind, he argued, was the seat of the soul – God-like and pure. The body, though, was very much of this world: profane, dirty and prone to corruption.

This idea was taken up enthusiastically by natural philosophers – those called scientists today – like Francis Bacon, Voltaire, David Hume, Immanuel Kant and Isaac Newton; by pioneering anatomists like Leonardo da Vinci and Andreas Vesalius; astronomers and mathematicians like Nicolaus Copernicus and Galileo Galilei and chemists like Robert Boyle and Robert Hooke. Each embraced the idea that the church could retain its interest in the mind and the soul, but the body could now be the focus of Enlightenment science.

The period of Enlightenment that swept through Europe during the 16th and 17th centuries radically challenged many centuries of superstition and faith-based medicine and brought with it a new interest in how the body functioned in health and illness. The body came to be understood as something that science might master and this quest for mastery of the body began with the study of anatomy.

The publication of *De Humani Corporis Fabrica* ('On the Fabric of the Human Body') by Belgian anatomist, doctor and artist Andreas Vesalius, created the first anatomical 'map' of the body. Prior to this point, understanding of the workings of the body had been limited by the church, which believed that God had not enclosed everything within the body, only for it to be opened up for examination (Turner 1996). Human anatomy quickly became a matter of huge public and scientific interest. Dissections became spectacles and anatomy lessons became celebrated in art (see e.g. *The Anatomy Lesson of Dr Nicholaes Tulp* (c. 1652) by Rembrandt and *The Reward of Cruelty* (1751) by Hogarth) (Samson 1999, p. 7). Connections between people's signs and symptoms in life and dissection findings on death suggested that illness was not the result of sin or a malign God, but lay entirely within the body of the sufferer – giving birth to pathological science and the idea of specific aetiology.

The Industrial Revolution also had a profound effect on the way people understood individual and collective bodies. Radical improvements in farming and manufacturing practices created surplus labour that forced people to leave the countryside and head to the cities, where a new mass of urban poor became politically active, giving rise to modern government and their desire to manage the population through technologies directed at people's bodies (legislation, planned work and leisure, surveillance etc. (Rose et al 2006)). Central to these activities were the professions that took on the work of governance. Doctors were particularly active in this role, developing epidemiological and statistical surveys of the population's health, offering solutions to public health problems, creating hospitals and regulated training institutions, and working assiduously to improve the health of people's bodies.

The idea of the body-as-machine became a powerful metaphor, particularly after the Industrial Revolution, when it was thought that it might apply not only to the function of various bodies, but to the machinery of production that had become necessary to fuel the growth of an economy. William Harvey described the 'pumping' action of the heart; Descartes compared the body to a clock and Baglivi identified pincers in the jaws, the stomach as a container, ducts in the arteries, filters in the bowels and bellows in the lungs (Samson 1999, p. 10). The musculoskeletal system was understood to be synonymous with an elaborate crane and soon, biomechanics – literally the study of the body-as-machine – became a key feature of modern medicine.

Notwithstanding these advances, medicine remained a relatively unsophisticated science until the start of the 20th century. Without antisepsis and antibiotics, many of the remedies for the ailments that physicians had discovered remained painful and often as dangerous as the disease itself. And without knowledge of placebo, most remedies were based more on guesswork than evidence of efficacy.

Investment in the medical sciences has grown exponentially over the last 100 years. Social medicine replaced theories of miasmas and humours with germ theory; public health medicine has dramatically reduced child mortality and instituted immunisation programmes around the world and war and new visuali-sation technology has brought radical advances in surgery and pharmacology has ended suffering and prolonged life for millions. Medicine's focus throughout has been on the body-as-machine and for this it has been both lauded and vilified.

Since the end of the World War II, medicine has been the focus of increasing criticism. This criticism stems from the power of doctors and their ability to define who is normal and who is abnormal. Prior to WWII, most people believed that the 'doctor knows best', but over time this belief has eroded. People have increasingly turned towards social medicine that deals not only with the body-as-machine, but the personal and social understandings of people's health and wellbeing and doctors are less interested in this. Medicine is not particularly interested in subjects like culture, history, linguistics, the arts, economics, politics, gender, kinship, social systems like healthcare, spirituality, disability, ethnicity and race, whereas much of our understanding of health in the last 50 years has come from these fields (Armstrong 1983; Fox 2012; Shilling 2012; Turner 2008; Hancock et al 2000; Williams 2003; Lupton 2012).

As a result, we have now entered a period of human history in which people – particularly those living in the West – are much less certain about what the body is, where it begins and ends and what might be possible in the future. All the accumulated knowledge of the last 3,000 years has not, it seems, given us greater confidence in our understanding of the body. It has merely shown humans to be immensely complex, idiosyncratic, adaptable and impressionable beings. Indeed, some postmodern philosophers are now arguing that even thinking about humans as 'beings' with 'identities' is misleading because it implies that humans are more stable than we really know them to be. Where once it was axiomatic that there were two clearly distinguishable genders – male and female – the idea that there are many different expressions of gender, sexuality and genetic inheritance has become more widespread. In the same way, other long-held distinctions between normal and abnormal, healthy and sick, able-bodied and disabled, and even alive and dead appear less certain.

And what used to be science fiction is increasingly becoming science fact, lead-ing some people to speculate that our historical view of the body may need a radical overhaul in the 21ˢᵗ century. How long before people can cheat death and preserve ourselves indefinitely (cryogenically or genetically)? How long before we routinely live beyond 100, with bodies that are endlessly regenerating? How long before someone replaces the legs they were born with, with prosthetic legs just because they can (Lilley 2013)? These fantasies are becoming a reality and they radically change our traditional view of what the body is and what it might become. This obviously has important implications for medicine, but it will also affect the role physiotherapy plays in society. What role does the body play in physiotherapy then?

I have argued in Chapter 3 that it was important for the founders of the physio-therapy profession to adopt an approach to practice that found favour with the medical profession. I believe that adopting a biomechanical view of the body was a powerful way to achieve this. What is also clear, however, is that training masseuses to view the body-as-machine served another, equally important purpose. If students could be trained to view the body-as-machine, it would be possible to teach them to touch bodies without thinking of the them as sensually. This would prove important for the profession's quest to rid legitimate massage practice of its association with decadence and licentiousness. How then did physiotherapy use the metaphor of the body-as-machine to develop its professional subjectivity and create the modern profession we know today?

Maintaining the body-as-machine

Throughout its history, physiotherapy has placed a biomechanical view of the body at the centre of its professional identity and this strategy has repeatedly served the profession well as it developed from a series of practices that caused public suspicion and medical scepticism, to a profession that would dominate the orthodox practices of physical rehabilitation in the 20th century. Had it not been for the masseuses' affinity with the body-as-machine, it is unlikely that they would have been so involved in the rehabilitation movement that began in earnest after World War I (Linker 2011). On their return from war, it is unlikely that they would have gained orthodox recognition in the nascent welfare state had it not been for their work on the bodies of patients recovering from the influenza, TB and polio epidemics of the inter-war years. Thus, when publicly-funded welfare state medicine became a major feature of the health systems of many developed countries after the 1930s, physiotherapy had already established itself as *the* pre-eminent provider of orthodox physical rehabilitation and so was the natural partner to medicine and nursing in the newly built state health systems.

Although it seems in poor taste to admit it, the physiotherapy profession has benefited greatly from many of the calamities that befell populations in the 20th century. And over the course of those 100 years, international membership grew from a handful of small, semi-autonomous practitioners to an international congress of over 300,000 members. What is truly remarkable over that time is how consistently and doggedly physiotherapists have retained fidelity with the idea of the body-as-machine.

This can be seen in any number of examples. As the profession grew in self-confidence, for example, members began producing books that would become standard texts for students learning how physiotherapy was meant to be practiced. Some of these text, like Edith Prosser's *Manual of Massage and Movement*, Noël Tidy's *Massage and Remedial Exercises*, E. Bellis Clayton's *Electrotherapy and Actinotherapy* and Joan Cash's various iterations of *Physiotherapy in Some Surgical Conditions; Textbook of Medical Conditions for Physiotherapists, Textbook of Orthopaedics and Rheumatology for Physiotherapists* and *Neurology for Physiotherapists* ran to many editions and reprints.[1] These texts help us trace the shifting trends in physiotherapy practice during the second half of the twentieth century. Noël Tidy's work provides possibly the longest account with the broadest scope and seeing the similarities and differences between the content in the first edition of the book in 1932 to the latest and the 15th edition of the book it might appear that much has changed (see Table 6.1).

Table 6.1 Tidy's *Physiotherapy* contents lists

1934 (2nd)	1961 (10th)	2008 (14th)
Tidy's Massage and Remedial Exercises	Tidy's Massage and Remedial Exercises	Tidy's Physiotherapy
Fractures: General considerations	Physiotherapy: General considerations	The responsibilities of being a physiotherapist
Fractures of the upper extremity	Fractures: General considerations	Musculoskeletal assessment
Fractures of the lower extremity	Fractures of the upper extremity	An introduction to fractures
Dislocations	Fractures of the lower extremity, pelvis and spine	Management of burns and plastic surgery
Sprains: Muscle injuries: Wounds and scars	Joint and muscle injuries	Physiotherapy in women's health
Treatment of the after-effects of injury: Stiff joints	Wounds and scars: Suppurative conditions: Burns and skin-grafts: Amputations	Biomechanics
Diseases of joints, synovial membranes and bones	Treatment of the after-effects of injury: Stiff joints	Osteoporosis
Diseases of the nervous system: General considerations	Diseases of the joints, synovial membranes, and bones	Physiotherapy in thoracic surgery
Diseases of the motor neurons	Diseases of the nervous system: General considerations	Cardiac disease
Diseases of the sensory neurons	Diseases of the motor neurons	Management of respiratory diseases
Other diseases of the brain and spinal cord	Diseases of the sensory neurons	Adult spontaneous and conventional mechanical ventilation
Lesions of the peripheral nerves	Other diseases of the brain and spinal cord	Cardiac and pulmonary rehabilitation
Neuritis and neuralgia. Cramp	Lesions of the peripheral nerves	Tissues inflammation and repair
Functional nervous diseases	Neuritis and neuralgia. Cramp	The physiotherapy management of inflammation, tissue healing and repair
Diseases of muscle	Functional nervous diseases	Neurological physiotherapy
Deformities of the upper and lower extremities	Disease of muscle	Massage

(Continued)

Table 6.1 (continued)

1934 (2nd)	1961 (10th)	2008 (14th)
Tidy's Massage and Remedial Exercises	*Tidy's Massage and Remedial Exercises*	*Tidy's Physiotherapy*
Deformities of the spine	Deformities of the upper and lower extremities	Exercise in rehabilitation
Constitutional diseases	Deformities of the spine	Electrotherapy
Diseases of the heart	Diseases of the respiratory organs	Pain
Diseases of the blood and lymph-vessels	Diseases of the heart	Common chronic inflammatory polyarthropathies
Blood diseases	Diseases of blood- and lymph-vessels:	Physiotherapy management of ankylosing spondylitis
	Diseases of the blood	The research process
Diseases of the respiratory organs	Constitutional diseases	Changing relationships for promoting health
Abdominal and pelvic conditions	Abdominal and pelvic conditions	Upper and lower limb joint arthoplasty
	Physiotherapy in surgical conditions	Physiotherapy for people with amputation
	Class-work. Children's classes. Treatment of the aged and chronic patients. Special methods	

The 1932 edition focuses a great deal on the three main clinical divisions in physiotherapy: musculoskeletal, neurological and cardiorespiratory (a distinction also picked up by Joan Cash and Bellis Clayton), whereas the 2013 edition has a broader scope, covering some other clinical specialties, some aspects of professionalism, research and some non-traditional approaches to healthcare. The focus also shifts from knowledge of pathology and treatment, to management. But notwithstanding these changes, the same reductive, objective, biomedical approach towards the body is maintained. Throughout the texts, the division of the body into systems is preserved; as is the emphasis on the need to identify and treat the specific aetiology that account for the patient's signs and symptoms; the therapist is defined by their role in physically managing the body of the patient as if it were a machine with dysfunctional parts or systems and we are encouraged to see that disease and illness reside within a physical body that can be understood with a detailed founding knowledge of its anatomy and physiology.

The same biomechanical approach to the body can be seen in the curricula of physical therapy programmes in all developed countries. The World Confederation for Physical Therapy, founded in 1951 from 11 original founder countries, published its guidelines for physical therapist professional entry level education in 2011 (World Confederation for Physical Therapy 2011). These guidelines acknowledge the curriculum diversity necessary in different countries, but set down that a physiotherapy curriculum should first include 'content and learning experiences in the biological and physical sciences necessary for initial practice of the profession (e.g. anatomy/cellular biology, histology, physiology, exercise physiology, exercise science, biomechanics, kinesiology, neuroscience, pathology, imaging and pharmacology)' (ibid).

In addition to this, the physiotherapy curriculum should include;

> content and learning experiences in the social/behavioural/technological sciences necessary for initial practice of the profession (e.g. applied psychology, applied sociology, communication, ethics and values, management, finance, teaching and learning, law, information communication technology (ICT), clinical reasoning, evidence based practice and applied statistics), including laboratory or other practical experiences.
>
> (World Confederation for Physical Therapy 2011)

In defining the physiotherapist's 'content and learning experiences in the clinical sciences', emphasis was given to 'content about the cardiovascular, pulmonary, endocrine, metabolic, gastrointestinal, genitourinary, integumentary (skin), musculoskeletal and neuromuscular systems and the medical and surgical conditions frequently seen by physical therapists'. The focus for patient 'management' was to emphasise 'patients/clients with an array of conditions (e.g. musculoskeletal, neuromuscular, cardiovascular/pulmonary, integumentary) across the lifespan and the continuum of care' (World Confederation for Physical Therapy 2011).

Notwithstanding the cursory mention of the more humanistic dimensions of practice, the guideline reiterates the importance of a biomechanical approach to the body. This privileging mirrors many of the graduate curricula found around the world that, like Tidy's Physiotherapy texts, show some signs of adaptation over time, but hold tightly to the core principles set down by the profession's founders over 100 years ago. The first year of the BSc (Hons) in Physiotherapy at the University of Brighton, for example, 'focuses on the core theory needed to start your career as a physiotherapist, such as anatomy, health psychology, medicine, exercise prescription, surgery, orthopaedics and research methods before you start clinical placements in year 2'. The BAppSci (Physiotherapy) at Sydney University in Australia begins with units in functional musculoskeletal anatomy, body systems, neuroscience and muscle mechanics and training (alongside, it must be said, an introduction to health, behaviour and society). And students in the Doctor of Physical Therapy programme at the University of St. Augustine in the USA study a curriculum in applied human anatomy, applied medical physiology, biomechanics, general pathology, musculoskeletal and therapeutic exercise in their first two trimesters, before moving on to modules that are governed entirely by a medical view of healthcare: child development, clinical neurosciences, gerontology, musculoskeletal and neuromuscular.

Taking examples from different programmes around the world is fraught with difficulty. There is a risk of oversimplifying what are sometimes quite subtle and nuanced curriculum variations, but also, physiotherapy programmes have grown dramatically in their size and configuration since moving into the higher education sector in the 1980s. Many universities now offer masters- and doctoral-entry programmes. Some are completed in two years, others in four. And there is little consistency within some of the larger countries, never mind across jurisdictions. Having said that, if one looks at any of the physiotherapy programmes offered around the world, one sees a remarkably consistent approach to the body (with the possible exception of some of the Scandinavian schools, a point I will return to later).

The same pattern can be seen in the content of the rapidly growing field of continuing professional, and post-qualification education. Here, most special interest groups and weekend courses focusing on developing skills of assessment and treatment in specific, biomedically-limited fields that are dominated by the many mid-range theories that now pervade the profession. One can become an expert in Maitland, McKenzie or Mulligan's approach to musculoskeletal management, for instance. None of these approaches, or any of their ilk, question the fundamental centrality of the body-as-machine to their practice. It is merely understood that a student of physiotherapy will accept this as a given.

Attempts to articulate a philosophy of physiotherapy have all sought to situate the profession within a larger cultural, historical, philosophical, psychological and social context, but all centre around the role the body plays in defining professional practice. Helen Hislop's Mary McMillan Lecture in 1975 (Hislop 1975) led the way with her vision of 'a great profession—one unified by shared values, shared beliefs, and shared attitudes' (Hislop 1975, p. 1069). Hislop's view was that pathokinesiology – or 'the study of anatomy and physiology as they relate to abnormal human movement' (1975, p. 1071) provided 'a theoretical base broad enough to afford a rational explanation of human motion disorders' (1975, p. 1071). Following Hislop, Cheryl Cott et al's 1995 Movement Continuum Theory criticised Hislop's model for being 'two-dimensional', and failing to 'reflect the interaction of individuals with society and with their environment' (Cott et al 1995, p. 88). By contrast, the Movement Continuum Theory situates movement at the heart of physical therapy practice. Here movement is seen as essential to life, occurring 'on a continuum from the microscopic level to the level of the individual in society' (Cott et al 1995, p. 89). And while Cott's model offers a more 'holistic' view of physical therapy, the biological body remains central[2]. A further attempt to define a conceptual framework for curriculum design in physiotherapy education (Broberg et al 2003) also attempted to imagine physiotherapy as a practice embedded in people's individual lived experiences and a broader social-cultural context, but began with the same founding principal that physiotherapy was bounded by its relationship to the body: 'The body is the starting point for physiotherapy'. And with no hint of irony; 'The body is the locus of the zest for life and is thus the basis for human existence and development' (Broberg et al 2003, pp. 163–4).

> In physiotherapy the interaction between the patient and the physiotherapist forms a "bodily meeting", in which the physiotherapist takes special responsibility for how the body is understood and thematized.
>
> (Broberg et al 2003, p. 164)

What is remarkable about the traces of philosophy applied to physiotherapy that are hidden within the research articles, textbooks, curricula and organisational arrangements of the profession of physiotherapy, is the almost complete lack of discussion about the body or its role in defining physiotherapy practice (Nicholls & Gibson 2010). Pick up any textbook used by undergraduate physiotherapy students, and you will find plenty of material on the body-as-machine, but little if any justification for this position. This is not the only body available to physiotherapists, yet it has been a constant factor in defining how physiotherapy may be thought and practiced over its long history. Given its remarkable 'centrality', one might ask why it is that the body has been so under-theorised. It would be hard to imagine psychologists not having a view on the nature of 'the mind' or architects debating the nature of space or buildings. So why has the body eluded physiotherapists' attention for so long?

The elusive body

The answer to this question is in some ways straightforward, but in other ways extremely complex. The more straightforward explanation is that viewing the body-as-machine excludes the possibility of thinking about the body otherwise. Physiotherapists have no need to learn about cultural, economic or social discourses of the body because their attention is on the physical form and function of the muscle, bone or joint before them. They have no need to explore the patient's spirituality, because this is irrelevant to the biomechanical basis of the patient's problems. Physiotherapists can effectively ignore social determinants of health, narrative explanations of individual suffering, and questions of knowledge and power that beset other professionals, because the body-as-machine is sufficient to the task of assessing, diagnosing and treating the patient's physical problems without the need for these 'polluting variables'. For those dimensions of health and illness that the body-as-machine does not address, there are others that the therapist can refer the patient on to (psychologists, counsellors, occupational therapists etc.).

The body-as-machine is an exclusive and totalising discourse that has served the profession extremely well over its history. But this rather simplistic explanation conveniently bypasses some deeper truths about physiotherapy that I would like to at least consider here; the first being that all experienced physiotherapists know that they will not survive in practice with a tool kit made up only of biomechanical 'hammers'. Most of the really good physiotherapists I have ever met learnt a long time ago that their training was woefully inadequate for their work and that they needed to find a way to engage meaningfully with the people who made up their practice. They learn that only a proportion of the patient's presenting problem stems from a biomechanical derangement, the rest being made up of a messy combination of complex subjective and interpersonal elements that often defies easy, even rational, explanation.

Many physiotherapists, at some point in their career, recognise that the body must be more than a machine and that the neat and tidy way the body is codified by their professional bodies, training schools and textbooks are the abstraction. But then this leaves them in a dilemma, because to treat the patient more holistically would imply moving beyond the limits of their professional identity. And so many either channel their energies into ever more sophisticated biomechanical reasoning (helped, all the time by the rhetoric of evidence-based medicine and continuing professional development), or they move incrementally away from physiotherapy and embrace more embodied modes of practice (Josephson et al 2015; Øberg et al 2015), struggling all the time to reconcile the differences between these approaches and sublimating the fear that their new approach constitutes a betrayal of their professional heritage.

Fortunately, there is enough support within the academy, within the literature and within the practices of other health professionals to sustain these maverick practitioners. A growing number of physiotherapists are undertaking higher-level study in departments of anthropology, cultural studies, philosophy and sociology and bringing this new learning back into the profession. The number of works they have produced for public consumption pale into insignificance when compared to the volume of biomechanical research undertaken by physiotherapists, but their work is all the more significant – in my estimation at least – because it asks fundamental questions about where physiotherapy has come from, where it is now and where it is going.

It is possible to glean three important principles from the studies of Gibson (2016), Setchell (2015), Dahl-Michelsen (2014), Sviland (2014), Sudmann (2009)

and others that may have a profound effect for future understandings of physiotherapy:

1   There is not just one kind of body, but many: the body is *multiple.*
2   Adopting the body-as-machine was a necessary response to social and political
     pressures faced by the early profession.
3   Should circumstances change, physiotherapy could make another pragmatic
     decision and adopt different views of the body (but only if physiotherapists
     know what other bodies are available).

If physiotherapists specialise in the body-as-machine, there must be other ways
to explain bodies that the body-as-machine does not address. There must be other
ways that do not strip the body of its sensuality – in the broadest sense of the word –
its affect; its culture, gender or ethnicity; other ways that engage with the spiritual,
collective or historical wisdom of people and other ways that do not divide the
whole up into body systems and structures (Sudmann 2009). Sociologists have
been exploring these other bodies for decades now and there are hundreds, possibly thousands of different interpretations that physiotherapists may choose to
engage with. Several influential texts have emerged over the last 20 years that have
provided powerful insights into previously taken-for-granted 'truths' about the
body (Scott & Morgan 2004; Shilling 2003; Mol 2002; Blackman 2008; Turner
2008; Cregan 2006; Shildrick & Mykitiuk 2005).
    Each of these texts explores the body 'multiple' (Mol 2002, p. 6) identifying the
many kinds of body now evident in society. Lisa Blackman, for example, identifies
dozens of different 'bodies': including the sociological, naturalistic, materialistic,
socially constructed, disciplined, gendered, sentient, somatically felt and posthuman
body (Blackman 2008). Chris Shilling devotes one chapter to each of seven distinct,
yet overlapping bodies (Shilling 2003). Kate Cregan's focus is upon the regulated
body; the bounded, abject body and the body of difference (Cregan 2006). Which
of these 'bodies' is available to physiotherapy then?

New bodies in physiotherapy

Although physiotherapists have been slower than others to theorise the body in all
its complexity and diversity, there are pockets of work that provide a starting point
for new ideas. Richard Darnell's thesis 'Corpus: The Philosophical Meaning of
Body in Physical Therapy' (Darnell 2007), for example, begins with an analysis of
the body-as-machine and concludes that the 'body as machine . . . is necessary but
not necessarily sufficient for the practice of physical therapy' (Darnell 2007).
Darnell devotes chapters to exploring how the body may be understood as a spiritual envelope, a tool, existence, a companion to the mind, sensorium, art form,
personal identity and as a historical, socio-cultural, legal and economic entity
(Darnell 2007). Darnell appeals to physical therapists to embrace more existential
understandings of the body[3], an idea that has been widely embraced by physiotherapists in Scandinavia, who have developed a large body of work exploring the

embodied nature of experience (see, e.g. Bullington & Fagerberg 2013; Bullington 2009, 2013; Øberg et al 2015; Standal & Engelsrud 2013; Bjorbaekmo & Engelsrud 2011; Groven & Engelsrud 2013).

Some physiotherapy researchers have focused less on the humanistic experiences of embodiment and more on some of the ways our bodies are the site of socio-cultural and political discourses (Gibson 2014; Gibson & Teachman 2012; Gibson et al 2009; Swain et al 2003; Corker & French 1999; Dahl-Michelsen 2015; Dahl-Michelsen & Solbrække 2014; Trede 2008; Trede & Higgs 2003; Rosberg 2006) or problematic moral judgements (Edwards et al 2011a, 2011b; Delany et al 2010). What is clear is that physiotherapists have much to offer this field. As highly educated, experienced practitioners, used to working on and with people's bodies, physiotherapists are in an ideal position to explore how the contemporary understanding of the body may develop in the coming years. To explore this, I consider three examples of bodies in pain, fat bodies and cyborg bodies.

Bodies in pain

Pain, like breathlessness, is now acknowledged as a largely subjective phenomenon that can only be understood by the person experiencing it. Physiotherapists work with people in pain every day across virtually every practice domain and immerse themselves in the daily machinations of people in pain, so one would think that they have much to offer as they struggle to develop collective understandings of the bodily expression and experience of pain. But physiotherapists have been somewhat reluctant to provide their own unique perspective, preferring instead to anchor their practice to powerful neuro-anatomical and physiological explanations of the phenomenon. These 'biological' explanations of pain promote the idea that pain can be objectively measured, resulting in the proliferation of pain scales, pain questionnaires and measurable pain variables. Unfortunately, these only provide part of the explanation for a person's experience of pain and people's uniqueness always seems to defy attempts to standardise approaches to the assessment, diagnosis and management of the phenomenon.

Pain remains elusive, which is clearly a problem for a profession so concerned with the way people live through their bodies. If physiotherapists cannot understand pain as well as, or even better than, other health professions, then a significant portion of the profession's social capital is lost. The problem remains though; pain is essentially subjective and it defies easy explanation. Elaine Scarry in her seminal book *The Body in Pain* wrote that:

> Whatever pain achieves, it achieves in part through its unsharability, and it ensures this unsharability through its resistance to language. 'English,' writes Virginia Woolf, 'which can express the thoughts of Hamlet and the tragedy of Lear has no words for the shiver or the headache. The merest schoolgirl when she falls in love has Shakespeare or Keats to speak her mind

for her, but let a sufferer try to describe a pain in his head to a doctor and language at once runs dry'.

(Virginia Woolf 1967, 'On Being Ill', in *Collected Essays*, Vol. 4, New York: Harcourt, p. 194, cited in Scarry 1985, p. 4)

In the same way, Arthur Frank, writing about his experience of cancer pain writes:

> Whether or not pain is the most difficult part of cancer to live through, it is probably the hardest to describe. We have plenty of words to describe specific pains: sharp, throbbing, piercing, burning, even dull. But these words do not describe the experience of pain. We lack terms to express what it means to live 'in' such pain. Unable to express pain, we come to believe there is nothing to say. Silenced, we become isolated in pain, and the isolation increases the pain. Like the sick feeling that comes with the recognition of yourself as ill, there is a pain attached to being in pain.

(Frank 2002, pp. 30–1)

The inability to effectively account for the complexity of pain, has led some physiotherapists to describe pain phenomenologically. Phenomenology explores the nature of 'being' (i.e. what it means to 'be' in pain, have MS or 'be' oneself), and how we make sense of our experiences. It has been a powerful influence on humanistic disciplines like nursing, midwifery, counselling and occupational therapy where whole branches of the discipline are devoted to it. Phenomenology is most developed in physiotherapy in Scandinavia and it is here that most of the current research into the phenomenology of pain is taking place (Bullington et al 2005; Lundberg et al 2007; Dragesund & Råheim 2008).

In 2003, Bullington and colleagues wrote that 'the pain experience is lived and constituted as chaos and disintegration, and that the healing process has to do with achieving a sense of meaning and coherence out of chaos' (Bullington et al 2003, p. 328). Treatment brought coherence because it reinstated a sense of 'whole' and overcame the reductive idea of the body-as-machine promulgated by a healthcare system dominated by biomedicine:

> [E]motions were experienced and accepted, memories could be brought together with associated feelings and body sensations, and the experience of self became connected temporally to the past and the future, as well as to the present life situation and significant others.

(Bullington et al 2003, p. 328)

As Bullington et al point out, therapy can restore a sense of wholeness to people fractured by chronic pain, but how can physiotherapists do this successfully if they view the body as a 'bothersome broken machine' (Bullington et al 2003, p. 328; Jones & Hush 2011)? Phenomenology holds the promise not only of a more holistic approach to pain, but also some critical insights into the limits of the profession's approaches to the body.

Fat bodies

One doesn't have to look far in the modern scientific literature to find evidence that body size is considered a major health problem[4]. Some have termed it an epidemic, others a crisis or a tsunami (Gard & Wright 2005), that will place unprecedented demands upon already overstretched healthcare services. Physiotherapists, like others, have been active in discussions about the proper way to manage body fat, concentrating on an understandable, but somewhat predictable approach that often relies on the simple formula of energy expenditure over energy consumption. Physiotherapists have become involved in the management of obesity primarily because so many large people have secondary health problems that complicate exercise prescriptions and require specialist input. Diabetes, peripheral vascular disease, respiratory compromise, poor aerobic capacity, low motivation and so on, all demand clinical experience and careful thought if a programme of activity is not to prove harmful. Physiotherapists are perfectly equipped to work in these areas. With their knowledge of the body's physiology in health and illness, and their experience in public health medicine, they know how to rehabilitate bodies, how bodies respond to exercise and training and how to recognise co-morbidities that may compound problems for the patient.

But obesity comes with a paradoxical problem for physiotherapists because so much of the problem is bound up in the person's self-image and current physiotherapy approaches are wont to ignore the existential aspects of obesity in favour of an emphasis on an idealised, normalised body. There is evidence that physiotherapists, like other health professionals, ascribe negative personality characteristics to obese people, thinking of them as lazy or lacking intelligence (Puhl & Heuer 2009) and this affects their attitudes towards the services they provide for patients and their demeanour towards them (Setchell et al 2014, 2016). In their recent study of weight stigma among physiotherapists, for instance, Setchell and colleagues found that 'the most common responses [from physiotherapists] were simplistic, implicitly negative and prescriptive advice. It was rare for responses to indicate a more complex consideration of weight or explicitly negative/stereotyping attitudes' (Setchell et al 2014, p. 161).

Because physiotherapists focus on an image of the biomechanical body – the kind of body represented in anatomy textbooks; devoid of culture, difference, history or personality – one might think that this would provide comfort for obese people who could obtain objective, judgement-free health advice from a professional whose only concern is to see the body-as-machine. This would surely be a profoundly liberating experience given the relentless stigmatising judgement that obese people experience from others during their long search for health. But recent evidence suggests that this is not the case. Rather, physiotherapists like others, are perpetuating negative discourses of laziness and low intelligence to justify the necessity of their input into this growing health 'crisis', while focusing on a normalised body that is the very object that many obese people have come to distrust and dislike. Certainly, a more thoughtful, nuanced, humane view of the body as a site of political contestation would be valuable here. As Setchell et al state, 'There may be value in physiotherapists reflecting on their own attitudes towards patients who are overweight' (Setchell et al 2014, p. 161).

Cyborg bodies

Over the next century, we are likely to see some remarkable transformations in our understandings of what the body is and what it can do, as advances in science and technology gleaned over the 20th century are applied not only to fixing problems with the body, but vastly enhancing its capability. Some suggest we are on the cusp of discovering how to arrest our bodies natural degenerative processes, allowing us to live significantly longer; that soon we will have drugs that vastly increase our ability to remember information and that we be able to have pros-thetic surgery not only to repair broken body parts, but to enhance the body parts we already have (Lilley 2013; Agar 2014).

Much of the transhumanism movement that has taken hold in recent years challenges our assumptions about our body's limits. 'The normal body' as a fixed, stable, universal ideal is certainly a fiction – (since who among us actually mirrors that image?) – but it is also a technology of constraint because it limits us to thinking about what our bodies might achieve if we were truly free to adapt and transform them to be a full expression of our imagination (Cohen & Weiss 2003). Prosthetic legs, for example, were a 20th century invention to help war veterans and others to regain a 'normal' gait pattern and thereby regain some of the ben-efits of having a normalised body. In recent years, biomechanical engineering has been applied to prostheses and it is now possible for amputees to compete along-side other 'able-bodied' athletes in international competitions. A person using prosthetic limbs now has a choice of different configurations to choose from: limbs for competition, limbs for walking, foreshortened limbs for everyday activ-ity and so on. How long before a person born with fully formed legs decides to have surgery to allow them to have new legs that can do so many more things? Why not have powered prostheses that allow you to bound the 10 km into work in 10 minutes?

These 'body projects' are no longer works of science fiction. All our experience of human history tells us that when technologies become available, it is not long before they are adopted and subverted. We can be sure then, that bodies will cease to exist in the way that we had once conceived them, and new (cyborg) bodies will emerge that maybe no longer need traditional therapies to sustain them (Haraway 2006). What does this mean for physiotherapists then, if they remain anchored to a 19th century vision of the body-as-machine?

Barbara Gibson and colleagues at the University of Toronto have been provoking us to think about questions like this in recent years. Gibson has used the postmodern theories of Gilles Deleuze and Felix Guattari to explore how we might imagine a future in which we are less concerned with developing people's independence, but focus instead on helping people to form meaningful assemblages with other human and non-human entities so that they enjoy health and wellbeing. This approach has forced Gibson and her colleagues to ask some difficult questions about rehabilitation. What harms do rehabilitation practitioners do to people in the name of rehabilitation, and why do societies value independence over enabling dependencies, not being the least of them (Gibson et al 2011, 2012; Gibson & Teachman 2012).

In 2012, Gibson and Teachman argued that practitioners valued some forms of mobility more than others, and discussions of 'the effects [of this] on clients, are largely absent in the profession' (Gibson & Teachman 2012, p. 480). The importance of this cannot be underestimated given that 'the social construction of disabled bodies as deficient can perpetrate an ongoing symbolic violence against disabled children and their parents' (Gibson & Teachman 2012, p. 480). Physiotherapists do not set out to exercise their power and authority to cause this kind of harm, in fact many would be mortified to think that their actions might have unforeseen, unimagined negative consequences. But the truth is perhaps that every action has multiple, sometimes unexpected, effects and it is likely that physiotherapists' affinity for the body-as-machine may be creating a number of conditions that may hamper the profession's progress in the coming years. If physiotherapists continue to pay little head to people's lived experience (as in chronic pain), stigmatise what they consider 'deviant' behaviour (as with obesity) or ignore the possibilities for radically different bodies in the 21st century, it is entirely possible that physiotherapy will lose its social capital and be replaced by practitioners who *are* more open to more diverse and inclusive ideas about bodies and what they can do and become.

Closing words

This chapter plays an important role in this book because it tries to explain so much about the problems now being faced by physiotherapy. The argument is a relatively simple one: that physiotherapy has benefited greatly from its affinity with the idea of the body-as-machine, but that this self-same idea is now constraining physiotherapists and restricting their growth. Thinking about the body-as-machine allows physiotherapists to address the concerns the public or the state might have for the legitimacy of its practice, but it can also prevent the profession from seeing people as a whole. It actively constrains physiotherapists from thinking about the cultural, economic, geographical, philosophical and social reasons why people experience poor health and puts them in a poor position now that people want so much more of these things when they look to their service provider.

Treating patient's bodies as machines has some important spin-off effects for the profession. It makes it hard for practitioners to engage in patient-centred care because so much of the profession's identity is bound to the knowledge that makes the profession distinct from the general public. Because of this, physiotherapists can find it hard to invert the traditional binary relationship between expert practitioner and patient and hand the power of decision-making over to its patients and communities. Treating the body-as-machine also makes it difficult for physio-therapists to move to population-based approaches to healthcare. Because the focus is on the body of the person beneath their hands, like surgeons, they have no mechanism that allows them to work with whole populations. Physicians have always offered mass screening programmes and whole population approaches to inoculation; there are nurses attached to each school and dentists offer yearly check-ups but few physiotherapists do this because their approach is to work with the body before them.

The same approach makes it difficult for practitioners to work inter-professionally; to share ideas and resources; to transcend professional boundaries and build func-tioning networks with the patient in the centre. Physiotherapists are territorial, always eager to define their 'point of difference' and envious of other professions' social standing. Rather than critique their professional culture, they concentrate on attempts to reinforce their autonomy and separation, enhance their 'brand image' and re-state the importance of the scientific study of the machinery of the body as the true calling of future practitioners, all the time robbing ourselves of the ability to think otherwise.

Fortunately, a few physiotherapists are breaking the mould and exploring physio-therapy at the margins of orthodox practice. Most of this work is challenging the idea of what the body means and where it might go in the future. This work cannot come soon enough though, because the idea of what the body is and what it might become is changing so rapidly now that there is a real risk that physiotherapists will be left behind. One only has to think of some of the advances in genetic therapy, body reassignment surgery, transformative pharmacology and haptic technologies taking place to realise that we are approaching an era in which the body can no longer be understood merely as healthy or sick, able-bodied or disabled. These traditional normative values are woefully inadequate in the face of the emerging world of trans-human health that is emerging.

And yet, physiotherapists have a privileged position in these transformations. They are trusted by the public and (currently) supported by the state; they are the primary providers of physical rehabilitation and have privileged access to patients in the public health system; they can use their touch to help and heal in a way shared by only a handful of other professions and they have a highly skilled, highly trained workforce that is increasingly asking questions about where the profession has come from, where it is now, and where it is going. For these reasons, among others, they should be satisfied. But in this chapter, I have argued that they will only transcend the profession's past and put ourselves on the road to a productive future if they first acknowledge that their traditional view of the body must change.

Over the course of the next two chapters, I explore some of the ways physio-therapy uses its approach to the body-as-machine to frame some important tenets of professional practice. Building on the disciplined approach to the body set up by the profession's founders, I look at how physiotherapists have used the ideas of posture and movement, function and rehabilitation to frame their professional identity.

Notes

1 Prosser, four editions from 1938–1958; Clayton, 12 editions from 1939–2008; Tidy, 14 editions from 1932-present. Cash's medical and surgical texts in multiple volumes from 1940–1987, orthopaedics 1984–1992 and neurological 1974–1986.
2 In a 'clarification' of the meaning of movement offered in the original paper by Cott et al, one of the paper's original authors proposed subdivisions of the broad concept of movement that could by applied to physiothearpy practice (Allen 2007). In the revised version, movement was reduced to a purely corporeal event; defined by dimensions like flexibility (the 'extent and ease of movement at joints'), strength (the 'force to propel or withstand against forces'), accuracy, speed, adaptability and endurance.
3 Existential ideas broadly concern our unique, subjective experiences of the world. It argues that human life is made unique by our 'being' in the world and cannot be understood scientifically or with grand theories about social causes.
4 The use of the term 'fat bodies' reflects a growing critical attitude towards the medicalisation of body size. This critical scholarship reclaims the language that has so long been used to marginalise people on the basis of their body comportment and contrasts with seemingly more medically acceptable terms like obese and overweight (Vigarello 2013).

References

Agar, N., 2014, *Truly human enhancement: A philosophical defense of limits*, MIT Press, Boston, MA.
Allen, D.D., 2007, Proposing 6 dimensions within the construct of movement in the movement continuum theory, *Physical Therapy*, 87(7), pp. 888–98.
Armstrong, D., 1983, *Political anatomy of the body: Medical knowledge in Britain in the twentieth century*, Cambridge University Press, Cambridge.
Bjorbaekmo, W.S. & Engelsrud, G.H., 2011, 'My own way of moving' – Movement improvisation in children's rehabilitation, *Phenomenology & Practice*, 5(1), pp. 27–47.
Blackman, L., 2008, *The body the key concepts*, Berg, Oxford; New York.
Broberg, C., Aars, M., Beckmann, K., Emaus, N., Lehto, P., Lähteenmäki, M.-L., Thys, W. & Vandenberghe, R., 2003, A conceptual framework for curriculum design in physiotherapy education – an international perspective, *Advances in Physiotherapy*, 5(4), pp. 161–8.
Bullington, J., 2009, Being body: The dignity of human embodiment, in L. Nordenfelt (ed.), *Dignity in care for older people*, Wiley-Blackwell, Chichester, UK, pp. 54–76.
Bullington, J., 2013, *The expression of the psychosomatic body from a phenomenological perspective*, Springer, Dordrecht.
Bullington, J. & Fagerberg, I., 2013, The fuzzy concept of 'holistic care': A critical examination, *Scandinavian Journal of Caring Sciences*, 27(3), pp. 493–4.
Bullington, J., Nordemar, R., Nordemar, K. & Sjöström-Flanagan, C., 2003, Meaning out of chaos: A way to understand chronic pain, *Scandinavian Journal of Caring Sciences*, 17(4), pp. 325–31.
Bullington, J., Sjöström-Flanagan, C., Nordemar, K. & Nordemar, R., 2005, From pain through chaos towards new meaning: Two case studies, *The Arts in Psychotherapy*, 32(4), pp. 261–74.
Cohen, J.J. & Weiss, G., 2003, *Thinking the limits of the body*, State University of New York Press, Albany, NY.
Corker, M. & French, S., 1999, *Disability discourse*, Open University Press, Buckingham, UK.
Cott, C.A., Finch, E., Gasner, D., Yoshida, K., Thomas, S.G. & Verrier, M.C., 1995, The movement continuum theory of physical therapy, *Physiotherapy Canada*, 47(2), pp. 87–95.

Cregan, K., 2006, *The sociology of the body mapping the abstraction of embodiment*, Sage, Thousand Oaks, CA.

Dahl-Michelsen, T., 2014, Sportiness and masculinities among female and male physiotherapy students, *Physiotherapy Theory and Practice*, 30(5), pp. 329–37.

Dahl-Michelsen, T., 2015, Curing and caring competences in the skills training of physiotherapy students, *Physiotherapy Theory and Practice*, 31(1), pp. 8–16.

Dahl-Michelsen, T. & Solbrække, K. N., 2014, When bodies matter: Significance of the body in gender constructions in physiotherapy education, *Gender and Education*, 26(6), 672–87, doi: 10.1080/09540253.2014.946475.

Darnell, R.E., 2007, *Corpus: the philosophical meaning of body in physical therapy, Theory and Practice*. Thesis.

Delany, C.M., Edwards, I., Jensen, G.M. & Skinner, E., 2010, Closing the gap between ethics knowledge and practice through active engagement: An applied model of physical therapy ethics, *Physical Therapy*, 90(7), pp. 1068–78.

Dragesund, T. & Råheim, M., 2008, Norwegian psychomotor physiotherapy and patients with chronic pain: Patients' perspective on body awareness, *Physiotherapy Theory and Practice*, 24(4), pp. 243–54.

Edwards, I., Delany, C.M., Townsend, A.F. & Swisher, L.L., 2011a, Moral agency as enacted justice: A clinical and ethical decision-making framework for responding to health inequities and social injustice, *Physical Therapy*, 91(11), pp. 1653–63.

Edwards, I., Delany, C.M., Townsend, A.F. & Swisher, L.L., 2011b, New perspectives on the theory of justice: Implications for physical therapy ethics and clinical practice, *Physical Therapy*, 91(11), pp. 1642–52.

Fox, N.J., 2012, *The body*, Polity, London.

Frank, A.W., 2002, *At the will of the body: Reflections on illness*, Houghton Mifflin, Boston, MA.

Gard, M. & Wright, J., 2005, *The obesity epidemic: Science, morality and ideology*, Routledge, Abingdon, Oxon.

Gibson, B., 2016, *Rehabilitation: A post-critical approach*, Taylor & Francis, New York.

Gibson, B.E., 2014, Parallels and problems of normalization in rehabilitation and universal design: Enabling connectivities, *Disability and rehabilitation*, doi: 10.3109/09638288.2014.891661.

Gibson, B.E. & Teachman, G., 2012, Critical approaches in physical therapy research: investigating the symbolic value of walking, *Physiotherapy Theory and Practice*, 28(6), pp. 474–84.

Gibson, B.E., Carnevale, F.A. & King, G., 2012, 'This is my way': Reimagining disability, in/dependence and interconnectedness of persons and assistive technologies, *Disability and Rehabilitation*, 34(22), pp. 1894–9.

Gibson, B.E., Darrah, J., Cameron, D., Hashemi, G., Kingsnorth, S., Lepage, C., Martini, R., Mandich, A. & Menna-Dack, D., 2009, Revisiting therapy assumptions in children's rehabilitation: Clinical and research implications, *Disability and Rehabilitation*, 31(17), pp. 1446–53.

Gibson, B.E., Teachman, G., Wright, V., Fehlings, D., Young, N.L. & McKeever, P., 2011, Children's and parents' beliefs regarding the value of walking: Rehabilitation implications for children with cerebral palsy, *Child: Care, Health and Development*, 38(1), pp. 61–9.

Groven, K.S. & Engelsrud, G., 2013, Allowing one's own bodily experience to "count": Elaborating on inter-subjectivity and subjectivity in phenomenological studies, *Journal of Education and Research*, 3(0), pp. 24–40.

Hancock, P., Hughes, B., Jagger, E., Paterson, K., Russell, R., Tulle-Winton, E. & Tyler, M., 2000, *The body, culture, and society: An introduction*, Open University Press, Buckingham, UK.

Hislop, H.J., 1975, The not-so-impossible dream, *Physical Therapy*, 55(10), pp. 1069–80.

Haraway, D., 2006, *A cyborg manifesto: Science, technology, and socialist-feminism in the late 20th century*, Springer, London.

Jones, L.E. & Hush, J.M., 2011, Pain education in physiotherapy: Guidance for curriculum reform. Journal of physiotherapy. *Journal of Physiotherapy*, 57(4), 207–8.

Josephson, I., Woodward-Kron, R., Delany, C., & Hiller, A., 2015, Evaluative language in physiotherapy practice: How does it contribute to the therapeutic relationship? *Social Science & Medicine (1982)*, 143, 128–36.

Lilley, S., 2013, *Transhumanism and society the social debate over human enhancement*, Springer, Amsterdam, Netherlands.

Linker, B., 2011, *War's waste: Rehabilitation in World War I America*, University of Chicago Press, Chicago, IL.

Lundberg, M., Styf, J. & Bullington, J., 2007, Experiences of moving with persistent pain: A qualitative study from a patient perspective, *Physiotherapy Theory and Practice*, 23(4), pp. 199–209.

Lupton, D., 2012, *Medicine as culture: Illness, disease and the body in Western society*, Sage, London.

Mol, A., 2002, *The body multiple: Ontology in medical practice*, Duke University Press, Durham, NC.

Nicholls, D.A. & Gibson, B.E., 2010, The body and physiotherapy, *Physiotherapy Theory and Practice*, 26(8), 497–509.

Øberg, G.K., Normann, B. & Gallagher, S., 2015, Embodied-enactive clinical reasoning in physical therapy, *Physiotherapy Theory and Practice*, pp. 1–9.

Puhl, R.M. & Heuer, C.A., 2009, The stigma of obesity: A review and update, *Obesity*, 17(5), pp. 941–64.

Rosberg, S., 2006, Empowering women through body awareness – a physiotherapeutic perspective on the body and women's stress related ill health. In W. Ernst & U. Bohle (eds.), *Naturbilder und lebensgrundlagen-konstruktionen von geschlecht*, LIT Verlag, Münster, pp. 86–106.

Rose, N., O'Malley, P. & Valverde, M., 2006, Governmentality, *Annual Review of Law and Social Science*, 2(1), pp. 83–104.

Samson, C., 1999, Biomedicine and the body, in *Health studies: A critical and cross cultural reader*, Blackwell, Oxford, pp. 3–21.

Scarry, E., 1985, *The body in pain: The making and unmaking of the world*, Oxford University Press, New York.

Scott, S. & Morgan, D. (eds.), 2004, *Body matters: Essays on the sociology of the body*, Falmer Press, London.

Setchell, J., Watson, B., Jones, L. & Gard, M., 2015, Weight stigma in physiotherapy practice: patient perceptions of interactions with physiotherapists. *Manual Therapy*, doi: 10.1016/J.MATH.2015.04.001.

Setchell, J., Watson, B., Jones, L., Gard, M. & Briffa, K., 2014, Physiotherapists demonstrate weight stigma: A cross-sectional survey of Australian physiotherapists, *Journal of Physiotherapy*, 60(3), pp. 157–62.

Setchell, J., Watson, B.M., Gard, M. & Jones, L., 2016, Physical therapists' ways of talking about overweight and obesity: Clinical implications. *Physical Therapy*, 96(6), 865–75.

Shildrick, M. & Mykitiuk, R., 2005, *Ethics of the body: Postconventional challenges*, MIT Press, Cambridge, MA.

Shilling, C., 2003, *The body and social theory*, 2nd ed., Sage, London.

Shilling, C., 2012, *The body and social theory*, Sage, London.

Standal, F. & Engelsrud, G., 2013, Researching embodiment in movement contexts: A phenomenological approach, *Sport, Education and Society*, 18(2), pp. 154–66.

Sudmann, T.T.T., 2009, *(En) gendering body politics, Physiotherapy as a window on health and illness*, Thesis.

Sviland, R., Martinsen, K. & Råheim, M., 2014, To be held and to hold one's own: narratives of embodied transformation in the treatment of long lasting musculoskeletal problems. *Medicine, Health Care and Philosophy*, 17(4), 609–24.

Swain, J., French, S. & Cameron, C., 2003, *Controversial issues in a disabling society*, Open University Press, Buckingham, UK.

Trede, F., 2008, *A critical practice model for physiotherapy practice: Developing practice through critical transformative dialogues*, VDM Verlag, Saarbrücken.

Trede, F. & Higgs, J., 2003, Re-framing the clinician's role in collaborative decision making: Re-thinking practice knowledge and the notion of clinician-patient relationships, *Learning in Health and Social Care*, 2(2), pp. 66–73.

Turner, B.S., 1996, *The body and society*, Sage, London.

Turner, B.S., 2008, *The body and society: Explorations in social theory*, Sage, London.

Vigarello, G., 2013, *The metamorphoses of fat: A history of obesity*, Columbia University Press, New York.

World Confederation for Physical Therapy, 2011, *WCPT guidelines for physical therapist professional entry level education*, available from www.wcpt.org/sites/wcpt.org/files/files/Guideline_PTEducation_complete.pdf, accessed 4 August 2015.

Williams, S.J., 2003, *Medicine and the body*, Sage, London.

7   Posture and movement

Introduction

It would be hard to imagine undertaking a critical history of physiotherapy without first considering 'the body', because the body is the principal object of the physiotherapist's gaze. It is the equivalent of the musician's instrument or the artist's canvas. But physiotherapists are neither surgeons nor pathologists, and they want to see the body moving, or at least prepared to move. And so, after the body comes posture and movement (what Judy Mead called physiotherapy's 'second core skill' (Mead 2003, p. 3)): two of the cardinal features that have differentiated physiotherapy thinking and practice for over a century. Whether you work in a child developmental centre, community private practice, in neurological rehabilitation or care of older adults, posture and movement underpin much of science and philosophy of physiotherapy practice and need to be explored if physiotherapists are to understand the role that these ideas have played in the profession's past, present and future.

Despite the fact that 'Most people are inclined to accept posture [and perhaps movement] as a natural and not particularly important aspect of the business of living' (Tucker 1960, p. 1), physiotherapists have seen them as central to their professional identity since the profession's inception at the end of the 19th century. A person's upright, erect, symmetrical posture had served as a visible sign of the natural development of normal human maturity for centuries and so became an obvious starting point for the assessment of physical illness and deformity. Eugenic concerns for racial degeneration added to the injurious effects of war, communicable diseases like tuberculosis and polio and degenerative conditions like arthritis gave physiotherapists the opportunity to demonstrate their skills of postural and movement analysis and treatment, and cemented the profession's relationship with medicine and the State. They were the foundation stones for the profession's approach to rehabilitation and the basis of their scientific inquiries after World War II. And they provided a way to distinguish physiotherapists from other competing professions. Posture and movement have represented the 'applied' arm of the body-as-machine, the body-as-*moving*-machine perhaps, and so are a vital component of any critical history of the profession.

In recent years, the movement has taken on symbolic significance for physiotherapists, with organisations ranging from small local practices to international organisations like WCPT adopting phrases like 'Movement for Life' and 'Physiotherapy is Movement' as marketing slogans to connect the profession with health funders, communities and key stakeholders. In a recent Editorial in the journal *Manual Therapy*, Gwendolen Jull and Ann Moore reviewed a range of contemporary definitions of physiotherapy and found movement at the heart of each of them (Jull & Moore 2013). Jull and Moore supported the American Physical Therapy Association's adoption of 'The Movement System' as its principal theoretical approach to practice, arguing that it is central to the profession's ongoing relevance and success (Jull & Moore 2013, p. 447). At the same time, Shirley Sahrmann pointed to need to '*own* the human movement system' (Sahrmann 2014, pp. 1040, my emphasis), claiming that 'movement is a key to optimal living and quality of life for all people of all ages that extends beyond health to every person's ability to participate in and contribute to society' (Sahrmann 2014, p. 1035).

It should be noted straight away, that Sahrmann and the APTA are not calling for physical therapists to command the entirety of human movement, per se, but only the 'physiological system that functions to produce motion of the body as a whole or of its component parts' (Sahrmann 2014, p. 1037). This is a very particular and much more restricted view of movement and it raises some important points that underpin the discussion in the rest of this chapter. Firstly, I want to argue that the adoption of 'The Movement System' as a fundamental principal in physiotherapy practice is really a restatement of the profession's long historical association with a biomechanical approach to posture and movement[1]. I want to show how physiotherapists have used their particular view of posture and movement to differentiate their practice from others who are also interested in bodily motion and thereby carved out a professional niche for themselves in orthodox healthcare. And I also want to continue an argument that I have made consistently throughout the book; that physiotherapists' biomechanical treatment the body-as-machine may have been valuable in the past, but may be a hindrance to the profession's growth in the future.

In many ways, the arguments set out in this chapter resonate with WCPT, APTA and many physiotherapy theorists who see movement as central to the future of the profession. What is less clear, however, is whether a deeper engagement with the physiology of movement will equip the profession for the challenges it now faces. The changing economy of healthcare; the need for activity-based solutions to many of the developed world's health priorities and the ongoing tensions around the costs of specialised publicly funded healthcare, all point to movement becoming an increasingly important health intervention in the future. Clearly, for physiotherapy to remain relevant as a healthcare profession in the 21st century, it must apply itself to people's 'optimal living and quality of life' (Sahrmann 2014, p. 1035). And if a patho-anatomical approach to posture and movement served the profession well in the past, a pathokinesiological approach *might* provide the answer to the profession's future. But it remains unclear how it will enhance the full range of scientific, humanistic, environmentally and socially holistic credentials of the profession on its own.

Looking beyond the biological confines of 'The Movement System' it is possible to examine physiotherapy's historic relationship with posture and movement, to trace some of its connections to cultural beliefs about the differences between humans and animals; to examine people's beliefs about posture and discipline and the physical and moral dimensions of erect, upright, 'normal' comportment and to consider the age-old connections made between people's attention, fitness, mental and physical health and wellbeing (Danielsson & Rosberg 2015; Danielsson et al 2016). It is perhaps surprising how little of this sort of scholarship has taken place in physiotherapy. As was the case with the previous chapter's focus on the body, I would argue that physiotherapists are primarily concerned with the practical application of a biological understanding of posture and movement and almost entirely uninterested in critical questions that ask why. On the one hand, this is a pity, because it ignores the rich history that has been operating parallel to the profession's scientific endeavours, but perhaps more significantly, the lack of interest in the deeper cultural, political and social relationships between physiotherapy, posture and movement hampers the ability to understand the present tensions facing the profession, and anticipate the profession's future.

Posture and movement are archetypical examples of the kinds of dual conditioning I mentioned at the beginning of Chapter 4 – where the critical power of an idea is often hidden from view, 'beneath the surface' as it were – providing the motive power to drive a profession in a particular direction. On the surface, physiotherapists engage in new techniques for assessing and treating postural and movement disorders, but these are not the things that significantly drive or shape their practice. We know this because methods of assessing and treating postural and movement disorders have changed little over the last century. Physiotherapy may now be entering a more sophisticated technological age, with new assessment tools like digital goniometers, accelerometers and 3D motion analysis, but these tools only provide a variation on the crude methods used to assess bodily deviation from midline and displacement over time that interested physiotherapists in the 1920s and 1930s. Similarly, the profession's treatment techniques are still based on the four cornerstones of physiotherapy: manual therapies, exercise, electro- and hydrotherapy.

Paradoxically, the *stability* of these approaches has been one of the profession's cardinal virtues; allowing the public, the medical profession and the State to develop confidence in the profession's constancy and reliability. So, constant innovations in practice have not been the driver of the profession's growth and development. Where the real innovation has happened has been in the way physiotherapy has applied its basic principles to the shifting cultural and social demands of the 20th and now 21st centuries. It is unlikely that physiotherapy would have retained an interest in exercise-based movement, for example, if it had not adapted its passive treatments and developed industrial scale exercise rehabilitation after WWI. Would it have been able to speak so authoritatively about posture, had it not responded to concerns about such clinically mundane things as scoliosis and flat feet, when called upon in the early part of the 20th century? Would it now be able to develop approaches around vocational rehabilitation if it hadn't had half-a-century of working with complex patients in rehabilitation centres, out-patient departments and pain clinics? When the significance of exercise- and activity-based rehabilitation to today's healthcare is considered, it becomes important to think about not only how the profession retained a historic connection with posture and movement, but also how physiotherapy's particular approach to these fundamental ideas shaped what it is now possible to say and do as a practitioner. This chapter attempts to tackle some of these questions.

I begin by exploring some of the cultural history of posture and movement, focusing on those things that affected people's beliefs about 'normal' postural 'attitude', including eugenic ideas about people's fitness, psychological interest in attention, problems caused by scoliosis and flat feet and the challenges of TB and infantile paralysis in the early part of the 20th century. I then spend some time looking at physiotherapy's historical relationship with remedial exercise and the profession's move away from 'passive' treatment. This brief introduction to the general history posture and movement allows physiotherapists to identify four key principles that can be used to better understand physiotherapy today. These look at posture and movement as spatial, temporal, self-referential and socio-political phenomena. I use these then to explore physiotherapy's approach to normal posture and movement, measurement and testing, and the ways physiotherapists are taught to 'read' the body. Finally, I focus on the ways posture and movement have shaped the physiotherapy profession, through its interest in 'purposeful' movement; the body-as-*moving*-machine, asking why physiotherapy has taken such a narrow view of the subject and what might be possible if it embraced a broader perspective.

Apart from providing a deeper critique of physiotherapy's relationship with posture and movement, I am trying to show that the biological aspects of these phenomena – so much valued and promoted by the APTA, WCPT and authors like Shirley Sahrmann – are neither their only, or their most significant dimensions. My aim is to show that the cultural, social and political aspects of posture and movement have always been much more important to physiotherapy than authors have previously credited, and that in the future physiotherapy must be much more aware of these things if it is to remain relevant. But to begin, I explore a little of the broader history of posture and movement and then locate physiotherapy within it.

A brief history of posture and movement

Posture, or 'relative position or arrangement of each portion of the body in relation to the adjacent body segment and in relation to the body as a whole' (Hines 1965), has been a concern and interest for natural philosophers and scientists throughout history. Consider the statues of Greek and Roman warriors and noblemen, for instance. Fredrick tells us that Roman orators were identified by their posture and gestures, and that 'There should be no unmanly softness of the neck, and the fingers should not make delicate gestures', that the orator will 'regulate himself with his entire torso by the vigorous and manly modulation of his upper body' (Fredrick 2002, p. 251)[2]. Figures and images of Christ with outstretched arms, Buddha sitting cross-legged or the protective stance of Vishnu, represent symbolic icons that have been used by all faiths and religions for millennia. Even the secular age has had its iconic images, most notably Leonardo da Vinci's Vitruvian Man, embodying the mathematical and scientific pursuit of 'man's' understanding and command of the natural world[3].

By the 19th century, Darwinian ideas of natural selection, a fascination with taxonomy and the uncovering of nature's mysteries, and sanitary science, with its concern to police the boundaries between nature and man, created an anatomical image of the human form as a static and analysable object (Armstrong 2002). This is the image of the body that came to be represented in so many anatomy text-books: male, Caucasian, naked, hairless, standing, arms externally rotated, almost Vitruvian. To all intents and purposes this was an image of a cadaver, or an ideal-ised body, a territory to be mapped. The suggestion offered by this image is that the normal body is consistent in its design and orientation; that one semimembra-nosus muscle is the same as any other, regardless of a person's lived experience, culture or history. Using this body map as its referent, medical science could explore deviations from the norm. The body could be passively manipulated into new, more desirable shapes (corsetry); it could be measured for minor deviation (scoliosis, flat feet) and could be used as a cultural marker of human development (from ape to human).

Following Darwin, enormous social capital was placed on the idea that humans had developed beyond their genetic ancestors and that this could be seen in their bipedal gait, the free use of their hands for manipulation and their higher con-sciousness. Humans did not crawl on their hands and knees, bellow or howl. Proof of man's elevation beyond his more primitive cousins could be seen in the fact that the ill, injured, mad and deformed often resorted to animalistic ways, and so the management of these tendencies was more than merely a medical interest. Managing people's posture and movement carried social and political significance because they were expressions of human sophistication and particularly the sophistication of Anglo-American culture.

Armstrong, Linker and others have argued that a scientific interest in posture – and particularly the posture of children – was a significant feature of 19th century medicine (Linker 2012; Armstrong 2002; Gilman 2014). Armstrong argues that posture 'addressed both internal and external aspects of body management', focusing attention on 'the internal alignment between body parts' and enabling 'the three-dimensional shape of the child's body to be turned towards and outside world' (Armstrong 2002, p. 39): posture reflected 'an attitude of the mind towards the body' (Tucker 1960, p. 1). Children's posture was of particular interest for two important reasons: Firstly, if a child's posture could be established or corrected while it was still 'impressionable, receptive, plastic and pliable' (Lloyd 1936, p. 207), then 'good' posture might be retained throughout adult life. Secondly, posture revealed the child's inner attitude and attention. Posture was more than simply a measure of the alignment of bodily structures, it spoke to the child's awareness of the outside world, and his preparedness for action[4].

Children's postures began to be examined in fine detail in the latter half of the 19th century. Fears for spinal and limb deformities caused by communicable diseases like tuberculosis, and concerns for children's increasing passivity brought on by improvements in education (which saw many more children sitting for long periods in the classroom), led many sanitary reformers to begin inspecting children's posture and instituting widespread preventative measures. The invention of military drilling without weapons in 1889 was quickly transferred from military to civilian life and rapidly adapted by children's health reformers and termed 'physical training' (Armstrong 2002, p. 38).

Standing to attention emphasised correct body alignment: neither slouching nor hyperextended (see 'Posture Wall Charts' in Linker 2012, p. 607). It also spoke to the child's alert state of mind and readiness to comply with instructions; 'Standing to attention was therefore the ideal posture, the point of highest perfection for body positioning and alertness to subsequent movement' (Armstrong 2002, p. 39)[5]. In this position, it was possible to assess the child's attitude: not only their physical attitude (the body's correct reaction to gravity), but also the child's mental attitude. Children that stood in a slouched, poorly toned fashion were of particular concern because their posture indicated that they were too relaxed and relaxation in the face of authority betrayed laziness or indifference that might have dire consequences in later life if the mature adult failed to follow orders or becomes defiant. So, although attitude began as an essentially 'physical' characteristic of the body, it became a pivotal part of the emerging discipline of psychology in the early 20th century as attention turned to people's instincts, motives and inner thoughts (Armstrong 2002, p. 72).

Posture became the 'litmus test for the healthy modern body of the perfect citizen' (Gilman 2014, p. 57) and created the conditions for the development of an 'entire sub-specialty . . . in which gymnastics defined and recuperated the body' (Gilman 2014, p. 57)[6]. Thanks to the work of Anders Ottosson and Thomas Terlouw, we have a reasonably clear idea how the physical therapies became significant here. In a series of recent papers, Ottosson and Terlouw have argued that much of what we know today as orthopaedic medicine derived from the work of 19th century physical therapists, most especially those educated in Sweden at the Royal Central Institute of Gymnastics (RCIG) under the auspices of Pehr Henrik Ling (1776–1839) (Ottosson 2005, 2010, 2011, 2015, 2016; Hansson & Ottosson 2015; Terlouw 2007b). Ling was not only interested in sport, physical culture and physical education, but was also a pioneer of a range of systematic educational and therapeutic gymnastics that, Ottosson argues, gave physical therapy its professional identity (Ottosson 2011, p. 88).

Reflecting the eugenic sentiments that often accompany ideas about gymnastics and physical culture, Ling founded the RCIG in 1813 to 'recreate some of the physical splendour that had previously distinguished the Swedish and Gothic people' (Ottosson 2011, p. 89). Heavily regulated and disciplined forms of gymnastics became an important vehicle for nations to regain their 'lost manliness and thereby restore the nation's defence' (Ottosson 2011, p. 90). Ling's programme featured four branches: pedagogical, military, medical and aesthetic gymnastics. Each served a distinct purpose, but all centred on a desire to discipline the body, gain control over movements, express the inner self through posture and movement and alleviate or cure suffering from illnesses like syphilis, rheumatism, hemiplegia, heart failure and tuberculosis (Ottosson 2011, p. 92). Ottosson argues that gymnastics represented perhaps Sweden's 'most successful cultural export of the 1800s' (Ottosson 2010, p. 1899). Given its impact in fields as diverse as architecture, sociology and cultural studies, education and healthcare, particularly orthopaedic medicine and physical therapy, and its influence on fellow gymnasiarchs like Jahn, Eiselen, Georgii, Branting and later Cyriax, Krusen and Mennell, it is hard to argue with Ling's legacy.

Social reformers like Ling saw posture as an 'essential precursor to movement' (Armstrong 2002, p. 40), but the control of movement was the real prize, because it was through movement that the person gained fluidity, engaged in the world, connected with others, acted for or against the greater will.

> Movement was therefore not a casual thing, even less an attribute that could be left at the mercy of 'natural' forces. It needed to be directed and managed, subsumed even, under some explicit inner and/or outer controls. Movement required order and guidance.
>
> (Armstrong 2002, p. 41)

Training children to move efficiently and with purpose became a focus of significant governmental and professional interest in the early 20th century, with training manuals, exercise textbooks, government policies and professional interventions all designed to develop techniques of body management through exercise and movement. Physical education in schools; the creation of formalised sports associations; the birth of heavily regulated and disciplined leisure activities like ballet, gymnastics and dance; and an increasing focus on 'active' therapies to replace the passive therapies of massage and manipulation became increasingly significant as the 20th century progressed.

Teaching the child to train his or her own movements efficiently created 'a virtuous circle linking body, mind and exercise', with 'the mind . . . trained to manage the movement of the body while movement, in its turn, had positive effects on the mind' (Armstrong 2002, p. 43). Central to this approach was a diverse network of professionals who readily accepted the opportunity to use their skills to promote what they saw as a social good. Teachers, physical training instructors, doctors, nurses and therapists monitored and regulated children's posture and movement, measuring every deviation (of mind and body) as the child grew to adulthood. Linker argues that even after antibiotics had significantly reduced the incidence of scoliosis caused by TB, American health reformers continued to promote the idea of 'a dangerous curve' and promote the widespread inspection of children through to adulthood (Linker 2012).

Gustav Zander, the inventor of many exercise machines that would be the precursor of today's gym equipment and himself a teacher of gymnastics at the RCIG in the mid-19th century, had learnt gymnastics as a way to cure scoliosis (Murphy 1995, p. 12). Zander realised that Ling's approach to gymnastics – which relied on almost constant attention from the instructor – was time-consuming, arduous and expensive. His solution was to draw on popular ideas about the industrialisation of movement (from steam railways, printing, mining and other devices), to develop a system that 'combined levers, wheels, and weights in a series of ingenious mechanical exercise machines that could be managed by patients with little or no assistance' (Murphy 1995, pp. 12–3; Terlouw 2007a). Zander coined the term 'mechanotherapy' and opened his own therapeutic institute in 1864, 'offering 27 different instruments for active exercise (the patient moved the machine), passive exercise (the machine moved the patient), and massage' (Murphy 1995, p. 13). Significantly, many of Zander's machines were adjustable and most allowed the attendant to monitor the patient's performance (Zander 1918). Zander's machines had an enormous impact on physical therapy from the 1880s through to the end of WWI (Hansson & Ottosson 2015; Fischinger et al 2009). Although Zander's machines were complicated and 'quite beyond the reach of any but the very few owing to the cost' (McKenzie 1916, p. 39), they did require less hands-on attention from an instructor and Zander argued they were more reliable than manual therapies (and therefore more scientific) (Hansson & Ottosson 2015, p. 12).

Zander's mechanotherapy highlighted an important tension in the management of people's posture and movement, particularly in the late 19th century. As I highlighted in Chapter 3, the market for physical therapies had grown exponentially since 1850, with doctors, unregulated bone-setters and masseurs, Swedish trained remedial gymnasts, osteopaths (after 1874), chiropractors (after 1894) and others flooding the marketplace, offering physical remedies to combat diseases and disorders that had only the loosest connection with mechanical medicine. Add to this, the list of agents interested in the assessment and management of 'normal' children and adults (physical training instructors, gym and dance teachers, scout leaders etc.) and you have an enormously competitive marketplace for ideas and approaches into which physiotherapists somehow found their place.

Physiotherapy prior to 1940 drew heavily on passive modalities: hands-on approaches, using massage and manipulations of the tissue in preference to exercise or gymnastics. In some ways, the founders of the physiotherapy profession turned away from Ling's gymnastic legacy preferring his approach to massage; popularised by the Dutch physician J.G. Metzger (1839–1909). Indeed, Swedish Remedial Exercises (SRE) were not promoted by the founders of the STM until 1909 and only then because of competition from a rival massage organisation (Barclay 1994, p. 59). 'Passive' treatments had been the custom for early members of the STM who primarily worked with private, fee-paying patients in their own homes. The advent of WWI and the overwhelming workload that accompanied it, however, forced the masseuses of the ISTM to reconsider their approach.

After 1914, there was a shift towards more active treatment, which served to make physical therapy more cost-effective (an important consideration during the Depression) and made patients more responsible for their own recovery. We are so familiar with the idea that we should all be responsible for our own health today that we forget, perhaps, that this was not always so. Prior to WWII, the prevailing discourse was that people were largely made ill by things that the State took responsibility for (see Chapter 4), and that treatment was something that people received quite passively, rather than took an active role within. One of the ways this culture gradually changed was through the more widespread use of exercise as a treatment modality.

Images from the 1920s and 1930s show an increasing interest in forms of group exercise (see, e.g. McIntosh 1952). Influential social movements like Muscular Christianity, Turnverein, community dancing, calisthenics, rhythmical gymnastics, drilling, marching and other forms of 'muscular bonding' (McNeill 1995) became highly visible symbols of national vigour and were used as propaganda against eugenic concerns for racial degeneration that rose almost to fever pitch in the early years of the 20th century. There were many prominent eugenicists[7], including H.G. Wells, Winston Churchill and George Bernard Shaw, who believed that racial deterioration could be stemmed by the selective breeding of 'superior' individuals (positive eugenics) and, in some cases, the prevention of breeding, or even sterilisation, of people who are considered weaker, defective or unsuitable (negative eugenics). Today many people consider these ideas abhorrent, but they had a powerful influence on people's beliefs about long-term illness and disability.

Physiotherapists were not immune to softer, but no less eugenic, ideas about racial degeneration and gymnastics, exercise and rehabilitation had long been fertile territory for discriminatory attitudes towards disability and difference (Pronger 2002; Snyder & Mitchell 2006). In the 1930s, when the Depression caused widespread human suffering, initiatives like the *Building the body beautiful* keep-fit movement targeted the physical development of white, English women and organisations like the *League of Health and Beauty* and the *League of Health and Happiness* were patronised and promoted by members of the CSMMG (Barclay 1994, p. 121). But perhaps not surprisingly, their 'mass demonstrations and eugenic overtones led to comparisons with Fascist Germany and Italy' (Barclay 1994, p. 121). There is no evidence that physiotherapy as a profession directly promoted eugenic ideals, but its desire to rehabilitate 'deformed' bodies and return the person to 'normal'; its highly disciplined and regimented approach to remedial exercise; its use of objective measurement and constant assessment of physical 'deviance' and its desire to be at the forefront of rehabilitation efforts to restore the physical strength of the population suggests that the physiotherapy profession in Europe and America was at least comfortable with many of these values (see Figure 7.1).

Having developed exercise from something done by individuals under the supervision of a therapist or gymnast in the late 19th and early 20th centuries, group movement became the norm in the 1930s and 1940s, helped by the necessity to

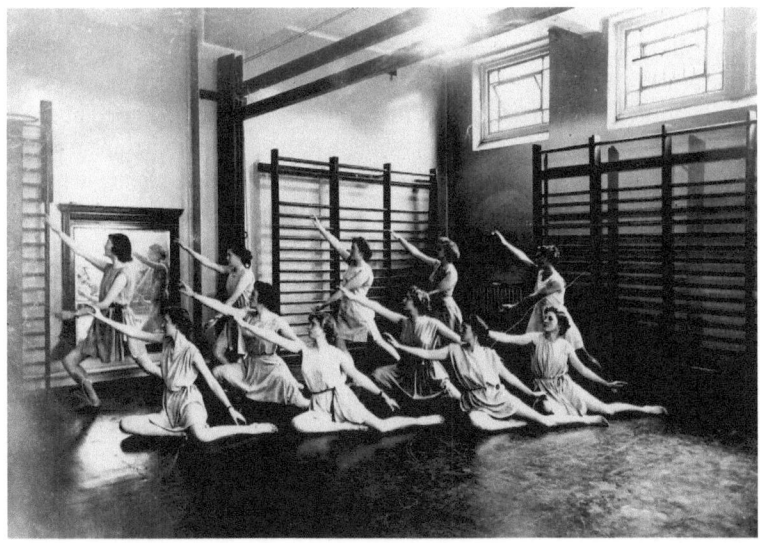

Figure 7.1 Physiotherapy students exercising, Ancoats Hospital, Manchester. Reproduced with the permission of The Chartered Society of Physiotherapy and the Wellcome Library, London.

rehabilitate large numbers of returned servicemen during WWII. As Licht argues, 'Each war during the past century has seen the increasingly greater use of restorative exercise, and World War II followed that pattern' (Licht 1978, p. 34). Part of the problem for physiotherapists was that their treatments had become increasingly associated with passive interventions given only at the beginning of a soldier's recovery:

> Physiotherapy is of great value for selected cases. It is a form of passive therapy and as such is given sparingly, because some patients are only too happy to lie at their ease on a couch and receive treatment which, for remedial purposes, is a poor substitute for their own activity.
>
> (Houlding 1943, p. 445)

William Tegner writes in the Forward to Dena Gardiner's book *The Principles of Exercise Therapy* that, '[t]he gospel of activity has been widely preached and the prescription of activity and movement has taken the place of the passive treatments so widely advocated before the second world war', and that 'passive treatments of inert patients making no effort to help themselves are regarded as possibly prolonging rather than cutting short invalidism' (Gardiner 1953, p. vii).

Physiotherapists were in direct competition with physical training instructors who, despite having no formal medical experience, offered servicemen opportunities for rehabilitation and restoration through group games, competition and active enjoyment (as well as considerable amounts of hard physical work), whereas the physiotherapist was seen as something of a soft option and servicemen tended to 'evade the physical training instructor for more pleasurable treatment at the hands of the masseuse' (Houlding 1943, p. 445).

Many doctors still preferred to have their patients to undergo remedial exercises under the guidance of a physiotherapist though because physiotherapists were still quite cheap to employ and they knew medical terminology, orthopaedic pathology and the detailed anatomy and physiology underpinning posture and movement. Thus, the inter-war years saw a slow and steady growth in physiotherapy and the creation of large massage departments, incorporating individual treatment spaces and large gymnasia running group classes for people with similar injuries and this model remains the basis of physiotherapy department design even today.

Physiotherapy's professional claim to be *the* provider of physical rehabilitation services after WWII rested largely on its ability to manage the patient's recovery from the moment of their injury or illness to their return to full fitness. To do this, physiotherapy needed to diversify and specialise in much the same way that medicine had become increasingly specialised and differentiated. No one therapist could manage patients in the intensive care unit, on the post-surgical orthopaedic wards or spinal injuries unit and then through to the out-patient department, gymnasium and community rehabilitation facility. This diversification was only made possible, however, because of the profession's historical affinity with therapies that were simple, heavily standardised but also incredibly adaptable. The 'passive' techniques colonised by the profession's founders could be easily adapted to the rapidly emerging acute care setting and work on posture, movement and exercise could be deployed in the gymnasium, rehabilitation centre and the home.

Although foundational texts on posture, movement and therapeutic exercise continued to be produced after WWII (see, e.g. Basmajian 1958; Brunnstrom 1972; American Academy of Orthopaedic Surgeons 1965; Hollis 1989; Galley & Forster 1982; Gardiner 1953, all of which ran through several editions from the 1950s to the 1990s), the predominant trend was for authors to apply the now standard biomechanical and physiological understandings of muscles and movements to clinical settings[8]. Authors also began to publish more journal articles and conference papers, focusing on more specialised and clinically applied subjects, and less on large volume encyclopaedic texts like Nöel Tidy's long-running *Massage and Remedial Exercises* series (Tidy 1937) that had been the standard form of theory development in the years before the war.

Of course, some of the principal drivers of change lay outside the physiotherapy profession. Economic and technological developments brought laboratory sciences into the profession; a growing critical mass of increasingly well-educated practitioners looking to specialise in cardiorespiratory, musculoskeletal, neurological and other fields; demands for greater evidence of efficacy and greater stability, protection and State sponsorship, all contributed to a growing desire to refine the profession's longstanding affinity with the body-as-machine. As new relationships and boundary tensions emerged between physiotherapy, medical and surgical specialists, occupational therapists, chiropractors, psychologists and others, the relationship between physiotherapy, posture and movement became more distinct, more refined and more nuanced.

Defining physiotherapy's approach to posture and movement

There are many ways posture and movement can be understood, examined and utilised. Physiotherapists long ago chose to focus on 'therapeutic treatment by systematic exercise of the organs forming the motor apparatus of the body' (Kleen 1918, p. 77). But this is only one way and it is not even the only *physical* way to understand posture and movement. Semantically speaking, posture can refer to one's *attitudes* and *inclinations*, *orientations* and *dispositions*; one's *reactions* to events in other people's lives; one's *outlook* on life based on our experiences and relationships; the things one *stands* for, the *positions* taken on matters of importance and *approaches* to things that have a *bearing* on one's welfare and wellbeing.

Likewise, the physical view of posture and movement can be viewed biomechanically, as Kleen does here:

> The skeletal muscles, which by their contraction convert the chemically stored elastic force into (heat) movement or positions; . . . bones, which act as levers for these movement; . . . joints, in which the movements take place round definite axes; . . . centrifugal motor nerve-elements, from which the motor impulses arise and are conducted; and . . . centripetal sensory nerve elements, upon which also the form and steadiness of the movement depend.
> (Kleen 1918, p. 77)

Movement is also a concept that extends well beyond the merely physical (Normann et al 2013). Movements can range from the imperceptible whirring of electrons around an atom and the microscopic osmotic flow of fluids across cell membranes, to the massive movements of fleeing migrants across state borders. There are other movements too that function as metaphors to help us understand complex ideas in emotive and meaningful ways: there are musical movements and films that move us; there are images of growth, progress and transformation; political movements and movements in economic market; relationship metaphors that are used to describe two parties coming together or drifting apart; gestures and signs; relocations and repositionings and psychological metaphors that describe people as driven or lives that are going nowhere.

Having explored some of physiotherapy's particular history of posture and movement at the beginning of the chapter, it is clear that a number of competing tensions influenced the profession's adoption of a biomechanical approach. The desire to associate closely with medicine; the profession's historical affinity with Swedish Remedial Exercise and the need to treat the body-as-machine not being the least of them. But before physiotherapists accept that this is the profession's legacy and take for granted that this necessarily represents physiotherapy's future, it is perhaps worth spending a moment considering some of the other ways physiotherapy educators, practitioners and researchers might understand posture and movement.

To begin with, posture and movement can be thought of as self-referential. In other words, they may be a visible outward expressions of a person's inner thoughts and attitudes, their personal circumstances, their beliefs and values. Pierre Bourdieu called this 'durable manner of standing, speaking and thereby . . . feeling and thinking' bodily 'hexis' (Bourdieu 1977, p. 93–4). Think of the way that the person on the subway in a smart suit or the hunched-over homeless person convey their personal circumstances through their posture and movement; the dancer trained to express feelings of love, hatred, anger and repose; the non-verbal communication of the scared patient or the sloppy anger of Friday night drinker. Society has long placed great value on the ability of some people to interpret these outward signs of one's inner disposition. Physiotherapists have traditionally distanced themselves from such existential analyses, however, preferring to see a lateral shift of the spine or torticollis as merely a mechanical derangement requiring a mechanical remedy. This has changed somewhat in recent years with educators and regulators at least recognising the importance of communication in the patient encounter (Winther et al 2014; Mendick et al 2015; Iversen et al 2008; Øien et al 2011; Wloszczak-Szubzda & Jarosz 2013; Duggan 2006). It is uncommon to find any discussion of the 'inner self' of the patient or therapist examined in much depth in the physiotherapy literature, however.

Posture and movement are also relational, in that they are always seen in the context of an 'other'. They always relate to something else, be it a moment in time or a fixed or mobile point in space – not just interstellar space, but also the space between people and things. They can refer to a person's immediate environment, when someone stands from sitting, for instance, or infer a posture or movement *towards* others, as in many contact sports. Thus, in talking about posture and movement, there is always an 'other' implied in any thought about displacement, transformation and change. Physiotherapists certainly concern themselves with a person's immediate environment when thinking about ground force reactions, the design of their treatment beds and the speed of a treadmill, and much of the therapeutic effect of treatment relies on the interaction of two or more objects working in sympathy (think of Brian Mulligan's approach to 'mobilisation with movement' approach or afferent firing from the skin to the higher cortex in pain 'gating', for example). Posture and movement therefore never operate in isolation and the object is always also subject to external facilitation and constraint – be it other people, slippery slopes or the pressure of time.

Unpacking this further, posture and movement are explicitly spatial and temporal. The way someone sits, leans against the wind or stretches out under the sun on a beach is an embodied response to their environment. These are spatial connections between the body and the objects and spaces that make up the world around us. Sometimes physiotherapists need to pay particular attention to these factors (when assessing a frail elderly person's safety in their home, for instance). At other times the external environment plays a more passive role (in the design of clinic spaces, for example). The external environment may also be other people, with their own physical, existential and social influences occupying the space around us. Some of these people are held close to us (both as physical entities, but also as memories) and others are figuratively kept 'at arm's length'. But when a person moves through this space, they unavoidably communicate with it, shape it and are shaped by it.

Posture and movement are also temporal, in as much as they change as time passes. This is not only the time measured in seconds (as in the Six Minute Walk Test or Timed Up and Go), but also the elastic time that flies by when people are late for work and drags when they are waiting for test results. Movement is maturational and physiotherapists have long concerned themselves with movement through the lifespan: children's increasing postural control, the ergonomic movement of workers and time spent in sedentary occupations have all drawn the attention of physiotherapists. In some ways, temporality is one of the defining features of physiotherapy. Physiotherapists ask their patients about their *past* medical history, assess their *present* function and work hard to reduce the *future* burden of poor health, dependence and disability.

Which brings me to the way that posture and movement may also be seen as socio-political. As I argued earlier in the chapter, there is a long history of the assessment, diagnosis of deviance and treatment of 'abnormal' posture and movement in order that the person can be returned to normal, functioning healthily, autonomous and independent. More than this, though, nation states have taken an active interest in creating 'environments' that allow their citizens to move. They support public education to allow people to develop skills to be successful in life and to be 'upwardly mobile'; they build transport networks to help people commute, footpaths and public parks to encourage recreation and support services as a safety net for times when normal life is on hold and people move from 'the kingdom of the well [to] the kingdom of the sick', becoming 'citizens of that other place', as Susan Sontag described it (Sontag 1977, p. 3). Physiotherapists have often managed to connect their particular view of movement with the State's interests in keeping people moving, suggesting that professional practitioners know that these discourses shape professional priorities as much, if not more, than any particular practice developments. This is, in essence, the dual conditioning I mentioned at the beginning of the chapter – the less visible but more powerful driver of physiotherapy's professional focus. I would argue that it is the self-referential, relational, spatial, temporal and socio-political dimensions of posture and movement that make them such powerful influences on people's sense of health and wellbeing, and that a broader view of these phenomena may hold a key to the profession's future.

Posture, movement and physiotherapy

Physiotherapy's approach to posture and movement begins, and ends to some extent, with the idea of the body-as-machine. Discussed at length in Chapters 3 and 6, physiotherapists have consistently defined their professional identity in reference to the anatomical, physiological and biomechanical body of the person at their fingertips. Whether it be an understanding of the neurophysiology of chronic pain or healing of an anterior cruciate ligament injury, physiotherapy defines itself and is defined by its relationship to the body of the person in front of them. This approach has helped it to distinguish itself from doctors, nurses, psychologists, occupational therapists, chiropractors, massage therapists, acupuncturists and many other allied professions. It has defined the profession's history and, perhaps, holds the key to its future.

As I have argued previously, central to physiotherapy's approach to posture and movement is the principal of normalisation. Here, bodies are assessed and referenced to a putative norm that states that humans are bipedal, erect animals, with a limited capacity to walk, run and jump and with ranges of movement specific to the species. Physiotherapists claim a special connection to some of this knowledge and use it to distinguish between what is pathological and what within normal tolerance. To be a physiotherapist is to know that the normal range of hip internal rotation in flexion is 45° and a significant asymmetrical reduction might indicate a capsular pattern and degenerative pathology. It is to know that this pattern might present with characteristic signs and symptoms, and that specific questions and tests can reproduce the problem and yield the specific aetiology through a process of deductive reasoning. To then have an armoury of treatment strategies to complete the cycle and allow for re-evaluation, reflection and planning, you have a complex interplay of competing knowledges that need expertise and skill to manage.

Physiotherapy is, therefore, far from being just a reductive, physical discipline: a pale imitation of biomedicine. On the contrary, physiotherapy's focus on the body-as-moving-machine does little to reduce the complexity of the challenge of assessing, diagnosing and treating postural and movement problems, in which 'things relate but [often] don't add up ... events occur but not within the processes of linear time, and ... phenomena share a space but cannot be mapped in terms of a single set of three-dimensional coordinates' (Law & Mol 2002, p. 1). Indeed, physiotherapists' ability to distinguish between normal and abnormal postures and movements has afforded them significant privilege, particularly over the last half century, and underpinned their recognition as primary diagnosticians; a privilege afforded to very few health professions.

One of the reasons why physiotherapists have been able to gain social capital for their work is that they make diagnoses not only of a person's abnormality, but also the social cost of illness, injury, disease, loss of functional independence and ability to participate in the meaningful activity. A person who stoops all the time or walks with a limp only attracts professional attention if their abnormality is likely to be a burden on themselves or others. Physiotherapy diagnoses are therefore as much about the *impact* of the person's abnormality, deviation or 'displacement' as they are about the physical features that make their posture or movement abnormal. Postures and movements that could be considered normal for some (the child that prefers to crawl, or the adult that likes to watch a lot of television, for example), are pathologised if they are thought to carry some social cost and physiotherapists, like other health professionals, are eager to take up this work of remediation. Therefore, although many of the bodily norms that physiotherapists deal with are relatively stable (range of movement, muscle function, basic physiological functions etc.), many of the social norms that define the profession's scope of practice are constantly in flux and it is a constant challenge for any profession to remain relevant in this shifting landscape.

Physiotherapists' ability to assess a person's deviation and displacement requires training in a wide range of techniques, and an enormous amount of time and energy is spent on developing, testing and disseminating new methods of assessment. Most physiotherapy methods of assessment attempt to make abnormal postures or movements more easily visible and easier to measure and record. Be it traditional methods of goniometry, the use of plumb lines to assess spinal deformity, or 3D motion sensors, somatosensory evoked potential or forced expiratory volume; the goal is to make the body's inner workings visible. Tests with the greatest fidelity to the body's 'natural' function carry the greatest weight because practitioners perceive that they remove the subjectivity from their judgement of that which is beyond their sight. This leaves them, as the professional, to make the judgement about the relevance of the pathological change. So, the physiotherapist's role is not to ascertain the degree of shift on the graph, per se, but rather the *significance* of the shift for the person's health and the likely downstream costs of that change[9].

Where there are no objective tests that can easily ascertain a deviation from the norm, therapists need to develop skills in the examination that, again, define their professional scope. There are no currently available mechanisms that can authentically and objectively reproduce a person's pain, which like breathlessness, can only really be understood as subjective phenomena. Pain makes people wince, grimace, limp and avoid postures and movements that physiotherapists learn to 'read'. The ability to observe bodily movement and distil a specific aetiology from these postures and patterns of movement, is one of the key skills possessed by expert practitioners. Pattern recognition can, of course, become formulaic, with people projecting older learnt patterns onto present problems from force of habit (Higgs et al 2008; Titchen, & Higgs 2001), but the ability to locate structural tension or laxity that may be causing outward malalignment, dysfunction or discomfort, has long been recognised as a cardinal capability for physiotherapy practitioners.

But many other health professionals also assess and treat the normalised body. Many use the same assessment tools and techniques, and many have to be able to 'read' the person's postures and movements in order to understand the inner workings of the body. These things do not *define* physiotherapy, per se. They are, however, used by physiotherapists to define the profession's particularly distinctive approach to the body that, on its own, says a great deal about the profession's identity. So, in what ways is it possible to distinguish a particularly 'physiotherapeutic' approach to posture and movement?

In Chapter 6, I argued that physiotherapy students have long been encouraged to view the body as docile, passive and inanimate – a lifeless entity akin to a cadaver, and that this was necessary to strip the body of its emotions, desires and sensuality so that they could treat the person dispassionately and rid the profession of any association with illicit touch or licentious behaviour. This construct of the body as 'cadaver', however, only really functions for representations of the *static* body – the kind of body students are introduced to in anatomy textbooks and pro-sections. It is inadequate, however, as a way of understanding and managing the moving body, because the moving body comes with self-referential, relational, spatial, temporal and socio-political connotations that are not present when the body is only viewed as a static machine. The extrapolation of the idea of the body-as-machine to the more complex problems presented by posture and movement have therefore always been a challenge to physiotherapists, who have sought to constrain, discipline and contain the body, and ensure that their practices are viewed as safe, visible and legitimate.

Perhaps for this reason, physiotherapy writers have consistently promoted the study of the physical properties of movement, particularly the mechanical properties of forces, levers, motions and moments (Palmer 1901; Despard 1916; Ellison 1898) (see Figure 7.2). Using these biomechanical principles, it was possible to take the image of the static, passive body and animate it using physical properties of movement that bypassed any concerns for the patient's 'vitality'.[10] Humanistic considerations, like a person's culture, personal feelings, likes and dislikes, sensitivities or passions, could be left to others (psychologists and psychotherapists especially), leaving the physical therapist to concentrate on the rigorous discipline of biomechanics.

A biomechanical approach to the body meant that the therapists could separate bodily actions from everyday functions, so that the focus fell on the role of the

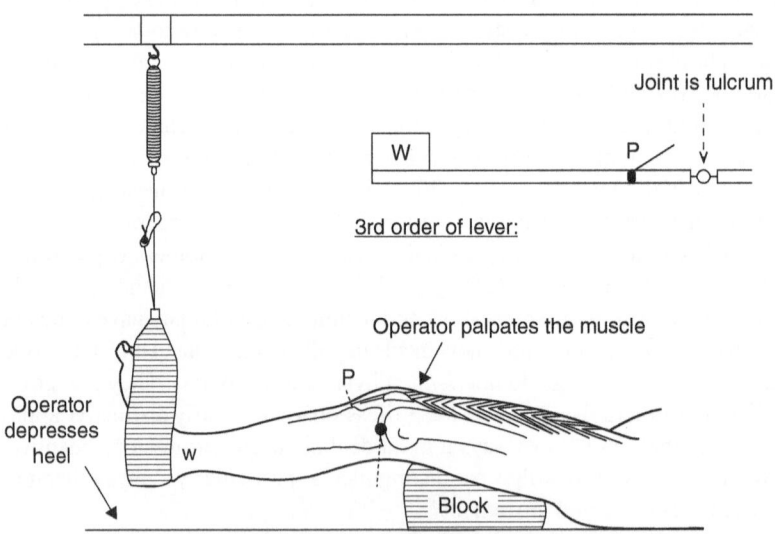

Figure 7.2 The 'model' patient – a biomechanical representation of forces applied to the lower limb. Guthrie Smith (1952) published by Elsevier.

biceps brachii in flexing the elbow and the 'purposeful' use of elbow flexion for eating and drinking, gesturing and dressing, and this became the domain of occupational therapists and others. Most physiotherapy texts that taught practitioners about posture and movement did so with few references to everyday functional uses for movement, preferring instead to refer to morphological features that facilitated and impeded movement (inert properties of tissues, muscle strength, flexibility etc.), normalised ranges of movement and pathologies in which these properties were manifested.

Consider five seminal texts taken from the last 100 years of posture and movement studies in physiotherapy: L.L. Despard's *Textbook of Massage and Remedial Gymnastics* (1916), Edith M. Prosser's *Manual of Massage and Movements* (1943), M. Dena Gardiner's *Principles of Exercise Therapy* (1953), P.M. Galley and A.L. Forster's *Human Movement: An Introductory Text for Physiotherapy Students* (1982, p. 1) and Margaret Hollis's *Practical Exercise Therapy* (1989). Each of these follows a similar structure, both biomechanical and kinesiological, focusing heavily on the structural mechanics of the body. Turn to any page, and you will find reproductions of bodies in motion. But this is not the motion of a parent hugging their child, a violinist in the midst of a recital or a crowd surging in the subway. This is the arm flexing and extending, the collinear forces acting on body segments and the external forces 'utilised to supplement the Force of Muscular Contraction' (Gardiner 1953, p. 40).

Consider how Galley and Forster introduce the subject of human movement to physiotherapy students:

> Efficient movement. Physiotherapy is involved in helping patients to move more efficiently as they seek to achieve a desired goal. An efficient movement is one that fulfills a specific purpose with economy of movement at the required speed.
>
> (Galley & Forster 1982, p. 118)

Or how Lewis describes postural training:

> Postural advice and education will help patients to have optimal ergonomics and facilitate everyday activities. 'Good posture' means recruitment of only the appropriate muscle fibres to limit fatigue and abnormal strains ensuing with pain.
>
> (Lewis & Porter 2003, p. 259)

Such descriptions are the embodiment of biomechanical reasoning: brusque, matter-of-fact and highly reductive. They convey the same kind of economy of writing seen in classic works of exercise science and kinesiology (see, e.g. Brunnstrom 1972; Basmajian 1958; Rasch & Burke 1978). But whereas these authors were unconcerned with the needs of any specific professional group, Prosser, Gardiner, Galley and Forster and others were writing specifically for physiotherapists, so when they used genderless stick figures to represent the therapist and patient; used fundamental and derived positions to discipline motion; or defined posture as,

> the attitude assumed by the body either with support during muscular inactivity, or by means of the coordinated action of many muscles working to maintain stability or to form an essential basis which is being adapted constantly to the movement which is superimposed upon it.
>
> (Gardiner 1953, p. 211)

There was some strategic significance given to the distinction between the body as *sensual* being and the mechanical moving assemblage of body parts that physiotherapists were supposed to see.

Seeing the patient in this way distanced the therapist from the lived experiences of their patients; it distinguished them from other caring professions who embraced the 'whole' person and it aligned them more closely with physicians and surgeons. It focused the therapist's attention on the individual patient or body in front of them, and it provided opportunities for endless re-analyses of its deviations from the anatomical textbook image that was the reference norm. The physiotherapy literature on movement has consistently reproduced this model, constructing the physiotherapist as a dispassionate witness to the intimate differences between each person's body. This was a body-as-*moving*-machine par excellence and no other profession has refined this image to the same degree.

The recent interest in the neuro-physiological control of movement seen in texts like Shumway-Cook and Woollacott's 2007 text *Motor Control*, show how these principles have been only marginally refined from early physiotherapy texts. Comparing *Motor Control* with L.L. Despard's 1916 *Textbook of Massage and Remedial Gymnastics*, for example, one sees that the only fundamental difference between the two is the amount of experimental research used to justify the approach. The therapists' focus on body-as-moving-machine remains, however, with the potentially more inclusive notions of posture and movement replaced by 'postural control' and the control of 'normal mobility', developed by people like Herman Kabot, Margaret Knott and Dorothy Voss, Margaret Rood and Karl and Berta Bobath. And while Shumway-Cook and Woollacott claim that 'few clinicians would argue the importance of posture and balance to independence in activities such as sitting, standing and walking' and that 'the ability to control one's body emerges from a complex interaction of musculoskeletal and neural systems' (Shumway-Cook & Woollacott 2007, p. 158), it may be possible to see that little has changed in the physiotherapist's privileging of the body-as-machine.

It is important here to acknowledge that this is perhaps one of the greatest achievements of physiotherapy: to have established so early a model that can transcend war, epidemic, economic depression, social transformation and resonate across so many international borders is a truly remarkable feat and one that *should* be acknowledged and celebrated. So perhaps an analysis of this sort helps to understand why physiotherapists have consistently chosen to retain their fidelity with a relatively narrow, but no less complex definition of posture and movement? Perhaps it explains why, given that posture and movement embrace such a wide range of concepts and ideas, physiotherapists have consistently defined their professional identity with reference to only those kinds of movement that are expressly biomechanical? Given the range of ways to understand posture and movement, it is telling that physiotherapists have consistently chosen *this* way and not one of the myriad other ways available to them.

This is not the first time these questions have been posed. In 1975, Helen Hislop described physical therapy as having 'a pyramidal structure which has its foundations in social and cultural needs' (Hislop 1975, p. 1075). She saw physiotherapy as part of a larger ecosystem, linking cells, with tissues, organs, systems, persons and family. Situating physiotherapy within this ecosystem, however, Hislop defaulted to the tacitly physiotherapeutic approach and proposed a pathokinesiological model of movement to restricted the profession to those aspects of the model that were expressly biomechanical. Similarly, in 1995, Cheryl Cott and colleagues argued that movement was essential to life, opening up the possibility of a much more inclusive idea of movement than had previously been possible. The authors followed, however, with the highly reductive explanation that movement 'involves a change of position of the body and its components' (Cott et al 1995, p. 88). In many ways, Cott et al provide the best explanation for physiotherapy's approach to posture and movement, by arguing that extrinsic factors *influence* movement (physical, psychological, social and environmental), even to the point of seeing movement as a continuum from the micro to the macro, but the focus for physiotherapy remained on movement as biomechanical displacement – movement as animated posture (Cott et al 1995; Allen 2007).

Some of the more recent writings on movement in physiotherapy have begun to challenge this reductive and restrictive view, however. Grete Barlindhaug, Nina Emaus and Nina Foss's recent article exploring 'Movements in a Broader Perspective' argues that, 'The patient's shape and movements embody the social structure, cultural values and the individual life story', and that physiotherapists should pay more attention to these aspects (Barlindhaug et al 2012, p. 85). Similarly, Camilla Wikström-Grotell and Katie Eriksson claim that physiotherapists have a long tradition of pragmatism when it comes to an understanding of movement, but that the 'need to deepen the understanding of a cumulatively developed theoretical concept of movement in PT [sic] remains' (Wikström-Grotell & Eriksson 2012, p. 429).

Wenche Bjorbækmo and Gunn Engelsrud's recent exploration of improvisational movement (Bjorbækmo & Engelsrud 2011), Veronika Williams and colleagues' metaphor of movement as a 'flowing stream' (Williams et al 2011) and Britt Normann et al's argument for physiotherapists to give greater emphasis to patients' contextual perceptions of movement (Normann et al 2013) all point to a sentiment now being echoed by WCPT and professional bodies around the world. This sentiment suggests physiotherapy may now be open to the idea of an expanded appreciation of posture and movement (Nicholls et al 2015). Whether this ever 'foment[s] revolution by inciting a "movement movement"' (Gibson 2016) or achieves the level of sophistication and theoretical depth and complexity of the writings of people like Couton, Doughty, Gros or Solnit (Doughty 2013; Solnit 2014; Gros 2014; Couton, & López 2009), remains to be seen.

Closing words

There are problems caused by rigid postures and a lack of movement and there are problems caused by laxity and too much movement, and these problems exist as much for professions as they do for patients. For reasons tied inextricably to the profession's long cultural history, physiotherapists have chosen to focus on biomechanical and kinesiological understandings of posture and movement at the expense of myriad other forms available to them. So now, when physiotherapists speak of a person's attitude, they are referring to their postural deportment rather than their bearing or manner towards authority; when they speak of inflexibility or instability, it is their hamstring muscles and their stepping strategies that they refer to. As with the profession's approach to the body-as-machine, this has been sufficient for many generations of physiotherapists and has seen the profession grow and prosper. But if healthcare is changing in ways that we have not seen before and people are demanding more from their health professionals than just technical competence, it may be that an expanded view of posture and movement hold the key to the future of physiotherapy. With physiotherapy's long history of interest and expertise in this area, the profession is well placed to lift its gaze from the body of the person in front of them and engage in a movement revolution.

Slowly, physiotherapists are starting to see the broader significance of posture and movement and are looking to fulfil the ideals of Hislop, Cott and others, who have long held out for physiotherapists to embrace a more inclusive vision of posture and movement (Wikström-Grotell & Eriksson 2012; Cott et al 1995; Hislop 1975). The profession still holds firmly to its biomechanical heritage, however, and has only shifted slightly in recent years to marry neurological understandings of sensorimotor function with more traditional anato-pathological approaches from musculoskeletal physiotherapy. The challenge is to find just the right amount of movement for the profession, so that it can embrace the ideas of posture and movement that are becoming more significant in the 21st century. In Chapter 8, I move further away from the static image of the body-as-machine, past the biomechanically reductive view of posture and movement, to consider how physiotherapy has come to relate to the functional body and the role rehabilitation has played in further defining the profession's professional purpose.

Notes

1 To reiterate a point made frequently throughout this book, I use the term biomechanical in the broadest possible sense here; referring to any approach that views the body-as-machine. Here, the term *biomechanical* incorporates neuro-physiological, kinesiological, patho-anatomical and physiological understandings of posture and movement.
2 For a very thoughtful review of the role that posture and movement played in ancient cultures and the shifts between the graceful poise of Greek social norms, through the

masculine muscularity of Roman culture and the saintly virtue associated with suffering and the rejection of the corporeal body seen in early Christianity, see Turner (1965, pp. 12–6).

3 For a comprehensive review of the etymology and use of the term posture thoughout history, see Gilman (2014). For a detailed history of therapeutic exercise, see Licht (1978).

4 I have used male pronouns in this part of the text to reflect the particular interest in male posture and movement in much of the literature of the time.

5 Demonstrating that cultural attitudes to correct posture are always changing, Hines states that the 'posture of attention (and tension) promoted as correct by the U.S. Army during World War I was considered incorrect during World War II' (Hines 1965, p. 486).

6 For a comprehensive overview of the kinds of gymnastics that formed the basis of physiotherapy practice in the 1920s and after, see Kleen (1918, pp. 77–161).

7 Eugenics was a popular idea, especially in the early 20th century. It was first developed by Francis Galton (1822–1911), Charles Darwin's cousin, who was something of a polymath, inventing questionnaires, correlation and regression statistics, and theories of perception.

8 There were some variations on this theme, including Barlow's notion of *postural homeostasis*, but these were largely isolated examples of more holistic thinking (Barlow 1952).

9 This point returns us to the principal of the physiotherapy paradox, where practitioners struggle to embrace the changing economy of healthcare in the 21st century because of their historical affinity with the body-as-machine. One could reasonably argue, however, that physiotherapy would not have progressed in the way it has without the ability to adapt to changing cultural, economic, political, philosophical and social discourses. So, does this not undermine my argument about physiotherapy's 'blindness' to other ways of viewing health and illness? I believe not. In Chapters 3–5, I argued that many events in the 20th century worked in the profession's favour, and that it benefited without needing to move greatly from the model set up by the profession's founders. I believe that the same approach will not be sufficient now and that physiotherapy must engage more thoughtfully with issues like the self-referential, relational, spatial, temporal and socio-political dimensions of posture and movement if it to understand and act on contemporary drivers of change in the profession.

10 In defining posture and movement, for example, Brooks argued that '"posture" means the static position of any part of the body, rather than just the description of a standing or sitting position of the whole body ... "Movements" are the transition from one posture to another' (Brooks 1986, p. 5).

References

Allen, D.D., 2007, Proposing 6 dimensions within the construct of movement in the movement continuum theory, *Physical Therapy*, 87(7), pp. 888–98.

American Academy of Orthopaedic Surgeons, 1965, *Joint motion: Method of measuring and recording*, Bishop and Sons, Edinburgh.

Armstrong, D., 2002, *A new history of identity*, Palgrave Macmillan, London.

Barclay, J., 1994, *In good hands: The history of the Chartered Society of Physiotherapy 1894–1994*, Butterworth Heinemann, Oxford.

Barlindhaug, G., Emaus, N. & Foss, N., 2012, Movements in a broader perspective – A study of women in a mountainous village in Nepal, *Advances in Physiotherapy*, 14(2), pp. 78–86.

Barlow, W., 1952, Postural homoeostasis, *Annals of Physical Medicine*, 1(3), pp. 77–87.

Basmajian, J.V., 1958, *Therapeutic exercise*, Williams & Wilkins, Baltimore, MD.

Bjorbækmo, W.S. & Engelsrud, G.H., 2011, 'My Own Way of Moving' - Movement improvisation in children's rehabilitation, *Phenomenology & Practice*, 5(1), pp. 27–47.

Bourdieu, P., 1977, *Outline of a theory of practice*. Cambridge University Press, Cambridge.

Brooks, V.B., 1986, *The neural basis of motor control*, Oxford University Press, New York.

Brunnstrom, S., 1972, *Clinical kinesiology*, F.A. Davis, Philadelphia, PA.

Cott, C.A., Finch, E., Gasner, D., Yoshida, K., Thomas, S.G. & Verrier, M.C., 1995, The movement continuum theory of physical therapy, *Physiotherapy Canada*, 47(2), pp. 87–95.

Couton, P. & López, J.J., 2009, Movement as utopia, *History of the Human Sciences*, 22(4), pp. 93–121.

Danielsson, L. & Rosberg, S., 2015, Opening toward life: Experiences of basic body awareness therapy in persons with major depression. *International Journal of Qualitative Studies on Health and Well-being*, 10, 27069.

Danielsson, L., Kihlbom, B., & Rosberg, S., 2016, 'Crawling out of the cocoon': Patients' experiences of a physical therapy exercise intervention in the treatment of major depression. *Physical Therapy*, 96(8), pp. 1241–50.

Despard, L.L., 1916, *Text-book of massage and remedial gymnastics*, Oxford University Press, London.

Doughty, K., 2013, Walking together: The embodied and mobile production of a therapeutic landscape, *Health & Place*, 24, pp. 140–6.

Duggan, A., 2006, Understanding interpersonal communication processes across health contexts: Advances in the last decade and challenges for the next decade, *Journal of Health Communication*, 11(1), pp. 93–108.

Ellison, M.A., 1898, *A manual for students of massage*, Bailliere, Tindall and Cox, London.

Fischinger, J., Fischinger, A. & Fischinger, D., 2009, Doctor Zander's medico-mechanical institute in Opatija, *Acta Medico-Historica Adriatica*, 7(2), pp. 253–66.

Fredrick, D., 2002, *The Roman gaze: Vision, power, and the body*, Johns Hopkins University Press, Baltimore, MD.

Galley, P.M. & Forster, A.L., 1982, *Human movement: An introductory text for physiotherapy students*, Churchill Livingstone, London.

Gardiner, M.D., 1953, *The principles of exercise therapy*, G. Bell and Sons, London.

Gibson, B., 2016, *Rehabilitation: A post-critical approach*, Taylor & Francis, New York.

Gilman, S.L., 2014, 'Stand up straight': Notes toward a history of posture, *Journal of Medical Humanities*, 35(1), pp. 57–83.

Gros, F., 2014, *A philosophy of walking*, Verso, London.

Guthrie-Smith, O.F., 1952, *Rehabilitation, re-education and remedial exercise*, Bailliere, Tindall & Cox, London.

Hansson, N. & Ottosson, A., 2015, Nobel Prize for physical therapy? Rise, fall, and revival of medico-mechanical institutes, *Physical Therapy*, doi: 10.2522/ptj.20140284.

Higgs, J., Jones, M.A., Loftus, S. & Christensen, N., 2008, *Clinical reasoning in the health professions*, Elsevier Health Sciences UK, London.

Hines, T.F., 1965, Posture, in S. Licht (ed.), *Therapeutic exercise*, 2nd ed., Waverley Press, Baltimore, MD, pp. 486–506.

Hislop, H.J., 1975, The not-so-impossible dream, *Physical Therapy*, 55(10), pp. 1069–80.

Hollis, M., 1989, *Practical exercise therapy*, Blackwell Scientific Publications, Oxford.

Houlding, R.N., 1943, Rehabilitation of injured air crews in Great Britain, in W.B. Doherty & D.D. Runes (eds.), *Rehabilitation of the war injured, a symposium*, Philosophical Library, New York, pp. 440–53.

Iversen, S., Marie Øien, A. & Råheim, M., 2008, Physiotherapy treatment of children with cerebral palsy: The complexity of communication within sessions and over time, *Advances in Physiotherapy*, 10(1), pp. 41–52.

Jull, G. & Moore, A., 2013, Physiotherapy's identity, *Manual Therapy*, 18, pp. 447–8.

Kleen, E.A., 1918, *Massage and medical gymnastics*, J. & A. Churchill, London.

Law, J. & Mol, A. (eds.), 2002, *Complexities: Social studies of knowledge practices*, Duke University Press, Durham, NC.

Lewis, R. & Porter, S.B., 2003, Physiotherapy in rheumatology, in S.B. Porter (ed.), *Tidy's physiotherapy*, Butterworth Heinemann, Edinburgh, pp. 241–72.

Licht, S., 1978, History, in J.V. Basmajian (ed.), *Therapeutic exercise*, Williams & Wilkins, Baltimore, MD, pp. 1–42.

Linker, B., 2012, A dangerous curve: The role of history in America's scoliosis screening programs, *American Journal of Public Health*, 102(4), pp. 606–16.

Lloyd, W.M., 1936, Health and physical education, *Medical Officer*, 55, pp. 207–8.

McIntosh, P.C., 1952, *Physical education in England since 1800*, Bell, London.

McNeill, W.H., 1995, *Keeping together in time: Dance and drill in human history*, Harvard University Press, Cambridge, MA.

Mead, J., 2003, The responsibilities of being a physiotherapist, in S.B. Porter (ed.), *Tidy's physiotherapy*, Butterworth Heinemann, Edinburgh, pp. 1–20.

Mendick, N., Young, B., Holcombe, C. & Salmon, P., 2015, How do surgeons think they learn about communication?: A qualitative study, *Medical Education*, 49(4), pp. 408–16.

Murphy, W., 1995, *Healing the generations: A history of physical therapy and the American Physical Therapy Association*, Greenwich Publishing, Lyme, CT.

Nicholls, D.A., Gibson, B.E. & Fadyl, J.K., 2015, Rethinking movement: Postmodern reflections on a dominant rehabilitation discourse, in K. McPherson, B.E. Gibson & A. Leplège (eds.), *Rethinking rehabilitation: Theory and practice*, CRC Press, FL, pp. 97–116.

Normann, B., Sørgaard, K.W., Salvesen, R. & Moe, S., 2013, Contextualized perceptions of movement as a source of expanded insight: People with multiple sclerosis' experience with physiotherapy, *Physiotherapy Theory and Practice*, 29(1), pp. 19–30.

Øien, A.M., Steihaug, S., Iversen, S. & Råheim, M., 2011, Communication as negotiation processes in long-term physiotherapy: A qualitative study, *Scandinavian Journal of Caring Sciences*, 25(1), pp. 53–61.

Ottosson A., 2005, Sjukgymnasten – vart tog han vägen?: En undersökning av sjukgymnastyrkets maskulinisering och avmaskulinisering 1813–1934, Göteborg University, Göteborg, Sweden.

Ottosson, A., 2010, The first historical movements of kinesiology: Scientification in the borderline between physical culture and medicine around 1850, *International Journal of the History of Sport*, 27(11), pp. 1892–919.

Ottosson, A., 2011, The manipulated history of manipulations of spines and joints?: rethinking orthopaedic medicine through the 19th century discourse of European mechanical medicine, *Medicine Studies*, 3(2), pp. 83–116.

Ottosson, A., 2015, One history or many herstories?: Gender politics and the history of physiotherapy's origins in the nineteenth and early twentieth century, *Women's History Review*, 25(2), pp. 296–319.

Ottosson, A., 2016, The age of scientific gynaecological masseurs. Non-intrusive male hands, female intimacy, and women's health around 1900, *Social History of Medicine*, 29(4), pp. 802–28.

Palmer, M.D., 1901, *Lessons in massage*, 1st ed., Bailliere, Tindall and Cox, London.

Pronger, B., 2002, *Body fascism: Salvation in the technology of physical fitness*, University of Toronto Press, Toronto, Canada.

Prosser, E.M., 1943, *Manual of massage and movement*, Faber and Faber, London.

Rasch, P.J. & Burke, R.K., 1978, *Kinesiology and applied anatomy*, Lea & Febiger, Philadelphia, PA.

Sahrmann, S.A., 2014, The human movement system: Our professional identity, *Physical Therapy*, 94(7), pp. 1034–42.

Shumway-Cook, A. & Woollacott, M.H., 2007, *Motor control: Translating research into clinical practice*, 3rd ed., Lippincott Williams & Wilkins, Philadelphia, PA.

Snyder, S.L. & Mitchell, D.T., 2006, Eugenics, in G. Albrecht (ed.), *Encyclopedia of disability*, Sage, Thousand Oaks, CA, pp. 624–5.

Solnit, R., 2014, *Wanderlust: A History of walking*, Granta Books, London.

Sontag, S., 1977, *Illness as metaphor*, Penguin, London.

McKenzie, R.T., 1916, The treatment of convalescent soldiers by physical means, *British Medical Journal*, 2(2902), 31–49.

Terlouw, T.J., 2007a, The rise and fall of Zander-Institutes in the Netherlands around 1900, *Medizin, Gesellschaft, und Geschichte*, 25, pp. 91–124.

Terlouw, T.J., 2007b, Roots of physical medicine, physical therapy, and mechanotherapy in the Netherlands in the 19th century: A disputed area within the healthcare domain, *Journal of Manual and Manipulative Therapy*, 15(2), pp. E23–41.

Tidy, N.M., 1937, *Massage and remedial exercises*, 3rd ed., John Wright & Sons, Bristol.

Titchen, A. & Higgs, J., 2001, Towards professional artistry and creativity in practice, in J. Higgs & A. Titchen (eds.), *Professional practice in health, education and the creative arts*, Blackwell Science, Oxford, pp. 273–90.

Tucker, W.E., 1960, *Active altered posture*, E. & S. Livingstone, Edinburgh.

Turner, M., 1965, *Faulty posture: It's effects and treatment*, William Heinemann Medical Books Ltd (Published in Association with The Chartered Society of Physiotherapy), London.

Wikström-Grotell, C. & Eriksson, K., 2012, Movement as a basic concept in physiotherapy – A human science approach, *Physiotherapy Theory and Practice*, 28(6), pp. 428–38.

Williams, V., Bruton, A., Ellis-Hill, C. & McPherson, K., 2011, The importance of movement for people living with chronic obstructive pulmonary disease, *Qualitative Health Research*, 21(9), pp. 1239–48.

Winther, H., Grøntved, S.N., Kold Gravesen, E. & Ilkjær, I., 2014, The dancing nurses and the language of the body: Training somatic awareness, bodily communication, and embodied professional competence in nurse education, *Journal of Holistic Nursing*, doi: 10.1177/0898010114561063.

Wloszczak-Szubzda, A. & Jarosz, M.J., 2013, Professional communication competences of physiotherapists – practice and educational perspectives, *Annals of Agricultural and Environmental Medicine*, 20(1), pp. 189–94.

Zander, E., 1918, Methods of medico-mechanical gymnastics, in E.A.G. Kleen (ed.), *Massage and medical gymnastics*, J. & A. Churchill, London, pp. 324–69.

8 Function and rehabilitation

Introduction

I have now explored three constructs that have fundamentally shaped the cultural history of physiotherapy. In Chapter 6, I looked at the particular way physiotherapists have understood the body and in Chapter 7, how physiotherapists have related to posture and movement. Although these constructs have obvious effects on the way physiotherapists practice and think, they are at the same time quite abstract, in that they do not really involve people – patients – living in the real world: going to school, doing their weekly shopping, tending their crops, driving their cars and reading their emails. So it is important now to move beyond the idea of the body-as-machine, and even beyond the body-as-moving-machine, to think about the body at work, rest and play; the person, not just a body, engaging in the normal activities of daily life: the neighbour, office worker, retired shopkeeper, grandmother; the patient struggling to recover from surgery, off work with lower back pain or convalescing after a fall; the disabled athlete, the wounded soldier, the sedated and ventilated child, the elderly man recovering from a stroke . . . In short, it is necessary to better understand the *person*.

Physiotherapy has often taken a very particular view of everyday life. Not wanting to abandon its biomechanical principles, it has viewed human flourishing from a distance; concerned more with the way the body moves through spaces and places than with the messiness and complexities of life itself. In keeping with their view of the body-as-moving-machine, physiotherapists have often been more interested in joint movements than social movements; postural stability and stepping strategies more than dancing. As Elizabeth DePoy and Stephen French Gilson put it:

> The legitimate scope of disability practice in rehabilitation is to restore, foster, or maximise function in a specified domain of professional concern . . . We use the term function here to reveal the normative stance of rehabilitation. That is, based in large part on longitudinal and exterior environment explanations, rehabilitation professions assume a desirable set of typical activities within age and role norms and only recently have included diversity patina variable in assessment and practice.
>
> (DePoy & Gilson 2011, pp. 178–9)

Perhaps the exception to this is the profession's interest in productive labour. Early in the profession's history, physiotherapy learnt a valuable and enduring lesson about the need to connect their practices to the economic and governmental imperatives of the time. In World War I, masseuses were asked to help rehabilitate thousands of returned servicemen and become part of the State machinery that developed into what we now know of as rehabilitation. Physiotherapists learnt from this experience that they could adapt their ideas of the body-as-machine to the organised reconstruction of bodies broken in battle. And from this, it was only a short step to realise that physiotherapy could be applied to the bodies of many others who were ill or injured, impaired and disabled. Physiotherapy made the transition so easily because it had already largely established its legitimacy. But it also had a practice model ideally suited to the governmental demands for productive human work. All physiotherapists needed to do was to develop the idea of the body-as-moving-machine and apply it to the world of work. The patient's body needed to be seen as a *functioning* machine.

In this chapter, I argue that the field of rehabilitation has been the location for some fundamental advances in physiotherapy. The need to rehabilitate injured servicemen in WWI has been credited with giving birth to the rehabilitation movement (McPherson et al 2015; Anderson 2011; Linker 2011, Wilson 1995), as well as initiating the formation of physical therapy professions in North America (Murphy 1995; Cleather 1995; Linker 2005). Rehabilitation provided the first experience of interprofessional practice for physiotherapists (as opposed to merely deferential referrals from doctors and working in parallel with nurses prior to WWI). It opened the door to practices focused on long-term and chronic conditions, and thus the possibility of longer contracts of employment and greater financial security for practitioners. Rehabilitation was the location where physiotherapists could address the social and economic costs of illness and injury, and thus prove to the State that it could be trusted when social insurance and national welfare systems began to emerge in the 1930s. It also instigated the now common interest in objective measurement and the assessment of treatment outcomes, which would, in turn, help the profession become research focused, evidence-based and concerned with the 'ends', not just the 'means', of assessment and treatment. In short, physiotherapists' concern for the body-as-*functioning*-machine has been both a necessary and highly significant influence on the profession's growth and development, and much of this advance has been made through rehabilitation.

Significantly, rehabilitation positioned physiotherapists firmly alongside the other orthodox health professions. In fact, it would be fair to say that physiotherapy *became* orthodox as a result of its inclusion in the burgeoning rehabilitation movement. Prior to World War I, the profession's focus, in Britain at least, was on the quest for legitimacy, critical mass and market closure. The profession's founders needed to establish that masseuses could be trusted to touch patients without fear of impropriety. They were determined to differentiate themselves from nurses, poorly trained masseuses and masseurs and prostitutes, and they were interested in creating a closed market for legitimate patient referrals by aggressively courting medical patronage. By 1914, the ISTM had spent 20 years fighting these battles and many had been won. With the outbreak of war and the astonishing demand created by battle injuries, physiotherapists were ready to leave behind the more parochial pre-war disputes for the greater good of the country. They showed, like many others at the time, a willingness to look outward; to answer a national call for help and in so doing put in place a new set of principles that would see the profession prosper for much of the rest of the century.

Being recognised as an orthodox health profession came with many benefits, not least state recognition, protective legislation, formal alliances with other orthodox health professions and access to patients in the public health system. But it also brought to the surface some underlying tensions. As a female-dominated profession, physiotherapy was seen as subservient to the male medical profession and early practitioners experienced the same kinds of gender discrimination as other female-dominated professions like nursing, teaching and administration. The profession's orthodox status also, ironically, situated the profession at odds with many disabled people. Although little criticism surfaced in the early years of the rehabilitation movement, physiotherapists and other allied health professionals have more recently been accused of living parasitically off disabled people (Swain et al 2003b); of focusing too much on pathology and impairments (Patston 2007; Hammell 2006) and not enough on disabling social conditions (Oliver 1998); of normalising and 'creating' deviance and disability (Corbett 1997) and of lacking patient-centred approaches to rehabilitation and treatment (Hammell 2013; Gzil et al 2007).

Tools like the International Classification of Function, Disability and Health (ICF) have become widely used models around which 'holistic' rehabilitation practices have emerged, and physiotherapists have been quick to embrace this particular model and its forerunner, the International Classification of Impairments, Disabilities and Handicaps (ICIDH), which was developed by the World Health Organization (WHO) in 1980[1]. The ICF is seen by many practitioners as the model around which all person-centred, holistic rehabilitation services should be wrapped (Solli & da Silva 2012; Escorpizo 2015). But it too has received considerable criticism among disabled people and disability activists (Abberley 1993; Pfeiffer 1998; Hurst 2000; Hammell 2006). Critics argue that it remains a system of classification that has assumed extraordinary power for 'othering' disabled people, for *creating* abnormality and identifying the body of the disabled person as the source of the problem, rather than cultural, economic, political and social causes that the public at large and the State bear the primary responsibility for (Hammell 2006).

It is not possible to answer the question of how physiotherapy has arrived at this point in its history, therefore, without considering how the profession adapted its objective, depersonalised view of the body, posture and movement, to the complexity and sociality of the functioning body, in order that it might become the world's leading provider of orthodox physical rehabilitation. So, in the remainder of this chapter, I explore the concepts of function and rehabilitation before offering a summary history of the rehabilitation movement as it has applied to physiotherapy in the 20th and 21st centuries. I will then look at some of the criticisms levelled against physiotherapists and others who advocate for functional rehabilitation, and tackle some of the costs and benefits of models like the ICF. Finally, I will look at the way the idea of the body-as-functioning-machine has influenced day-to-day physiotherapy practice. To begin with, then, I will explore some of the different meanings ascribed to function and rehabilitation.

What are function and rehabilitation?

It is possible to see from the broad spread of literature published over the last century that physiotherapists have a very specific definition in mind when they explore the idea of function. They are most often referring to what a body part can do, how it can move and what it can achieve. They are concerned primarily with what is called the primary biological function of the body (Neander 1991; Ariew et al 2002; Bigelow & Pargetter 1987). Unlike occupational therapists, they are seemingly less concerned with the way that a function affects a person's life roles (as a parent, office worker or carer, for example). Equally, they have given little attention to the task made possible by the particular bodily function. By this, I mean that physiotherapists have traditionally been less concerned with a person's ability to safely drink a cup of hot coffee and have been more concerned with their ability to fully flex their elbow and maintain good shoulder muscle stability. This is not to say, of course, that physiotherapists are entirely disinterested in these things, only that this has not historically been a large focus for their work.

Before I focus too closely on the physiotherapy view of function, it may be important to bear in mind that the concept of function extends well beyond the biological and social tasks and roles of patients, and infers any specific outcome brought about by a specific agent. So, it is possible to talk about the function of the heart, for example, being to pump blood around the body. This does not assume that this is the heart's only function or significance, since hearts can fail and be broken; it merely links a structure with an 'end'. In the same way, a hammer can be said to function as a tool to strike nails into wood. (It certainly does this better than a hot water bottle would.) It is possible to say then that something is implied or inherent in the structure of objects that predisposes them to certain functions.

Functions have been described as normative, meaning that they refer to a baseline standard 'from which actual traits can diverge' (Neander 1991, p. 454), and that they point to a future action or event that may or may not eventuate. Part of the problem with people's understanding of function is that it assumes that we have a heart, for instance, *because* we need to pump blood around our bodies. It assumes that there is a goal or endpoint inherent in the structure of the thing doing the functioning (White 1973). As if the biceps had been 'designed' to flex the elbow. But as Bigelow argued:

> The future outcome may be, in many cases, nonexistent. A structure may never be called upon to perform that function. The function of a bee's sting, for instance, is relatively clear; yet most bees never use their stings. Likewise teeth may never pulp food, just as nutcrackers may never crack nuts.
>
> (Bigelow & Pargetter 1987, p. 181)

So describing a function cannot entirely explain the character of the object performing the task (especially when it is more complex than a nutcracker). Functions lack causal, explanatory power, and this is particularly true when people talk about the functions of such complex assemblages as human beings. Not surprisingly perhaps, the function has come to mean many things when it is applied to people and it has become the subject of a great deal of thought and scholarship over the last century (White 1973; Preston 2013; Ariew et al 2002; Bigelow & Pargetter 1987). Social scientists explore the functionalism of social order; mathematicians use functions to help derive equations and predict outcomes; architects study function and form; philosophers explore the function of language and the mind (Wouters 2005). Physiotherapists study the function of the static and moving body.

Physiotherapists are concerned with functional movements and abilities; the purposeful, deliberate, productive movements in service of a particular role or task and the capacities and demands placed on the body in performing its everyday actions. There is a strong link here between function and rehabilitation. The WHO's definition of rehabilitation states that it involves 'the combined and coordinated use of medical, social, educational and vocational measures for training or retraining the individual to the highest possible level of functional ability' (World Health Organization 1969). Thus, function and functional ability lie at the very heart of rehabilitation. Unfortunately, the function becomes complex and messy when it applies to people. Just because an object *can* function in a particular way does not mean that it *will*. Every physiotherapist knows that the capacity for the optimal function does not necessarily equate to the reality of people's actual performance, and ideal function will all too often be influenced by people's less-than-optimal desires and needs (Cott et al 1995). And so, rehabilitation becomes fraught with difficulties, challenges and complexities that cannot be explained purely mechanistically.

Which raises a very important point for physiotherapists, because some of the mechanistic ways that have been used to explain how the body works in illness and injury may fail to take into account some of the subtle, subjective and complex reasons why patients sometimes ignore or resist health professionals' desire to see them achieve optimal function. Just because the quadriceps muscle *can* overcome a certain load in principle, for instance, does not mean it *will* in practice. The danger here is that mechanistic interpretations can presume a lack of effort or motivation on the part of the patient, or imply some malign intent. Thus, a patient in pain but with no visible signs of lower back injury on MRI, may be assumed to be malingering. And the person who has passed all of their biometric tests may be treated less empathically if they now feel the need to walk with a cane.

The tension that exists between what a body is capable of doing and what a person will do illustrates where the biomechanical idea of function reaches its limit, and the expertise of practitioners like physiotherapists become all important. In some respects, physiotherapists and others are needed simply *because* people defy the predictive logic of functionalism that is often applied to bodies.

Throughout the history of the profession, physiotherapists have shown their true worth when they have managed to achieve goals and outcomes that did not always follow the predictive simplicity of functional logic. It is interesting to reflect, therefore, on the energy and effort applied to the science of physiotherapy in recent years and how much of that has sought to establish the objective, value-neutral, predictive, evidence-based 'truth' of physiotherapy's effectiveness and how much has looked at what is required after biomechanical function has reached its explanatory limits. Perhaps the field of rehabilitation offers one of the best examples of this tension at work.

Like function, rehabilitation is prospective, future-orientated and, hence, teleological. Its focus is on a different future; a future that is privileged on the notion of a return to normal – either the norm for the person, or a socially-mandated norm. As Barnes argues, rehabilitation:

> . . . takes as its starting point the potential for reconstruction of the body and self after acquiring an impairment. While rehabilitation remains within a broad personal tragedy approach, it breaks new ground in laying emphasis on the possibility for a 'second chance'.
>
> (Barnes & Mercer 2003, p. 82)

Although physical rehabilitation is very diverse, with no clear single theoretical approach (Whyte 2008; Siegert et al 2005), it is inextricably linked to function and functional imperatives and offers the promise of recovery from personal tragedy. It would be extremely uncommon for a physical rehabilitation programme not to place functional movements and functional ability at the centre of its operational structure. Similarly, physiotherapists and others involved in physical rehabilitation work hard to ensure that patients accept the necessity of privileging functional goals and work hard to focus the patient's attention on the necessity of returning to 'normal'. In this way, the roles of functional rehabilitation appear to be to enable and empower, to reintegrate and facilitate a return to participation and to foster autonomy and independence.

Of course, there is a strong economic imperative underpinning physical rehabilitation. People with long-term injuries and chronic illnesses are often unable to contribute to the national economy; they are frequently in need of social welfare and subsidised medical expenses; they draw on the support of their family and friends that, in turn, affects *their* ability to be economically productive. Not surprisingly then, rehabilitation plays an important economic role in returning people to work at the lowest possible cost (Fadyl 2013). Autonomy and independence are therefore more than just worthy aspirations for the patient. They are also vital outcomes for society and critical interests of any health professional who wants to retain the State's support and patronage.

> Disablement makes an important contribution to the ideological crisis surrounding health and welfare in capitalist societies . . . because disabled people, being both deserving and expensive, pose a crisis of legitimacy for the

State in those capitalist societies which seek to be both profitable and civilised at the same time.

(Williams 1991, p. 517)

Beth Linker argues that this economic imperative largely explains the reasons why reconstruction aides (the forerunners of physical therapists) were established in America and Canada in WWI (Linker 2011). Economic drivers also help explain the intimate connection between physical rehabilitation and the development of outcomes measures, classification systems and taxonomies of impairment, handicap and functional capacity. All of these attempt to establish the person's level of disability in order that goals can be established and teleological predictions made as to the likely outcome of rehabilitation. At their most basic level, tools like the ICF, QALYs, DALYs and the myriad outcome measures now used in rehabilitation are human cost/benefit analyses that put the therapist on the side of the assessor and positions the patient as the one being 'weighed and measured'.

The economic imperative to return people to work or independent self-care has become pervasive, taken for granted and largely unquestioned by physiotherapists. But other professionals working in and around healthcare have challenged such assertions. Many people working in the mental health sector, for example, reject the idea of rehabilitation, arguing that ideas of recovery and insight are much more patient-centred, achievable and personally meaningful goals for patients (Finkelstein 2001; Halleck, & Witte 1977; Deegan 1988). Others have argued that the productive, ableist, normalising rhetoric of physical rehabilitation is actually harmful to the social relationships that now exist between disabled people and rehabilitation professionals (French 1994; Gibson 2016). Such questions remind us that we cannot adequately define rehabilitation without considering its economic social function. And we cannot think about the drive to normalisation, the need for people to be productive or the idea that chronic illness and disability are problems to be overcome without thinking about how these are underpinned by ideas of cost and value (Iezzoni 1996).

Although it has not been common for physiotherapists to debate or theorise such things, they have unknowingly been critical agents in furthering the connection being made between a person's social 'value' and their physical capacity. Having accepted the challenge of rehabilitating soldiers, disabled children, polio victims and others, physiotherapists were given access to patients in the public healthcare systems and the security of income that came with being government employees; they were allowed to treat patients over extended periods without needing direct charging; they were given protective legislation and support for training and they were given elite status as one of a handful of orthodox health professionals. In return, they addressed the government's health priorities, measured the efficacy of their interventions (in economic terms like return to active duty/work) and provided the justification for governments to show that the State was actively working for the health, wealth and happiness of the population. These are profoundly significant achievements, not only for the physiotherapy profession, but also for the development of healthcare in the 20th century. Creating the new field of rehabilitation also created new subjectivities for therapists and disabled people. It established healthcare systems that had not previously existed and created new ways of working. It defined a new vocabulary, replacing old language (spastic, handicapped, crippled) with new, less stigmatising phrases (optimal health, participation, engagement). It created powerful new subjectivities and social roles for disabled people and therapists, and generated debates around access to services, human rights and social responsibilities. These have been pivotal in shaping physiotherapy over the last century. How then, did this come about?

Physiotherapy and the history of rehabilitation

The history of rehabilitation in many ways mirrors the history of physiotherapy. In both cases, practices that would later be synonymous with physiotherapy and rehabilitation had already existed for many years. In physiotherapy, these were massage, electrotherapy, remedial gymnastics and hydrotherapy, and people have always sought to return people to active work or productive life (Krusen 1941; Gritzer & Arluke 1985). It is unlikely that there was a time, for instance, when it was not vital to return injured workers back to the fields, factories and forges. But a desire to return people and the presence of a few local doctors and healers does not constitute rehabilitation. So, like physiotherapy, we can only consider rehabilitation as a discrete entity when it became formalised, organised, professionalised and systematised, and whereas this process began for physiotherapists in the last decade of the 19th century, the process began for rehabilitation with the outbreak of World War I (McPherson et al 2015; Gritzer & Arluke 1985). As Anderson argues, '[W]e see the beginning of rehabilitative therapy . . . in the cooperation between doctors, voluntary associations or charities and the War Office' (Anderson 2011, p. 44).

Prior to 1914, the greatest group in need of any form of rehabilitation were those with acquired or congenital impairments. Poverty and poor nutrition, the presence of disfiguring communicable diseases, a lack of workplace safety and a lack of an effective medical system led to high rates of infant malformation and widespread disability, chronic pain and premature dependence. Despite repeated attempts to support this population, most notably through charitable aid and 'Poor Law' legislation (Lucey & Crossman 2014), the problem of disability remained a potent drain on national resources. In the absence of formal health and welfare services, attempts to manage disability centred on the family and the local community and, in some cases monasteries, asylums and rudimentary hospitals funded largely by benefaction. Where a family had some private wealth, a disabled child or invalided relative could be cared for. But the medical services available were piecemeal and haphazard, relying on sometimes frightening and brutal treatments like purging, poisoning, restraint and isolation (Baynton, & Davis 2013; Borsay 2005; Nielsen 2012; Stiker 1999).

Frank Krusen, one of the foremost historians of physical medicine, wrote in 1941 that 'Physical therapy is at once the newest and the oldest field of medical practice' (Krusen 1941, p. 9). The physical therapy commonly associated with the physiotherapy profession was once very much the province of medical specialists like Gilbert, Herschel, Charcot, Krueger, Jallabert, Duchenne and Preissnitz. Even some of the most famous scientists of modern history made contributions to physical therapy: Isaac Newton and Humphrey Davy's experiments with light; Benjamin Franklin, Nikola Tesla and Guillaume Duchenne's studies of electricity and Pehr Henrik Ling and John Harvey Kellogg's work on exercise, forming part of a renaissance of interest in the machinery of the body throughout the 17th, 18th and 19th centuries (Krusen 1941).

What makes these practices of physical medicine and therapy 'rehabilitative', however, is a concern for the social cost of long-term illness and disability and the availability of mechanisms – physical, economic, political and social – to better manage the 'burden' of disability. Prior to the Industrial Revolution, most disabled people were dispersed throughout the country, largely invisible to the State, which saw no real need to intervene to centralise care and support. Following the Industrial Revolution the necessity to develop a country's economic and political power became a major consideration, particularly for European and North American states. Now, the ability of a country to prosper depended on the capacity of its population to labour and fight, and a whole population of disabled people became a very visible sign of the country's weakness and vulnerability.

Prior to World War I, Nation States had a largely disorganised approach to rehabilitation. There were few surveys to assess the scale of the issue, little legislation to centralise disability support and little nationalised healthcare to enable a wide variety of care facilities and services to develop (Stiker 1999). The emphasis remained very much on public health measures to reduce accidents and disease with little established support for formal rehabilitation. Beth Linker shows how the decision to organise formal rehabilitation services in America was as much an economic decision as a therapeutic one. Following the American Civil War, the victorious soldiers of the Union were told that the 'grateful people will not hesitate to sanction any measures having for their object the relief of soldiers mutilated … in the effort to preserve our national existence' (President Andrew Johnson, quoted in Linker 2011, p. 2). But by 1916, it was estimated that 'the United States had spent over $5 billion on Civil War pensions, an amount that exceeded the price of the actual war' (Linker 2011, pp. 2–3). Clearly, some form of economic and social rehabilitation had become necessary, if only to relieve the burden of responsibility now weighing so heavily on the State.

Perhaps not surprisingly, given the cost of war reparations, the ongoing burden of overseas conflict, the growing problems of urban disease and poverty and a growing sense of State responsibility, attitudes towards society's 'dependents' – however noble – began to change. By the early part of the 20th century, Nation States began to weigh the cost of ongoing support and, drawing on Protestant virtues of hard work and independence, began to promote the idea that disabled people *wanted* opportunities to contribute to society, and wanted to cast off the 'bondage of idleness and despair' (Linker 2011, p. 3). The idea that all 'men' were capable of making a productive contribution to society, underpinned the creation of legislation like the 1916 *National Defense Act*, the 1918 *Soldier Rehabilitation*

Act and the 1920 *Vocational Rehabilitation Act* in America and the creation of the Ministry of Reconstruction in Britain, which created vocational training programmes, sheltered workplaces and employment assistance schemes to help injured soldiers return to civilian work (Bitter 1979, pp. 15–6). As Prime Minister David Lloyd George argued in 1917; 'you cannot maintain an A1 Empire with a C3 population' (Barclay 1994, p. 69)[2]. During a frantic period of social reform surrounding WWI, war veterans, crippled children, infirm elderly and those with long-term congenital or acquired injuries and illnesses were swept up in a wave of welfarist legislation that sought to redefine the nature of dependence and disability. Progressive reformers saw rehabilitation as a way to 'cope, economically, morally, and militarily, with the fact that millions of men had been lost to the war' (Linker 2011, p. 4).

Initially, much of the managerial responsibility for establishing rehabilitation programmes was given to the relatively small, unfashionable group of orthopaedic surgeons who, at the time, had only limited experience experimenting with childhood spasticity, scoliosis, fractures and other mechanical disorders. The need to cope with the overwhelming demand for acute and long-term care of the many thousands of injured servicemen created the need for a much more complex network of services. Importantly, it was this demand that provided the impetus for much of the North American physical therapy system today. As Beth Linker says:

> Rehabilitation legislation . . . led to the formation of entirely new, female-dominated medical subspecialties, such as occupational and physical therapy. The driving assumption behind rehabilitation was that disabled men needed to be toughened up, lest they become dependent of the state, their communities, and their families. The newly minted physical therapists engaged in this hardening process with zeal, convincing their male commanding officers that women caregivers could be forceful enough to manage, rehabilitate, and make an army of ostensibly emasculated men manly again.
>
> (Linker 2011, p. 6)

By 1919, at least 120,000 soldiers had passed through the American rehabilitation programme and such was the success of the scheme in returning men to active duty or productive occupations outside of the military that rehabilitation was considered a 'resounding success' (Linker 2011, p. 8).

Progress following WWI was slower, partly because of economic depression and the necessity to focus on other social health problems like influenza, polio and TB epidemics. As well as economic resources being spread more thinly, there was little available central funding to support the growth of professions like physiotherapy and occupational therapy, and for much of the inter-war years, the physiotherapy profession grew slowly. Progressive reformers also fought against the slow centralisation of healthcare, arguing that it might encourage people to be dependent, rather than developing people's sense of their own capacity for self-help. Welfarist legislation and the outbreak of World War II, however, reinvigorated calls to coordinate rehabilitation services, encouraged by the kinds of stable service offered by the doctors, nurses and masseuses, who had come to form the backbone of rudimentary rehabilitation services in many countries around the world.

Although the number of physiotherapy members of the CSMMG in Britain rose from 3,641 to 15,118 between 1918 and 1945, and there were some significant developments in organised healthcare, growth in other countries continued more slowly (Barclay 1994; Bentley & Dunstan 2006; Murphy 1995), physiotherapists continued to struggle for recognition – not least because they were the 'only medical service comprising both genders' (McMeeken 2015, p. 53). Pay rates remained low, competition from untrained massage therapists continued, and the profession's organising bodies were dominated by doctors. Physiotherapy remained largely also female dominated. Addressing the Society on 'Physiotherapy and the State' in January 1946,

> British Minister of Health Aneurin Bevan praised the members' work and promised to do all he could 'to assist in the development of physical medicine in this country'. He expressed concern about the shortage of physiotherapists, particularly men for heavy work in industry.
>
> (Barclay 1994, p. 153)

Bevan reported that 'only half [of] the Society's 14,500 members were active' and with fewer than 1,000 men it looked 'almost like a matriarchy' (Barclay 1994, p. 153). By comparison with nurses, 'who received two salary increases in 3 years . . . and were clothed, fed, housed, given pocket-money and training fees' (Barclay 1994, p. 177), physiotherapists received a 'miserly pittance' (Barclay 1994, p. 177). Similarly, in America, reconstruction aides fought for recognition. A survey conducted by the APA in 1940, showed that it had only 1,077 members, of which 493 currently worked in civilian hospitals and clinics, 154 in schools, 94 in physician's offices, 87 in private practice, 79 in facilities devoted to crippled children, 66 with the Visiting Nurse Associations and United States Public Health Service, nine with industrial organisations and 37 with the military – a notably small number given America's impending involvement in WWII (Murphy 1995, p. 106). Notwithstanding these impediments, physiotherapists built on the principles that had served them so well in the years leading up to WWI, using the new demands of the inter-war years to establish some new systems and structures that would not only consolidate their status, but would lay the foundations for the profession's focus on function and rehabilitation today.

The rapid growth of rehabilitation in the inter-war years necessitated five important developments in physiotherapy practice that might not have happened otherwise. These were:

1 The establishment of physiotherapy as an orthodox profession
2 The license to treat long-term illness, injury and disability
3 The new relationship created between therapist and patient
4 The drive to classification and categorisation
5 The move to active treatment

Exploring these in more detail, the establishment of physiotherapy as an orthodox health profession, or one that was firmly aligned with the operations and goals of the State, can be seen in the profession's role alongside doctors and nurses during both world wars. Physiotherapy's emerging orthodoxy can be seen in protective legislation created around the profession, like the 'gift' that Murphy called the 1935 *Social Security Act* (Murphy 1995, p. 99); the government-funded construction of large new physiotherapy departments (Stanton Woods 1943);[3] the favoured status given to those working with communicable diseases like infantile paralysis and polio (Murphy 1995, p. 95) and their incorporation into nationalised systems like the NHS, which almost extinguished private practice in England after 1950 (Barclay 1994, p. 207)[4]. McMeeken (2015) argues that physiotherapy's 'graduation to professional status with the health and medical services and at governmental level was assisted greatly by the relationships developed with serving medical men of influence'. Through these connections, physiotherapists were promoted as 'one of the leading pioneers in the development of the rehabilitation idea' (McMeeken 2015, p. 67).

Orthodox status came with some significant benefits, not least legal protections, centralised funding (paid for through general taxation), support for training and the competitive advantage that came with the State's tacit support for the profession's ways of thinking and practising. Orthodox status threw physiotherapy into its first interprofessional working relationships, building on the profession's traditional deference to medicine, with an array of new working relationships negotiated with nurses, occupational therapists, physical trainers and others. Physiotherapists became part of a large industrial rehabilitation machinery for the first time, and had to learn skills of delegation and resource distribution that had not been required before. History suggests that physiotherapists largely succeeded in adapting to these challenges, because the lessons learnt with the development of large-scale rehabilitation programmes transferred directly to the new national health systems that developed with the welfare reforms of the 1940s, 1950s and 1960s. In essence, as Julie Anderson argues, physiotherapists had learnt that 'rehabilitation could be applied to any given set of circumstances' (Anderson 2011, pp. 178–9).

The second development in physiotherapy practice relates closely to the profession's orthodox status, and it involves the shift from the masseuses' focus on acute and short-term treatments, to the management of long-term disability. Prior to the development of widespread rehabilitation programmes, masseuses were poorly paid for short-term physical therapies, usually delivered in the homes of those who could afford massage, passive treatment or electrotherapy (Barclay 1994). Occasionally, masseuses were employed at spa resorts or other therapeutic centres, but the vast majority of practitioners were independent, competing in a vast marketplace of other physicians, bone-setters, chiropractors and osteopaths, nurses and midwives, masseurs, electrotherapists and gymnasiarchs. With the advent of formal rehabilitation, and the acceptance of physiotherapists as *the* respected provider of physical rehabilitation services, practitioners gained immediate access to patients who would return for repeated appointments, sometimes over the course of many weeks or months. With care now funded centrally, there was no need to collect fees from patients, treatment could be provided purely on clinical grounds and the question of what the patient could afford was effectively removed. New therapeutic hierarchies were needed that differentiated categories of disability and stages of recovery and new therapeutic locations were required. Physiotherapists could concentrate on specific categories of illness or injury and could choose to work in the acute or longer-term rehabilitation sectors. This would pave the way for the kinds of specialisation that would later develop as a critical mass of therapists entered the profession after WWII.

Thirdly, the creation of large physiotherapy departments at the heart of the rehabilitation centre quietly overturned the relationship between therapist and patient. This mirrored a similar change that had occurred in medicine in the 19th century (Armstrong 1995). To begin with, patients now presented to the therapist, rather than the other way around, creating some radical possibilities for professional growth. But more than this; in return for the creation of comprehensive and highly expensive rehabilitation services, it was expected that patients would 'do their bit' and actively contribute to their own recovery. Although many quickly came to feel that free rehabilitation was the least they should expect given that they had fought for their country, or been made ill or injured through no fault of their own, patients were expected to attend appointments, commit to a programme of rehabilitation and make every effort to return to productive work or active duty (see the classic idea of the 'Sick Role' defined by Talcott Parsons (Parsons 1951)). In effect, patients were put into a position of enforced dependence on the services that society had generously provided. The complex tensions that subsequently emerged around the respective social roles taken up by disabled people and health professionals became the source of intense criticism. What is clear is that physiotherapists had no difficulty adopting a dominant, authoritative position and their efforts to discipline injured servicemen and others proved that they were ready to manage the 'pathetic mangled remains of shattered humanity' that now populated many rehabilitation departments (Anderson 2011, p. 51).

The fourth significant development in physiotherapy related to the necessity to classify and categorise impairments and disabilities so that the right care could be delivered at the right time to the right person. As rehabilitation services became more complex and dispersed, national, and sometimes international, classification systems were needed. Prior to 1950, most classification systems focused on assessments of functional incapacity, with the degree of disability measured by the percentage of the bodily impairment. Crude measures of 'time to recovery' were used as substitutes for the cost of care and basic measures of task performance were taken. But without much in the way of formal note taking, or a research culture to encourage people to record accurately, instrumental measurement remained piecemeal. Following WWII, 'men trained in modern business techniques, and who understood the impact of wasted man hours, entered the Services, and used their expertise to improve levels of efficiency, in line with theories of efficiency and man management. Rehabilitation was', as Anderson makes clear, 'the perfect setting for [these] theories to be played out' (Anderson 2011, p. 94).

Finally, one of the ways in which the prodigious number of people requiring rehabilitation could be managed was to shift from the traditional emphasis upon passive, labour-intensive treatments like massage and electrotherapy, towards group exercise. Perhaps because of Molly McMillan's experience with 'physical culture and corrective exercises' (Murphy 1995, p. 43), American physical therapists readily took to exercise as a mainstay of early rehabilitation. This was not the case in Britain, however. Despite the fact that in 1919, people like Major Souttar of Netley described 'machines to exercise 12 men at once which could be made from old packing cases and pulleys for 30 [shillings]' (*JISTM* 1919, p. 257), most members of the STM still favoured 'hands-on' techniques like massage and electrotherapy, and took a long time to adopt therapeutic exercise and return to the model of remedial gymnastics offered by Ling in the 19th century (see Figure 8.1). When they did place more emphasis on exercise after 1916, it retained an individualised focus. Olive Guthrie-Smith's work on slings and suspension, for example, required individual therapists to work with individual patients. Similarly, most texts that show Swedish Remedial Exercises (SRE) being practiced after 1918, emphasise one-to-one treatment (Prosser 1938; Vance 1936; Cutter 1934; Tidy 1932). It was not until WWII, under pressure from physical trainers, that British

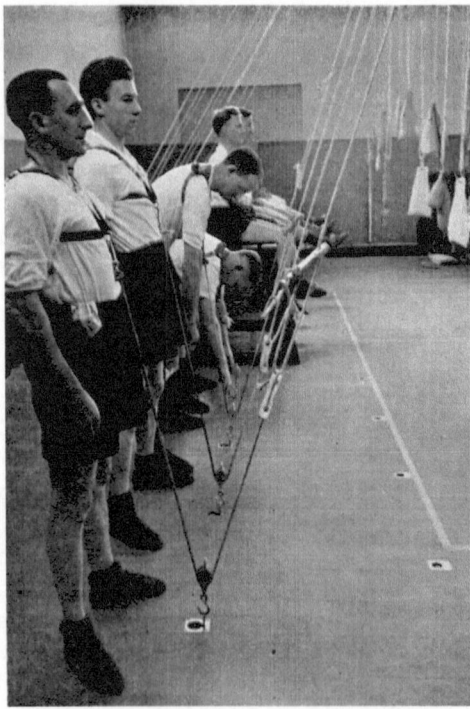

Figure 8.1 Group exercise at Berry Hill Hall. Guthrie Smith (1952) published by Elsevier.

physiotherapists adapted to the need to treat large groups of people simultaneously (Anderson 2011).

The significance of these five developments on today's physiotherapy practice cannot be overstated. Not only did these changes set the foundations for many of the clinical developments that were to follow, but evidence suggests that they were much more significant in shaping physiotherapy's scope of practice and social standing than any subsequent clinical development. To all intents and purposes, physiotherapists still draw on the same ideologies and practice modalities that they have always done. Techniques of tissue mobilisation and manipulation, therapeutic exercise, electro- and water-based therapies still underpin the majority of clinical approaches. And while physiotherapists have a battery of new methods of assessment and treatment and a whole array of outcome measures, journal articles and clinical manuals, any review of clinical texts from the 1920s, 1930s and 1940s will show that their approach to practice has remained remarkably consistent since then.

What *has* changed, however, is the context and location in which physiotherapy has operated. Becoming an orthodox profession granted physiotherapy extraordinary privileges. It also came with some demands that have been willingly accepted by physiotherapists but are not unproblematic. First and foremost, have been the demands to measure the effectiveness of their interventions. Although it is common to think of outcome measures as a relatively recent development (Stokes 2011), they are by no means new and the effectiveness of physiotherapy has been scrutinised by governments and other funders ever since the profession gained the formal support of the State[5]. But the recent development and extension of measurement thinking, in and around healthcare, is creating unprecedented levels of tension and, ironically, adding to people's uncertainty about the effectiveness of interventions. Perhaps these tensions can be best understood by examining the contested role that the ICF now plays in shaping physiotherapy practice in rehabilitation.

The classification of function and disability

Prior to the 1980s, most measures of therapeutic benefit used in rehabilitation were largely crude measures of functional capacity. Measures like range of movement and muscle strength, combined with simple, but relatively unreliable tests of task competence could be found in most clinical centres and the few standardised measures available (the Barthel Index, the Sickness Impact Profile and the Mini-Mental State, for example) were used in some specialist centres, but were far from widespread (Haigh et al 2001). Measures of work readiness, like the General Aptitude Test Battery, personality inventories and vocational interest measures had been common psychological batteries for many years (Bitter 1979), but rehabilitation texts prior to 1980 primarily concentrated on methods of assessment and treatment, common pathologies and, occasionally, the structural make-up of rehabilitation services rather than well defined, sensitive, reliable and valid tests. In Krusen, Kottke and Ellwood's seminal *Handbook of Physical Medicine and*

Rehabilitation (Krusen et al 1965), for example, not one of the 725-pages is devoted to outcome measures and although the concept of patient evaluation runs through the entire book, the focus is on the physician's clinical assessment, based on classical diagnostic techniques.

Physiotherapists working in rehabilitation had no profession-specific outcome measures, in part because their outcomes (recovery of movement and function, task improvement and return to work) were 'global' objectives shared by the whole rehabilitation team. With the exception of Australia, which granted first contact status to its physiotherapists in 1976 (Bentley & Dunstan 2006, p. 204), physiotherapy was still only offered after medical referral and so the impetus to account for the physiotherapist's contribution to rehabilitation was limited. And although physiotherapists had been actively researching their therapeutic efficacy for many years, the quality of their clinical trials remained low. Outcome measures certainly were used to assess the results of rehabilitation, especially measures of quality of life. Pioneering grounded theorist Anselm Strauss, for instance, explored the quality of life of people with chronic illness (Strauss 1975), while Campbell, Converse and Rodgers' pioneering text on *The Quality of American Life* (Campbell et al 1976) devoted large sections to the 'experience of work'. The whole culture of outcome measurement changed, however, with the development of the ICIDH.

Designed to complement the International Classification of Diseases (ICD) – which, since its inception in 1893, concerned itself with the causes of congenital disorders, acquired illnesses and injury – the ICIDH considered the *consequences* of impairment, disability and social disadvantage (de Kleijn-de Vrankrijker 1995). Published in 1980, the ICIDH created a 'common framework and a common language enabling better understanding and communication', it structured 'a certain area, thus facilitating policy formulation, data collection, statistics and documentation of information' (de Kleijn-de Vrankrijker 1995, p. 109). The benefits and possibilities of the ICIDH were immediately apparent to those working in rehabilitation. Its ability to connect the impairments that were at the heart of the acute medical management to ensuing disabilities increased the likelihood that well-conducted studies might show which interventions were effective and which were not. Added to this, the ability to link these outcomes to the handicap, or social disadvantage, allowed the patient's experience to influence what had previously been a medically-led process.

The ICIDH unquestionably privileged the medical view of disability, however. With 1009 items concerned with impairment, 338 items relating to disability and only 72 focusing on social disadvantage, it is perhaps easy to see in hindsight why many disabled people railed against its popularity among health professionals and researchers. The ICIDH presumed that disability was caused by handicap; that if you were blind, per se, this was the cause of your disability and social disadvantage. Disabled people and disability rights activists argued, however, that it was our attitudes and lived environments that caused disability, and that if we had not created a world that, at best, served the needs of the majority of people considered 'normal' and at worst actively marginalised others, people would experience much less 'disability'. The ICIDH effectively entrenched the idea that impairment caused disability and so social disadvantage and handicap were attributed to personal (bodily) flaws (Hammell 2006, p. 17). It took no account of the fact that 'many diseases, illnesses and injuries are produced by wars, violence, abuse, land-mines, poverty, malnutrition, unsafe work practices, pollution and through the unequal distribution of resources' (Hammell 2006, pp. 17–8). As Pfeiffer argued in 1998, 'when half the world goes to sleep hungry and hundreds of thousands of people face death every day, the ICIDH-2 (ICF) is pointless' (Pfeiffer 1998, p. 519).

The ICIDH and ICF that followed in May 2001, became the territory for a pro-longed and bitter conflict between disabled people and rehabilitation practitioners, who adopted the classification tools with remarkable enthusiasm (Hammell 2006, p. 19). Many disabled people argued that the ICIDH/ICF perpetuated disability and questioned the rights of doctors, physiotherapists and others to pronounce on questions of quality of life; 'determining where [disabled people] can park their cars . . . and whether they are capable of working' (Hammell 2006, p. 19). Finkel-stein called it 'able-bodied chauvinism' (Finkelstein 1999, p. 23).

At the heart of the criticism lay the power that the tools gave to health profes-sionals to classify and normalise ill and injured people; people with long-term illnesses; people displaying 'anti-social behaviours' and different world views; indigenous and minority groups that did not value social independence and isola-tion in the way that many in the West did; victims of workplace accidents, birth 'defects' and acquired illness and especially disabled people. Much of this power, and the source of much of the criticism, referred to the role that normalisation played in the ICIDH and ICF.

I discussed the way that physiotherapists and other orthodox health profession-als have traditionally normalised the body in Chapter 6. Normalisation has been a key feature of biomedicine since the 19th century (Wolfensberger et al 1972; Vehmas, & Watson 2016; Moll & Cott 2013; Gibson & Teachman 2012; Gibson 2014; Pickard 2011; Hansen, & Philo 2007; Guyton 1971). It refers to the need to distinguish between those who are healthy and those who are sick; those who are mad and those who are sane. It is important to remember here, that the ICIDH and ICF are simply classification systems, albeit rather ambitious international classi-fications of function, disability and health. They are, nonetheless, systems designed to enable health professionals to classify people's level of impairment, functional ability and level of social participation. They are designed to follow the biomedical principles of objectivity and value-neutrality closely, while folding into the tool a range of more nuanced economic, social and cultural contexts, political and legal considerations. Notwithstanding this ambition and complexity, the ICIDH and ICF remain tools used primarily for classifying the consequences of injury and illness.

The ICIDH and ICF are, therefore, primarily tools for health professionals. As Karen Whalley Hammell argues, 'they do not have any inherent benefit for those being coded and classified' (Hammell 1998). While it is perfectly reasonable to argue that through such classification systems disabled people's needs have been identified, which has, in turn, allowed for services to be provided and resources directed towards people's care and support, critics have argued that this has come at considerable cost: '[T]he ICF fosters a view of disabled people as catalogues of deficits and deprivations rather than as people with various abilities and resources' (Hammell 2006, p. 18). The ICF pays little, if any, attention to the environmental and social determinants of health – things that are known, through extensive high quality evidence, to be perhaps the greatest causes of long-term illness and disability (see, e.g. Davidson 2014; Keleher & MacDougall 2011; Baum & Fisher 2014; Marmot et al 2008). The ICF promotes the idea that disability is a medical issue and a problem to be overcome. This marginalises other ways of understanding the experience of disability and places enormous power in the hands of those who control and administer the classification system and benefit from its adjudications.

This might be acceptable if the ICF confined medical interventions to purely medical matters, but it gives medical professionals enormous power to pronounce on people's quality of life and, to define this, again, in medical terms. Like their sister measures, QALYs and DALYs, the ICIDH and ICF legitimate and codify the belief that the quality of one's life is defined by one's medically-assessed health status (Hammell 2006, p. 26). Perhaps it is not surprising then that many disability rights activists have vehemently critiqued the use of these tools and the practitioners who use them. Rachel Hurst has argued that no other marginalised group in society has experienced such intrusive scrutiny as disabled people (Hurst 2000) and David Pfeiffer believes that the ICF represents proof that healthcare professional 'are part of the advantaged class' who will always value their social status and power over the voices of disabled people (Pfeiffer 2000, p. 1079).

As part of the orthodox public healthcare system, physiotherapists are very much seen by disabled people as part of the 'advantaged class' and practitioners have used tools like the ICIDH, ICF, QALY and DALY as justification for their therapeutic interventions. Tools that classify (ab)normality carry with them an implicit need to fix or remedy what is abnormal and physiotherapists have long traded on their purported ability to return people to normal. This ability has its origins in the very first data that was captured on the return to active duty of soldiers injured in battle in WWI. Jean Barclay, for instance, describes how one early rehabilitation centre constructed in Eastbourne in 1915 had 32 masseuses and masseurs treated 20–25 patients a day. To manage the enormity of the work, each masseuse would have four patients under treatment at any one time ('two perhaps on heat treatment, a third on ionisation or interrupted current with a metronome and a fourth being massaged'). Through this system, an average of '580 patients were discharged each month, of whom 80% were considered fit enough to return to the front, 7% were unfit for general service; 6% were transferred to Command Depots, and 7% returned to hospital' (Barclay 1994, p. 66).

Physiotherapists showed long ago that they were able to meet the challenge of returning people to active duty and vocational competence (Holmes 2007), but a number of authors have asked a more fundamental question about their role; a question that is rarely ever asked by physiotherapists themselves: why is it that rehabilitation necessarily follows on from the classification of someone as 'disabled'? Why is it, for instance, that once an assessment tool identifies some-one as 'special', they are not paraded through the streets, celebrated and given special civic privileges? Why is it necessary to reject their existing self-image, capability and form, while insisting that they should 'develop' into something 'other'? Why is the idea of returning the person to 'normal' – an idea with a much more fluid and changeable history than we would like to believe – so important? Why is it so important that people 'develop'? Why is independence, and not dependence, the goal? These questions form not only the backbone of a great deal of critical scholarship for many writers in disability studies, but perhaps even more significantly, they are now questions being asked by physiotherapists and rehabilitation scholars themselves.

These questions have recently been posed by Barbara Gibson in her book *Reha-bilitation: A Post-Critical Approach* (Gibson 2016). Gibson, a physiotherapist working in rehabilitation, asks some radical and fundamental questions about rehabilitation and the part that professions like physiotherapists are playing in its design and delivery. In this book and elsewhere, Gibson asks why we construct disability as a 'lack' of something rather than a normal variation; why we use a 'medical model' when its focus is on 'fixing' the disabled body; why we privilege upright, bipedal walking and why we have such a limited view of mobilities, par-ticularly in an age when movement is seen in so many different forms (Gibson 2006, 2014; Gibson et al 2007, 2009, 2010, 2012; Gibson & Teachman 2012).

In many ways Gibson's critique resonate closely with those of people like Thomas Abrams (2014, 2016a, 2016b), Sally French (French & Swain 2008; Swain et al 2003a, 2003b), Dan Goodley (Goodley 2014; Goodley et al 2015; Goodley & Runswick-Cole 2014), Karen Whalley Hammell (2004, 2015a, 2015b), Annmarie Mol (Law & Mol 2002; Mol 2002), Christina Papadimitriou (2008a, 2008b), Margrit Shildrick (Shildrick 2009; Price & Shildrick 1998; Shildrick & Price 1996), Myriam Winance (Winance 2006, 2014; Winance et al 2010) and others. These authors echo Ivan Illich's classical description of the mid-twentieth century the 'Age of Disabling Professions'; an age when people had problems, experts had solutions and scientists measured imponderables such as 'abilities' and 'needs' (Illich 1977). As physiotherapist Sally French argues;

> Disability was perceived by the state and by the medical profession and ther-apists as being a problem located within the individual. This was harmful to disabled people as it placed the emphasis on changing *them* rather than on adjusting the physical and social environment to accommodate their needs.
>
> (French & Swain 2008, p. 49)

Physiotherapists, along with other orthodox health professions, helped to make disabled people less visible in the community and helped to remove the stigma associated with visible displays of deviance (French & Swain 2008, p. 50). They treated children's rickets with ultraviolet light rather than championing the need for access to better food, reductions in poverty and better living conditions for children. And they successfully avoided 'social unrest among large groups of disaffected men' (French & Swain 2008, p. 47), when they returned from war. Seen in these terms, it is not unreasonable to see physiotherapists are very much on the orthodox medical side of the ledger; working to meet the needs of the State, constantly striving to remain relevant, using rehabilitation (and, by extension, disabled people and people with long-term injuries and illness) as their subject matter in an ongoing quest for social capital.

This is not to say, of course, that physiotherapists and other rehabilitation professionals are ill-meaning, manipulative and callous. Far from it. Many, many disabled people's lives have been turned around by the kindness, skill and dedication of physiotherapists and others who have worked tirelessly to help people live more comfortable, capable and satisfying lives. What it does do, however, is to remind us, first and foremost, that physiotherapy is an organ of the State and that its continued relevance relies on its ability to respond to governmental concerns, even if these place the needs of disabled patients second (Bourke 1996). It reminds us that there may be subtle, perhaps unseen drivers of physiotherapy practice that can be opposed to those of the profession's patients (French & Swain 2008, p. 47). And that physiotherapists' 'entrenched practices' of impairment-based rehabilitation (Gibson 2016, p. 137), have perhaps masked the fact that 'the rehabilitation professions are not apolitical and that the rehabilitation process is often irrelevant, meaningless and useless' for disabled people (Hammell 2006, p. 5). Why then has rehabilitation been such a powerful driver of physiotherapy practice and how has physiotherapy used it as a vehicle to shape its current professional identity? To answer this question, I need to return to the idea of the body-as-moving-machine I left in Chapter 7.

Function, rehabilitation and physiotherapy

In the previous chapter, I discussed how it had been necessary to develop an approach to the moving body; an approach that was consistent with the idea of the body-as-machine, but took into account the fact that the kinds of bodies seen by physiotherapists could not be understood only as the object of passive treatments, but that an approach to the moving body was also necessary. Adopting specific approaches to posture and movement gave physiotherapists the opportunity to widen their field of interest and apply their biomechanical lens to a broader range of practices. This was what I called the idea of the body-as-*moving*-machine.

The idea of the body-as-moving-machine also had its limitations, however. Although it was sufficient as a way to codify many of the more dynamic physiotherapy interventions, it did not extend far enough into the realm of people's everyday lives to be meaningful to patients. Its emphasis on a detached, depersonalised approach to treatment took no account of the fact that the patient before the therapist was not simply assemblages of body parts, but was, in fact, a real person, with their own social roles and occupations, leisure interests, passions and desires, values and beliefs. This was a radical realisation for the profession's leaders and occurred as the profession became embroiled in the first struggles to establish rehabilitation systems after WWI. In hindsight, it may be possible to see that without an approach to practice that made a direct connection with people's everyday lives, physiotherapy would not have been able to establish itself much beyond a small, marginal organisation. Physiotherapy's relatively passive approach to the body-as-machine might have satisfied the medical profession, but it would not have been able to command the respect and support of the State and thereby benefit from the century of legislative and financial support.

I would argue that rehabilitation gave physiotherapy its ultimate purpose: to return people back to work and meaningful activity. It showed that massage, mobilisation and movement, electrotherapy, hydrotherapy and gymnastic exercise could be more than just as an indulgence of the luxuried classes. It gave physiotherapists longer and more secure employment and spoke to government health priorities, like the need to return injured servicemen to The Front; the need to give disabled children as much independence as possible and the need to manage the sequelae of long-term injuries and illnesses. Physiotherapists did this not by rejecting the body-as-machine idea, but rather adapting it to the body's capacity for function. Importantly, this was far from the idea of the embodied, holistic, socially constructed person many physiotherapists explore today (Sivertse & Normann 2014; Sviland et al 2012; Covington 2015; Standal & Engelsrud 2013; Bullington 2009a, 2009b; Nicholls & Gibson 2010). This was not the idea of a 'person' at all, as much as a functioning body: a body engaged in, so called 'normal', purposeful activity; working, playing sport, attending school and doing housework. The person's individual history, personal experiences, culture, social networks, beliefs and values were not considered. Even the person's age was only relevant in as much as it provided a context for the age-related norms as a confounding variable in the assessment of the person's functional performance. This was an animated image of the body-as-machine. In effect, a body-as-*functioning*-machine.

Borrowing once more from the legacy of Pehr Henrik Ling and the graduates of the Royal Central Institute of Gymnastics, physiotherapists adopted a rigid system of normalised movement patterns as the basis for their approach to functional movement and rehabilitation. This approach would be the cornerstone of movement therapies in physiotherapy for the next half-century and relied on what were called 'fundamental' and 'derived' positions. The principal consideration for physiotherapists was how to define, capture and delimit functional movement. Physiotherapy was no place for freeform, expressive movement. This could not be assessed and measured. It served no clear purpose and, worse still, resonated with ideas of pleasure and sensuality that were anathema to the profession. Functional movements needed to be governed and the therapeutic manipulation of the movement needed to be under the control of the therapist.

The use of fundamental and derived positions drew directly from the work of the RCIG in the 19th century, with its emphasis on pedagogical and, especially, military gymnastics. They were divorced from everyday social activities such as walking, sitting on the bus, or leaning at the bar. They were 'fundamental' positions from which all other movements, and importantly muscle actions, could be derived.

They were defined by the body's 'attitude'; its position relative to the ground or the apparatus that the therapist positioned the body upon. Almost every basic body position that could be used as the starting point for therapeutic movement had a description which the therapist learnt to apply with precision. For example, L.L. Despard, in her 1916 *Text-Book* [sic] *of Massage and Remedial Gymnastics*, describes the Standing Fundamental Position as follows:

- Heels together.
- Feet forming an angle of not more than 45°.
- Knees fully extended.
- Hips fully extended.
- Head erect and chin slightly drawn in.
- Shoulders held well back and drawn down.
- Arms hanging by the sides.
- Fingers not fully extended.
- Palmar surface of the hand in contact with the lateral side of the thigh.
- This position innervates all the muscles of the back of the neck, the back, extensors of the leg and thigh, and others. It expands the chest and maintains the pelvis in a *correct* position.

(Despard 1916, pp. 226; emphasis preserved)

Starting positions such as these provided the template from which a number of 'derived' positions and subsequent movements could be performed (see Figure 8.2).

Although these approaches to the functional movement have now been super-seded, they remained the most common and familiar way for physiotherapists to learn SRE for the next 5o years (Kleen 1918; Prosser 1938; Guthrie-Smith 1952)[6]. Using simplistic, gender-neutral stick figures or formally staged photographs, all the pleasure and sensuality of movement has been removed. Everything is control and technique. Notably, none of the physical therapy texts used by doctors from the time incorporated this approach, since physiatrists were not engaged in the kinds of mass rehabilitation performed by the rehabilitation aides and physiother-apists (Stewart 1925; Stafford 1928; Sampson 1923).

The value of such approaches in the early days of the rehabilitation movement were that they offered a system that could be communicated, trained and assessed easily; they could be taught to massed ranks of new students coming for training; they could be used on large groups of recovering servicemen (see Figure 8.3) and they could be scaled up so that only one instructor was needed for many patients. They resonated with the profession's desire to move away from 'passive' treat-ments like massage and electrotherapy; they enhanced the therapists 'power' over the patient, who became the active subject of the therapist's gaze and they differ-entiated the therapist further from doctors and nurses.

SRE allowed every functional movement to be defined by categories of body position. Every action could be analysed for its ability to locate the body in space and the body work involved in each movement could be calculated as a sum of forces. They provided the same consistency, measurability and objectivity as

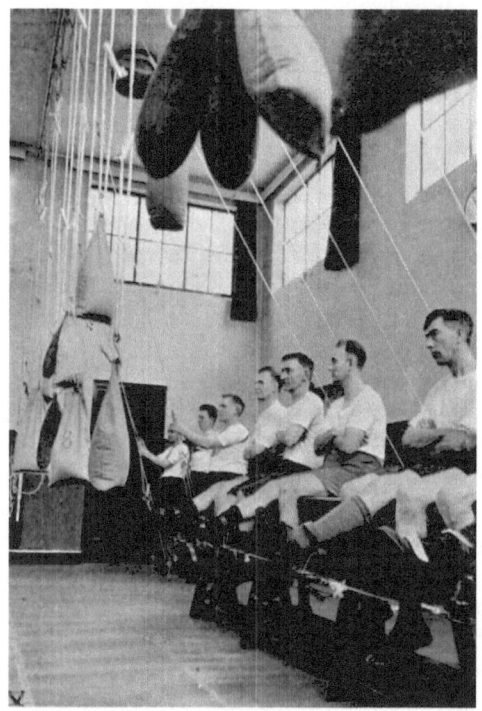

Figure 8.2 Group exercise. Guthrie Smith (1952) published by Elsevier.

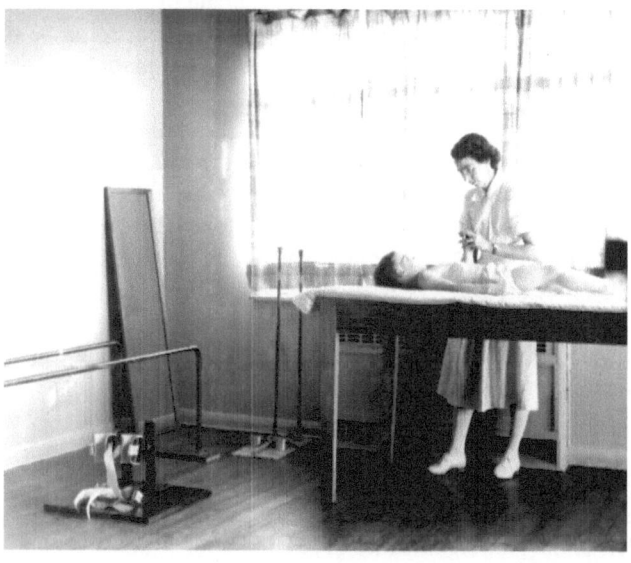

Figure 8.3 Image showing standard treatment bed. Author's personal collection.

electrotherapy, but transferred the responsibility for the work to the patient, who was increasingly expected to 'own' his recovery. SREs distracted the kinds of unregulated, free movement that people engaged in in everyday life, from the public sphere, and recast them 'in the neutral language of science . . . transforming [them] into [a] *technical* problem for the sole attention of specialists and experts' (Hook 2003, p. 610).

Although sounding somewhat old-fashioned now, the use of fundamental and derived positions in SRE gave physiotherapists their first profession-specific vocabulary and provided the foundations for language that still pervades physiotherapy today. Accessory joint mobilisation and Mobilisation with Movements (MWM) undertaken by manipulative therapists, active and assisted muscle work in spinal cord injury, associated movements seen in recovery from stroke, the ergonomic assessment of time and motion, constraint-induced movement therapy and exercise rehabilitation all resonate with the same principles established by physiotherapists in the inter-war years[7].

From the 1950s onwards, specialisation brought new approaches to functional movement. Paediatric, cardiorespiratory, water-based, sports and neurological physiotherapists were particularly interested in exploring new forms of therapeutic exercise and movement but in many ways, the twin principles of regulated movement and biomechanical function remained the basis of the body-as-functioning-machine. This is no more evident than in the growth in assessment measures and tests developed by the profession. Prior to 1980, the focus of assessment concentrated on tests of physical flexibility (Harris 1969), assessments of motor performance (Stockmeyer 1965), prognostic tests of nerve excitability (Snow 1940), tests of functional performance (Smith 1954) and tests of muscle function (Graham & Kramer 1954). In some cases, these tests were idiosyncratic to physiotherapy, but measures always referred back to a biomechanical standard that could be referenced to a medical standard. They also reinforced the notion that physiotherapy could be objective, value-neutral and scientifically credible: an ideal that very much resonated with the therapist's approach to the body-as-functioning-machine.

After 1980, there was a dramatic increase in the number and diversity of tests, ranging from measures of mobility, physical activity, impairment and impact scales, measures of satisfaction and quality of life (Stokes 2011). Not only do physiotherapists have to account for their assessment and treatment strategy, but in many jurisdictions they are primary healthcare providers. As first contact professionals, physiotherapists are increasingly being asked to account for their efficiency and effectiveness, and most are now battling to defend their hard-won orthodox status and privileged state-support. The profession's traditional approach to function and rehabilitation, which sought to locate the cause of disability in the patient's physical impairment, is being increasingly challenged and more personally-relevant and socially connected justifications for the continued support of physiotherapy are being sought.

The key to understanding the significance of rehabilitation in physiotherapy lies in the fact that it showed that physiotherapists could work in service of the State: that physiotherapists were willing to use their skills of physical assessment and treatment to address the health problems of returned servicemen, children with polio and cerebral palsy; the elderly suffering the effect of strokes, Parkinson's disease and multiple sclerosis; people with chronic arthritis, amputees and those recovering from joint surgery. But physiotherapy could also now be relevant to coal miners, office workers and stay-at-home parents. It was a therapy amenable to the entire population. In effect, physiotherapy turned from being 'inward' to 'outward' facing.

The rehabilitation movement saw physiotherapists adapt quickly to the work demands of the WWI treatment units and showed that physiotherapy's own model of practice was malleable and infinitely scalable, however many therapists were needed to meet demand. Training was efficient; therapists were proficient; practitioners knew their place and were suitably deferential to doctors; they showed little political militancy and they were safe and could be trusted. Almost without needing to alter a single principle set down by the profession's founders, physiotherapists were able to connect into national pressure to take responsibility for people's health and wellbeing, and this connection between the profession and the State would become the driving influence shaping physiotherapy practice for the next 100 years. The question being posed now, though, is whether the adaptations made by the profession in the past will be sufficient for the population in the future.

Closing words

In this chapter, I have argued that physiotherapy's approach to the rehabilitation of functional movement, which began in WWI, created a practice template that defined the profession for the next 100 years. Broadly, it comprised four elements:

1   A focus on the body-as-functioning-machine, connecting 'modern' physiotherapy practice with the lessons learnt from its past while also giving the therapist a distinctive professional focus.
2   An attention to assessment, particularly that which identifies physical impairment and evaluates outcomes.
3   A practical purpose in applying transformative treatment to restore normal function and ability, without the need for the movement to be necessarily 'purposeful'; rather the focus was on movements that conformed to anatomical and physiological norms.
4   A constant teleological attention towards the goal of practice, which was to serve the interests of the State and to adapt the first three principles to prevailing health concerns.

From these four basic principles, it is possible to see that rehabilitation has clearly had a profound effect on physiotherapy's present ways of thinking about and practising physiotherapy. In this chapter, I have argued that this is as much to do with the way physiotherapy is situated within the social world of healthcare as it is to do with any radical change in the nature of physiotherapy practice itself.

Rehabilitation has created opportunities for growth and social capital that were unimaginable while the profession concentrated on individual, fee-paying patients, largely being treated in their own homes. The model that existed for physiotherapy practice prior to 1914 would never have seen the kinds of growth in numbers (and thereby, influence), seen in physiotherapy over the last century. Fortunately for the profession at large, physiotherapy was, once again, in the right place at the right time. Having proven its legitimacy in the 20 years before WWI, masseuses rapidly became pivotal in the government's reconstruction efforts in the years following the war and maintained their influence as publicly funded healthcare became a national issue in the 1930s and 1940s. After WWII, the profession's focus turned to greater specialisation, technological development and a greater focus on outcome measures and research, but the main assessment and treatment modalities remained largely the same.

Perhaps the greatest influence rehabilitation has had in physiotherapy, however, is in the way it positioned physiotherapy in relation to the State. Realising that state service provided opportunities to grow the profession and receive reliable financial and legislative support, physiotherapists moved to establish their profession as a key arm in government rehabilitation efforts. Significantly, this meant adopting approaches, techniques and ideologies that positioned them in complex and difficult relationships with disabled people and critics of orthodox rehabilitation. The emphasis physiotherapists placed on the external, third-party assessment and validation of impairment, function and participation through tools like the ICF; the importance the profession gave to taxonomic classification and statistical distribution of 'normal' function and the power to apply statistically-based judgement that it claimed for itself, have proven to be problematic for many of the patients that physiotherapists claim to serve.

Significantly, '[t]he opposition expressed by disabled people to the ICIDH and ICF classifications has been in stark contrast to their almost universal and uncritical acceptance by researchers' (Hammell 2006, p. 19). This is, perhaps once again, an expression of the physiotherapy paradox because few physiotherapists are really aware of much of this criticism and little of it ever makes its way into physiotherapy discussions of the costs and benefits of the latest assessment techniques, therapeutic interventions or outcome measures. This may be because physiotherapists want to retain their professional status and social capital as the provider of orthodox physical rehabilitation services, and to achieve this it is felt that the profession needs to demonstrate its efficacy by identifying and normalising the functional capacities of ill, injured and disabled people. If this is the case, then the field of physical rehabilitation provides a perfect platform for that work. But the approach currently taken by physiotherapists is a model based on deficits; on the artificial 'othering' of people by virtue of their physical (in)capacity; the labelling of people as disabled based on externally determined physical impairments and the relative ignorance of the environmental and social factors that are significant for disabled people themselves. Time will tell whether physiotherapists can adapt, once again, to the changing needs of the population and the State and retain its privileged status and social capital.

In the section that follows, I bring together a range of arguments from the previous eight chapters, to consider how the history of the profession and its approach to important concepts like posture and movement, function and rehabilitation are influencing present-day education, practice, regulation and research. I then move to close the book with a final chapter asking whether we are, indeed, experiencing the end of physiotherapy.

Notes

1 For an excellent overview of the the the ICF, see Bickenbach (2012).
2 During World War I, soldiers were graded from A1 (the most suitable for physical training) to C3. Someone graded C3 would have a significant disability that would make them suitable only for clerical or sedentary work (see McDermott 2011).
3 The pressure of work generated by the need to rehabilitate large numbers of casualties from WWI has been discussed in Chapter 4. The need for improved post-war facilities and new departments is illustrated by these two accounts from Murphy (1995);

> Base Hospital #8 [was] a 20,000-bed hospital complex located in the little village of Saveney, near Nantes. Here 30 PTs put in 14-hour days, six and seven days a week, as wave after wave of orthopedic cases were brought in from distant hospital field stations to be stabilized before being sent home. In November 1918, Saveney reconstruction aides clocked 3,440 treatments; in December, 5251 treatments. The heavy work load continued to grow as 1919 began. In January PTs delivered care to 6,568 patients; in February 6,528; in March, 4,333; and in April, 4,218. Much of the work carried on in the overseas hospitals was 'massage of fractures,' according to PT and head aide Susan Hills.
>
> (Murphy 1995, pp. 59–60)

> And "While the overseas physical therapy reconstruction aides had rendered important service behind the battle lines, it was only when the bulk of orthopedic cases were brought home and distributed to specialized hospital centers that the Physiotherapy Division of the Reconstruction Department came into its own. In the two years following the Armistice, state-side reconstruction aides gave some 86,000 disabled soldiers more than 3 million treatments".
>
> (Murphy 1995, pp. 60–1)

4 To fully understand the power of the National Health Service on the structure and design of the physiotherapy profession, it is worth reflecting on the rhetoric put forward by the British Minister of Health Aneurin Bevan at the time.

> When asked about private practitioners – 'whose prospects looked bleak', Bevan replied that 'he would not stop anyone who "wished to buy the services of a doctor or the services of a physiotherapist, or to buy the services of an osteopath, or a nature healer, herbalist, or Christian Scientist' but that he was 'quite frankly more concerned about the fate of the millions of people who needed treatment than about the physiotherapists themselves'.
>
> (Barclay 1994, p. 153)

5 See, for example, the measures of return to active duty and rates of return to work used during and after WWI and II to justify further spending on physical rehabilitation (Lanska 2016; McDougall 1943; Johnstone 1943; Linker 2007; Anderson 2011; Elsey 1997; Eldar & Jelić 2003; Verville 2009; Carden-Coyne 2007; Linker 2011).
6 Physiotherapy's more recent daliance with pilates offers an insight into the ways that fundamental and derived positions continue to infleunce practice. Tellingly, Joseph

Pilates developed his approach to rehabilitation by using bed springs as resistance devices while he was a prisoner of war in WWI. In a nod to the desire to control movement, Pilates called his method 'contrology' (Pilates & Miller 1945).

7 For a clear indication of how fundamental and derived positions have influenced rehabilitation outcome measures, see the ICF categorisation of mobility as: d410 Changing basic body position; d415 Maintaining a body position; d420 Transferring oneself; d450 Walking; d455 Moving around and d460 Moving around in different locations (Stokes 2011, p. 57).

References

Abberley, P., 1993, Disabled people and 'normality', in J. Swain, V. Finkelstein & S. French (eds.), *Disabling barriers – enabling environments*, Open University, London, pp. 107–15.

Abrams, T., 2014, Flawed by Dasein?: Phenomenology, ethnomethodology, and the personal experience of physiotherapy, *Human Studies*, 37(3), pp. 431–46.

Abrams, T., 2016a, Cartesian dualism and disabled phenomenology, *Scandinavian Journal of Disability Research*, 18(2), pp. 118–28.

Abrams, T., 2016b, *Heidegger and the politics of disablement*, Palgrave Macmillan, London.

Anderson, J., 2011, *War, disability and rehabilitation in Britain: 'Soul of a nation'*, Manchester University Press, Manchester.

Ariew, A., Cummins, R. & Perlman, M., 2002, *Functions: New essays in the philosophy of psychology and biology*, Oxford University Press, Oxford.

Armstrong, D., 1995, The rise of surveillance medicine, *Sociology of Health & Illness*, 17(3), pp. 393–404.

Barclay, J., 1994, *In good hands: The history of the Chartered Society of Physiotherapy 1894–1994*, Butterworth Heinemann, Oxford.

Barnes, C. & Mercer, G., 2003, *Disability*, Polity Press, Cambridge, UK.

Baum, F. & Fisher, M., 2014, Why behavioural health promotion endures despite its failure to reduce health inequities, *Sociology of Health & Illness*, 36(2), pp. 213–25.

Baynton, D.C. & Davis, L.J., 2013, Disability and the justification of inequality in American history, in *The disability studies reader*, Routledge, New York, pp. 17–33.

Bentley, P. & Dunstan, D., 2006, *The path to professionalism: Physiotherapy in Australia to the 1980s*, Australian Physiotherapy Association, Melbourne, Australia.

Bickenbach, J.E., 2012, The international classification of functioning, disability and health and its relationship to disability studies, in N. Watson, A. Roulstone & C. Thomas (eds.), *Routledge handbook of disability studies*, Routledge, London, pp. 51–66.

Bigelow, J. & Pargetter, R., 1987, Functions, *The Journal of Philosophy*, 84(4), pp. 181–96.

Bitter, J.A., 1979, *Introduction to rehabilitation*, Mosby, St. Louis, MO.

Borsay, A., 2005, *Disability and social policy in Britain since 1750: A history of exclusion*, Palgrave Macmillan, Basingstoke.

Bourke, J., 1996, *Britain and the Great War*, Reaktion Books, London.

Bullington, J., 2009a, Being body: The dignity of human embodiment, in L. Nordenfelt (ed.), *Dignity in care for older people*, Wiley-Blackwell, Chichester, UK, pp. 54–76.

Bullington, J., 2009b, Embodiment and chronic pain: Implications for rehabilitation practice, *Healthcare Analysis*, 17(2), pp. 100–9.

Campbell, A., Converse, P.E. & Rodgers, W.L., 1976, *The quality of American life: Perceptions, evaluations, and satisfactions*, Russell Sage Foundation, New York.

Carden-Coyne, A., 2007, Ungrateful bodies: Rehabilitation, resistance and disabled American veterans of the first world war, *European Review of History/Revue Européenne d'Histoire*, 14(4), pp. 543–65.

Cleather, J., 1995, *Head, heart and hands – The story of physiotherapy in Canada*, Canadian Physiotherapy Association, Toronto, Canada.

Corbett, J., 1997, Independent, proud and special: Celebrating our differences, in L. Barton & M. Oliver (eds.), *Disability studies: Past, present and future*, The Disability Press, Leeds, pp. 90–8.

Cott, C.A., Finch, E., Gasner, D., Yoshida, K., Thomas, S.G. & Verrier, M.C., 1995, The movement continuum theory of physical therapy, *Physiotherapy Canada*, 47(2), pp. 87–95.

Covington, J.K., 2015, Developing a professional embodiment of movement: A situational analysis of physical therapist clinical instructors' facilitation of students' emerging integration of movement in practice, Doctoral thesis, North Carolina State University, Raleigh, NC.

Cutter, I.S., 1934, History of physical therapy and its relation to medicine, in *Principles and practice of physical therapy*, W.F. Prior, Hagerstown, MD, pp. 1–115.

Davidson, A., 2014, *Social determinants of health: A comparative approach*. Oxford University Press, Oxford.

Deegan, P.E., 1988, Recovery: The lived experience of rehabilitation, *Psychosocial Rehabilitation Journal*, 11(4), p. 11.

DePoy, E. & Gilson, S.F., 2011, *Studying disability: Multiple theories and responses*, Sage, Los Angeles, CA.

Despard, L.L., 1916, *Text-book of massage and remedial gymnastics*, Oxford University Press, London.

Eldar, R. & Jelić, M., 2003, The association of rehabilitation and war, *Disability and Rehabilitation*, 25(18), pp. 1019–23.

Elsey, E., 1997, Disabled ex-servicemen's experiences of rehabilitation and employment after the first world war, *Oral History*, pp. 49–58.

Escorpizo, R., 2015, Summary and way forward: Doing more of ICF in physical therapy, *Physiotherapy Research International*, 20(4), pp. 251–3.

Fadyl, J.K., 2013, Re-working disability: A Foucauldian discourse analysis of vocational rehabilitation in Aotearoa New Zealand, Doctoral thesis, Auckland University of Technology, Auckland, NZ.

Finkelstein, V., 1999, A profession allied to the community: The disabled peoples trade union, in E. Stone (ed.), *Disability and development: Learning from action and research on disability in the majority world*, The Disability Press, Leeds, pp. 21–4.

Finkelstein, V., 2001, The social model of disability repossessed, *Manchester Coalition of Disabled People*, Manchester, UK, pp. 1–5.

French, S., 1994, The disabled role, in S. French (ed.), *One equal terms: Working with disabled people*, Butterworth Heinemann, Oxford, pp. 47–60.

French, S. & Swain, J., 2008, *Understanding disability: A guide for health professionals*, Elsevier/Churchill Livingstone, Edinburgh.

Gibson, B.E., 2006, Disability, connectivity and transgressing the autonomous body, *Journal of Medical Humanities*, 27(3), pp. 187–96.

Gibson, B.E., 2014, Parallels and problems of normalization in rehabilitation and universal design: Enabling connectivities, *Disability and Rehabilitation*, 10.3109/09638288.2014.891661.

Gibson, B.E., 2016, *Rehabilitation: A post-critical approach*, Taylor & Francis, New York.

Gibson, B.E. & Teachman, G., 2012, Critical approaches in physical therapy research: Investigating the symbolic value of walking, *Physiotherapy Theory and Practice*, 28(6), pp. 474–84.

Gibson, B.E., Young, N.L., Upshur, R.E. & McKeever, P., 2007, Men on the margin: A Bourdieusian examination of living into adulthood with muscular dystrophy, *Social Science & Medicine (1982)*, 65(3), pp. 505–17.

Gibson, B.E., Darrah, J., Cameron, D., Hashemi, G., Kingsnorth, S., Lepage, C., Martini, R., Mandich, A. & Menna-Dack, D., 2009, Revisiting therapy assumptions in children's rehabilitation: Clinical and research implications, *Disability and Rehabilitation*, 31(17), pp. 1446–53.

Gibson, B.E., Nixon, S.A. & Nicholls, D.A., 2010, Critical reflections on the physiotherapy profession in Canada, *Physiotherapy Canada*, 62(2), pp. 98–100, 101–13.

Gibson, B.E., Carnevale, F.A. & King, G., 2012, 'This is my way': Reimagining disability, in/dependence and interconnectedness of persons and assistive technologies, *Disability and Rehabilitation*, 34(22), pp. 1894–9.

Goodley, D., 2014, *Dis/ability studies: Theorising disablism and ableism*, Routledge, London.

Goodley, D. & Runswick-Cole, K., 2014, Becoming dishuman: Thinking about the human through dis/ability, *Discourse: Studies in the Cultural Politics of Education*, 37(1), pp. 1–15.

Goodley, D., Runswick-Cole, K. & Liddiard, K., 2015, The DisHuman child, *Discourse: Studies in the Cultural Politics of Education*, 37(5), pp. 770–84.

Graham, M.A. & Kramer, H., 1954, Revised method for obtaining atrophy-hypertrophy measurements, *Journal of the American Physical Therapy Association*, 34, p. 557.

Gritzer, G. & Arluke, A., 1985, *The making of rehabilitation a political economy of medical specialization, 1890–1980*, University of California Press, Berkeley, CA.

Guthrie-Smith, O.F., 1952, *Rehabilitation, re-education and remedial exercise*, Bailliere, Tindall & Cox, London.

Guyton, A.C., 1971, *Basic human physiology: Normal function and mechanisms of disease*, W.B. Saunders Company, Philadelphia, PA.

Gzil, F., Lefeve, C., Cammelli, M., Pachoud, B., Ravaud, J.F. & Leplege, A., 2007, Why is rehabilitation not yet fully person-centred and should it be more person-centred?, *Disability and Rehabilitation*, 29(20–21), pp. 1616–24.

Haigh, R., Tennant, A., Biering-Sørensen, F., Grimby, G., Marincek, C., Phillips, S., Ring, H., Tesio, L. & Thonnard, J.-L., 2001, The use of outcome measures in physical medicine and rehabilitation within Europe, *Journal of Rehabilitation Medicine*, 33(6), pp. 273–8.

Halleck, S.L. & Witte, A.D., 1977, Is rehabilitation dead?, *Crime & Delinquency*, 23(4), pp. 372–82.

Hammell K.W., 1998, From the neck up: Quality in life following high spinal cord injury, doctoral thesis, University of British Colombia, Vancouver, Canada.

Hammell, K.W., 2004, The rehabilitation process, in M. Stokes (ed.), *Physical management in neurological rehabilitation*, Elsevier, Edinburgh, pp. 379–92.

Hammell, K.W., 2006, *Perspectives on disability & rehabilitation: Contesting assumptions, challenging practice*, Churchill Livingstone/Elsevier, Edinburgh.

Hammell, K.W., 2013, Client-centred practice in occupational therapy: Critical reflections, *Scandinavian Journal of Occupational Therapy*, 20(3), pp. 174–81.

Hammell, K. W., 2015a, Client-centred occupational therapy: The importance of critical perspectives, *Scandinavian Journal of Occupational Therapy*, 22(4), pp. 237–43.

Hammell, K.W., 2015b, Quality of life, participation and occupational rights: A capabilities perspective, *Australian Occupational Therapy Journal*, 62(2), pp. 78–85.

Hansen, N. & Philo, C., 2007, The normality of doing things differently: Bodies, spaces and disability geography, *Tijdschrift voor Economische en Sociale Geografie*, 98, pp. 493–506.

Harris, M.L., 1969, Flexibility: Review of the literature, *Physical Therapy*, 49, p. 591.

Holmes, J., 2007, *Vocational rehabilitation*, Blackwell, Oxford.

Hook, D., 2003, Analogues of power: Reading psychotherapy through the sovereignty – discipline–government complex, *Theory & Psychology*, 13(5), pp. 605–28.

Hurst, R., 2000, To revise or not to revise? *Disability & Society*, 15(7), pp. 1083–7.

Iezzoni, L.I., 1996, *When walking fails: Mobility problems of adults with chronic conditions*, University of California Press, Berkeley, CA.

Illich, I., 1977, *Disabling professions*, Marion Boyars, London.

JISTM, 1919, Editorial, *Journal of the Incorporated Society of Trained Masseuses* (May).

Johnstone, R.T., 1943, Industrial participation in the rehabilitation of the war wounded, in W.B. Doherty & D.D. Runes (eds.), *Rehabilitation of the war injured, a symposium*, Philosophical Library, New York, pp. 541–7.

Keleher, H. & MacDougall, C., 2011, *Understanding health: A determinants approach*, Oxford University Press, Australia.

Kleen, E.A., 1918, *Massage and medical gymnastics*, J. & A. Churchill, London.

de Kleijn-de Vrankrijker, M.W., 1995, The international classification of impairments, disabilities, and handicaps (ICIDH): Perspectives and developments (Part I), *Disability and Rehabilitation*, 17(3–4), pp. 109–11.

Krusen, F.H., 1941, History of physical therapy, in *Physical Medicine: The employment of physical agents for diagnosis and therapy*, W.B. Saunders, Philadelphia, PA.

Krusen, F.H., Kottke, F.J. & Ellwood, P.M., 1965, *Handbook of physical medicine and rehabilitation*, W.B. Saunders, Philadelphia, PA.

Lanska, D.J., 2016, *War neurology*, Karger Publishers, Basel.

Law, J. & Mol, A. (eds.), 2002, *Complexities: Social studies of knowledge practices*, Duke University Press, Durham, NC.

Linker, B., 2005, The business of ethics: Gender, medicine, and the professional codification of the American Physiotherapy Association, 1918–1935, *Journal of the History of Medicine and Allied Sciences*, 60(3), pp. 320–54.

Linker, B., 2007, Feet for fighting: Locating disability and social medicine in First World War America, *Social History of Medicine*, 20(1), pp. 91–109.

Linker, B., 2011, *War's waste: Rehabilitation in World War I America*, University of Chicago Press, Chicago, IL.

Lucey, D.S. & Crossman, V., 2014, *Healthcare in Ireland and Britain from 1850: Voluntary, regional and comparative perspectives*, Institute of Historical Research, London.

Marmot, M., Friel, S., Bell, R., Houweling, T.A. & Taylor, S., 2008, Closing the gap in a generation: Health equity through action on the social determinants of health, *The Lancet*, 372(9650), pp. 1661–9.

McDermott, J., 2011, *British military service tribunals, 1916–1918: 'A very much abused body of men'*, Manchester University Press, Manchester.

McDougall, J.B., 1943, Problems involved in the rehabilitation of the disabled in England, in W.B. Doherty & D.D. Runes (eds.), *Rehabilitation of the war injured, a symposium*, Philosophical Library, New York, pp. 607–13.

McMeeken, J., 2015, Australian physiotherapists in the First World War, *Health & History*, 17(2), pp. 52–75.

McPherson, K., Gibson, B.E. & Leplège, A., 2015, Rethinking rehabilitation: Theory, practice, history – and the future, in K. McPherson, B.E. Gibson & A. Leplège (eds.), *Rethinking rehabilitation: Theory and practice*, CRC Press, FL, pp. 3–206.

Mol, A., 2002, *The body multiple: Ontology in medical practice*, Duke University Press, Durham, NC.

Moll, L.R. & Cott, C.A., 2013, The paradox of normalization through rehabilitation: Growing up and growing older with cerebral palsy, *Disability and Rehabilitation*, 35(15), pp. 1276–83.

Murphy, W., 1995, *Healing the generations: A history of physical therapy and the American Physical Therapy Association*, Greenwich Publishing, Lyme, Connecticut.

Neander, K., 1991, The teleological notion of function, *Australasian Journal of Philosophy*, 69(4), pp. 454–68.

Nicholls, D.A. & Gibson, B.E., 2010, The body and physiotherapy, *Physiotherapy Theory and Practice*, 26(8), pp. 497–509.

Nielsen, K.E., 2012, *A disability history of the United States*, Beacon Press, Boston, MA.

Oliver, M., 1998, Theories in healthcare and research: Theories of disability in health practice and research, *BMJ*, 317(7170), pp. 1446–9.

Papadimitriou, C., 2008a, Becoming en-wheeled: The situated accomplishment of re-embodiment as a wheelchair user after spinal cord injury, *Disability & Society*, 23(7), pp. 691–704.

Papadimitriou, C., 2008b, It was hard but you did it: The co-production of work in a clinical setting among spinal cord injured adults and their physical therapists, *Disability and Rehabilitation*, 30(5), pp. 365–74.

Parsons, T., 1951, *The social system*, Free Press, New York.

Patston, P., 2007, Constructive functional diversity: A new paradigm beyond disability and impairment, *Disability and Rehabilitation*, 29(20–21), pp. 1625–33.

Pfeiffer, D., 1998, The ICIDH and the need for its revision, *Disability & Society*, 13(4), pp. 503–23.

Pfeiffer, D., 2000, The devils are in the details: The ICIDH2 and the disability movement, *Disability & Society*, 15(7), pp. 1079–82.

Pickard, S., 2011, Health, illness and normality: The case of old age, *BioSocieties*, 6(3), pp. 323–41.

Pilates, J.H. & Miller, W.J., 1945, *Return to life through contrology*, Christopher Publishing House, Boston, MA.

Preston, B., 2013, *A philosophy of material culture: Action, function, and mind*, Routledge, New York.

Price, J. & Shildrick, M., 1998, Uncertain thoughts on the disabled body, in J. Price & M. Shildrick (eds.), *Vital signs: Feminist reconfigurations of the biological body*, Edinburgh University Press, Edinburgh, pp. 224–49.

Prosser, E.M., 1938, *Manual of massage and movement*, 1st ed., Faber and Faber, London.

Sampson, C.M., 1923, *Physiotherapy technic: A manual of applied physics*, C.V. Mosby, St. Louis, MO.

Shildrick, 2009, *Dangerous discourses of disability, subjectivity and sexuality*, Palgrave Macmillan, Basingstoke, UK.

Shildrick, M. & Price, J., 1996, Breaking the boundaries of the broken body, *Body and Society*, 2(4), pp. 93–113.

Siegert, R.J., McPherson, K.M. & Dean, S.G., 2005, Theory development and a science of rehabilitation, *Disability and Rehabilitation*, 27(24), pp. 1493–501.

Sivertsen, M. & Normann, B., 2014, Embodiment and self in reorientation to everyday life following severe traumatic brain injury, *Physiotherapy Theory and Practice*, pp. 1–7.

Smith, L.K., 1954, Functional tests, *Journal of the American Physical Therapy Association*, 34, p. 19.

Snow, W.B., 1940, Electrical testing of muscles and nerves, and determination of its value in prognosis and treatment, *Journal of the American Physical Therapy Association*, 20, p. 358.

Solli, H.M. & da Silva, A.B., 2012, The holistic claims of the biopsychosocial conception of WHO's international classification of functioning, disability, and health (ICF): A conceptual analysis on the basis of a pluralistic-holistic ontology and multidimensional view of the human being, *Journal of Medical Philosophy*, 37(3), pp. 277–94.

Stafford, A.M., 1928, *A handbook of physio-therapy*, Medical and Surgical Publishing Company, Chicago, IL.

Standal, F. & Engelsrud, G., 2013, Researching embodiment in movement contexts: A phenomenological approach, *Sport, Education and Society*, 18(2), pp. 154–66.

Stanton Woods, R., 1943, Rehabilitation in the British emergency medical service, in W.B. Doherty & D.D. Runes (eds.), *Rehabilitation of the war injured, a symposium*, Philosophical Library, New York, pp. 416–23.

Stewart, H.E., 1925, *Physiotherapy: Theory and clinical application*, Paul B. Hoeber, New York.

Stiker, H.J., 1999, *A history of disability*, University of Michigan Press, Chicago, IL.

Stockmeyer, S., 1965, Pattern for evaluation in the assessment of motor performance, *Physical Therapy*, 45, p. 453.

Stokes, E.K., 2011, *Rehabilitation outcome measures*, Churchill Livingstone, Edinburgh.

Strauss, A.L., 1975, Chronic illness and the quality of life, in *Chronic illness and the quality of life*, Mosby, St. Louis, MO.

Sviland, R., Råheim, M. & Martinsen, K., 2012, Touched in sensation – moved by respiration, *Scandinavian Journal of Caring Sciences*, 26(4), pp. 811–19.

Swain, J., French, S. & Cameron, C., 2003a, *Controversial issues in a disabling society*, Open University Press, Buckingham, UK.

Swain, J., French, S. & Cameron, C., 2003b, Practice: Are professionals parasites?, in *Controversial issues in a disabling society*, Open University Press, Buckingham, UK, pp. 131–40.

Tidy, N.M., 1932, *Massage and remedial exercises in medical and surgical conditions*, 1st ed., John Wright & Sons, Bristol.

Vance, E.B.M., 1936, Physiotherapy in the treatment of injuries in general and orthopaedic practice, *British Medical Journal*, 1(3914), pp. 53–7.

Vehmas, S. & Watson, N., 2016, Exploring normativity in disability studies, *Disability & Society*, 10.1080/09687599.2015.1120657.

Verville, R., 2009, *War, Politics, and philanthropy: The history of rehabilitation medicine*, University Press of America, Lanham, MA.

White, L., 1973, Functions, *Philosophical Review*, LXXXII, pp. 139–68.

Whyte, J., 2008, A grand unified theory of rehabilitation (we wish!), The 57th John Stanley Coulter Memorial Lecture, *Archives of Physical Medicine and Rehabilitation*, 89(2), pp. 203–9.

Williams, G.H., 1991, Disablement and the ideological crisis in healthcare, *Social Science & Medicine (1982)*, 32(4), pp. 517–24.

Wilson, H.C., 1995, *Physiotherapists in war*. Honor C. Wilson, Adelaide.

Winance, M., 2006, Trying out the wheelchair: The mutual shaping of people and devices through adjustment, *Science, Technology & Human Values*, 31(1), pp. 52–72.

Winance, M., 2014, Universal design and the challenge of diversity: Reflections on the principles of UD, based on empirical research of people's mobility, *Disability and Rehabilitation*, 36(16), pp. 1334–43.

Winance, M., Mol, A., Moser, I. & Pols, J., 2010, Care and disability: Practices of experimenting, tinkering with, and arranging people and technical aids, in *Care in practice. On tinkering in clinics, homes and farms*, Transcript Verlag, pp. 93–117.

Wolfensberger, W.P., Nirje, B., Olshansky, S., Perske, R. & Roos, P., 1972, *The principle of normalization in human services*. National Institute on Mental Retardation, Toronto.

World Health Organization, 1969, WHO expert committee on medical rehabilitation, Technical Report Series, No. 419, available from http://apps.who.int/iris/bitstream/10665/40738/1/WHO_TRS_419.pdf, accessed 18 July 2016.

Wouters, A., 2005, The function debate in philosophy, *Acta Biotheoretica*, 53(2), pp. 123–51.

Part III

9 Implications for education, practice, regulation and research

Introduction

In this third section of the book, my task is to bring together the concepts, ideas and questions from the first nine chapters and answer the question 'so what?' Having detailed the evidence in support of my argument that the conditions that were once so favourable to physiotherapy's growth and expansion are now threatening its future, I need to look at how these tensions are playing out in the places and ways that physiotherapy is taught, practiced, regulated and researched.

In this chapter, I return to one of the book's key arguments and argue that the physiotherapy paradox is affecting physiotherapy's curricula and methods of teaching and learning, the most mundane aspects of everyday practice, the profession's values and ideals and its aspirations to be an evidence-based, orthodox and significant healthcare profession. While the tensions now being experienced by the profession have their roots in the seemingly abstract changing economy of healthcare, the effects are being felt in hospital departments and community-based private clinics each and every day. The evidence is increasingly clear that if profession's like physiotherapy wish to remain relevant and significant in healthcare services of the future, they must adapt to the opportunities and threats now confronting them. Fortunately, clear signs are appearing that some physiotherapists are increasingly aware of the ruptures taking place across the entire field of health and social care and there is a sense that everyone now understands that the future holds something different from the image of physiotherapy that was constructed in the late 19th century and operationalised in the 20th. Many physiotherapists are engaging with professional debates and discussions about their professional futures, be it at local branch meetings, national policy forums or international conferences.

Notwithstanding this growing awareness, my argument throughout has been that physiotherapy creates a kind of casual docility in its practitioners who are taught to ignore all of the 'other' causes of health and illness, focusing only on the body-as-machine; taking a dispassionate, detached and value-neutral view of the world and the people within it; de-sensualising what are otherwise highly 'sensual' human encounters so that physiotherapy practice can be considered legitimate, orthodox and safe. These strategies have been enormously significant in shaping the profession's past. Indeed, it is unlikely that the profession would have made it into the 20th century had it not been for these approaches. But the self-same strategies that have been embedded so deeply in the ways of thinking about and practising physiotherapy are now threatening to have the opposite effect, by reducing the profession's relevance to the public and the State; undermining its authority; limiting its influence and marginalising through normalisation those that the profession purports to serve. So, this book is particularly directed towards those physiotherapy practitioners who have been deliberately trained *not* to think about such things, and have not had the opportunity to reach into a world beyond their profession and sense the challenges and opportunities that now reside beyond their clinic door.

In this chapter, I explore four locations where the tensions currently surrounding physiotherapy are operating: in education, practice, regulation and research. Most readers will identify with at least one of these and perhaps more. I tackle some of the challenges facing lecturers and students as they try to prepare for the uncertainty and instability of future practice. I look at the ways that practitioners are having to change as a result of external pressures that they are ill equipped to deal with and argue – perhaps counterintuitively – for the benefits of regulation and against professional autonomy. Finally, I look at the remarkable expansion in clinical research, perhaps the biggest growth area in physiotherapy over the last two decades, and explore how this is shaping physiotherapy's future. To begin with, though, I want to return to the place where physiotherapy practice begins – in the colleges and universities where proto-therapists are moulded to meet the demands of future practice.

Education

In 2005, I wrote an article with my colleague Dr Peter Larmer titled 'Possible Futures for Physiotherapy' (Nicholls & Larmer 2005). In the paper, we argued that physiotherapy education had arrived at a crossroads: that the profession was unprepared for the future; that the population's needs had changed; that physiotherapy had largely remained the same and that it was up to physiotherapy schools, in their role as progenitor of the next generation of practitioners, to do something about it. Acknowledging that 'Physiotherapy is a first class profession with a strong heritage and a distinctive brand identity', we argued that it might not 'retain this status if it fail[ed] to address the challenges of healthcare reform of the future' (2005, p. 59). We proposed four possible responses, each of which carried positive and negative implications for the profession:

1   Watching and waiting;
2   Returning to the body-as-machine;
3   Complete renaissance;
4   Integration of old and new.

A summary of the advantages and disadvantages of each position laid out in the we can be seen in Table 9.1.

Table 9.1 Possible models for physiotherapy development

	Model	Rationale	Possible Advantages	Possible Disadvantages
1	Watching and waiting	No dramatic changes would be made to the direction, philosophy or strategies employed by physiotherapists. Political changes would be monitored for their potential impact upon the profession and significant change would be limited to material content and specifics of education and practice, without the major philosophical changes advocated by some new health policy rationalities. Changes would be permissible as long as they correlated with the philosophical tenets of the profession; namely the 'body-as-machine'.	Watching and waiting would give the profession time to accommodate to changes in health care and decide its best course of action. This would allow for a period of critical reflection upon the influences of health care policy, both nationally and internationally. Physiotherapists have been reluctant to explore the philosophical basis of their practice – possibly because they have felt secure in their identity, and this would not be challenged by this option.	Cycles of change are slow (most notably in education) and change may happen without us. Legislative change may force us to be reactive rather than proactive. Conversely, it could see the profession stagnate, appear intransigent or reactionary. We could become isolated and weakened by our lack of responsiveness and we could find others encroaching more and more on territory that we could rightfully claim as our own. We could easily be portrayed as having an 'old-world' view of health.
2	Enhancing the body-as-machine	This option would see a strengthening of the biomechanical base that established physiotherapy as a distinctive and highly regarded profession in the health sector. It would involve an outright rejection of some of the more liberal health policy initiatives in favour of a strengthening of core physiotherapy values of 'body-as-machine'. It would value the historical relevance of a profession that has remained relatively true to its founding beliefs in the face of major social and political change. It would argue that the profession will outlive current health care policy predilections and offer an authentic model of professional practice built on over a century of health care experience.	It reinforces physiotherapy's strong profile. Physiotherapists remain a visible presence and offer patients a service with distinct parameters. It builds on a health care philosophy that is well established. It reinforces a highly marketable, authoritative practice philosophy and it relies on a longer history than the current political opinion. It would be easy for physiotherapists to identify, market and position themselves in future health care services, and it would provide a clear message that health care practices need not be at the mercy of contemporary political rhetoric.	As a model of health, the 'body-as-machine' is universally criticised for its ability to depersonalise health care. Physiotherapy has become diverse and is struggling to maintain coherent connections with its heritage; many colleagues may see a move back to body-as-machine as regressive. It may also be seen as conservative and intransigent in the face of strong evidence that the health care marketplace has changed. If contemporary political opinion becomes established, we will have been left behind or displaced by other health disciplines aggressively marketing for areas we have relinquished.

(Continued)

Table 9.1 (continued)

	Model	Rationale	Possible Advantages	Possible Disadvantages
3	Rejecting the body-as-machine	Here physiotherapists acknowledge that the health care environment requires a new approach. The traditional technical rationalism of physiotherapy would be rejected, possibly for a new 'holistic' approach, or one directly in line with prevailing health policy. Physiotherapists adopt a more flexible 'generalist's' approach to rehabilitation. This acknowledges that the health care environment demands a new approach from physiotherapists. This would represent a renaissance for the profession involving the adoption of practice philosophies entirely new to physiotherapy.	Brings physiotherapy into line with other professions looking to develop population-based models of health and disability. It has the advantage of positioning physiotherapy as a responsive, proactive professional group able to respond to the new legislative environment. Physiotherapists would be confident in their ability to contribute effectively, and in many cases lead, rehabilitation services. It would open physiotherapy to new possibilities – social, political, cultural, environmental, psychological dimensions of health and illness that have been a problem for the body-as-machine focus of the past. It would be more inclusive to the diversity of modern physiotherapy practice.	Physiotherapy would effectively lose its unique identity and becomes one of a number of generic health workers. It might hypothetically result in the disappearance of physiotherapy as a discrete profession. Physiotherapists would need to adopt philosophies previously alien to them. Inter-professional rivalries might be exacerbated due to the further blurring of boundaries between professions. It would also force us to separate the new profession from its discrete heritage. In effect, we would migrate to new territory. Physiotherapy might be seen as professionally weak, in not resisting the current political fashion.
4	Integration	This would involve bringing the strengths of physiotherapy into a more 'holistic', population-based approach to health care. Amplifying the biomechanical basis of our curricula and placing it in the context of the enormous potential offered by the health care environment of the future. It rejects the need to see the various models of health care as discrete and argues for the integration of social, political, cultural, environmental, psychological and biological philosophies of health. It would involve a complete revision of the basis of physiotherapy education and an enormous investment in the development of people equipped to facilitate new modes of learning.	Brings the best of the body-as-machine and integrates it into a more holistic model of health. Physiotherapists have the potential to become the 'complete' rehabilitation worker. This would inevitably lead to the development of therapists with a much greater scope for diversification and the potential to become a key player in the rehabilitation work of the future. It would equip therapists with a much more holistic appreciation of the patient's health problems and enable them to address a much greater array of problems. It would encourage a more critical perspective upon physiotherapy and relate well to the academic development of physiotherapy as a profession.	Curricula may become overloaded. Differences between philosophies of health may present a confused model of physiotherapy. It would be a considerable shift in the nature of physiotherapy education. Some content currently taught would have to be lost to accommodate a mass of new material. A diverse, complicated, theoretically dense undergraduate degree may force us to consider alternative models of education (e.g. graduate entry). Philosophically, it might be more difficult to locate the logical centre of physiotherapy practice – since there would be a shift to problematize the body-as-machine, whilst at the same time retaining much of this content. There is the distinct possibility of confusion as well as overload.

Although we presented four possible responses, we knew that Option 4 – the integration of the old and the new – was the one most likely to enhance the profession's social capital, serving the needs of the public, the profession *and* health funders into the future (Nicholls et al 2009a). Deciding to have a more inclusive curriculum and actually implementing it though, are two quite different things. Many physiotherapy education programmes around the world have attempted new curriculum designs, but few have shown signs of significant deviation from the norm. Indeed, most are remarkably similar. Despite significant cultural and regional variations, physiotherapy programmes around the world bear all the hallmarks of curricula stretching back to the early part of the 20th century. With a strong Anglo-American influence; a systems-based, linear, heavily assessed programme of study and relatively standard progression from biomechanical theory to clinical practice, few programmes, despite their exit qualification, show signs of radical variation. Finding exemplars to guide us to a new curriculum, therefore, proved harder than we had first thought. Some of the reasons for this became clear as we began the process.

Our first challenge was to develop a curriculum that incorporated new and, in many cases, unfamiliar material. We knew no way to successfully 'blend' this new material into the traditional 'core' physiotherapy subjects and had few exemplars to help us manage the transition. We quickly realised that there was no easy fit between the biomechanical sciences and subjects drawn from the humanities, philosophy and sociology. Most were unfamiliar subjects for our teaching staff who were mainly experts in their respective clinical fields and so confident in their subject areas. But they, themselves acknowledged that they had little to offer when it came to subjects like embodiment, cultural studies and social theory. We tried bringing in non-physiotherapy lecturers to teach the new material, or freed up teachers with broader interests to teach the new material. Perhaps unsurprisingly, it proved difficult for these people to assert themselves in teams of highly experienced colleagues who had a long history of teaching physiotherapy traditionally. The teachers struggled to assert their material and gain the credibility long afforded to subjects like patient assessment, orthopaedics and exercise rehabilitation. Their content was often subtly and often unknowingly undermined by some of the senior staff who perhaps resented giving up space in the curriculum to this new material. They argued persuasively that the traditional 'core' physiotherapy subjects were being increasingly squeezed and the students were not being well prepared for clinical practice.

We found that many of our teachers struggled to move away from traditional approaches to teaching and learning. Most of our physiotherapy lecturers had come into teaching as experienced clinicians or researchers and few had a strong background in educational theory and practice. Most were employed because they were experts in neurological physiotherapy, for example, not because of their deep knowledge of Dewey, Freire or Vygotsky. Naturally, they saw that their role as specific to their area of clinical specialty: they were a champion for cardiorespiratory physiotherapy, paediatrics or women's health. Perhaps they too saw the influx of new non-clinical material as a threat to their ability to represent their subject speciality.

And so, as curriculum space became increasingly competitive, lecturers pushed for more time for their material, arguing that there was now not enough space for the students to learn all they needed.

As our curriculum became more and more unwieldy, and the demands on the students grew, symptoms of a curriculum under stress became evident. But lacking the depth of knowledge of educational theory, principles and practice we struggled to know what to do. Complaints came in from students who were struggling to balance the demands of the programme with the need to remain mentally and physically healthy, the need to work and have some sort of social life. Staff complained that the students were not as resilient as they used to be, or that they lacked the educational preparation. We toyed with new mechanisms to short circuit the necessity for deep, slow learning, including higher entry requirements and hot-house qualifications (where students complete their course in a shortened time by foregoing traditional summer breaks), but decided against moving to a masters- or doctoral-entry programme that had become increasingly common in Australia, North America and the UK. Perhaps in this instance, our desire to cling to traditional approaches to learning over-rode our desire to follow the example set by our colleagues overseas.

This is not to say, however, that our curriculum experiment was not a success. We learnt many things and engaged in a six-year long conversation around physiotherapy curricula. We explored ways of integrating the best of the old with some new approaches to practice, learning and teaching. And the staff committed thousands of hours to providing the best possible learning experience for the students. There was no doubt, however, that staff often defaulted to traditional modes of delivery (lectures, tutorials and practical demonstrations) when faced with the volumes of content that they believed the students should learn. And despite some real innovations in content delivery (including the development of apps for mobile devices), the predominant pedagogy in our programme remained didactic, with content 'delivered' to students in what Paulo Freire called a process of 'banking' (Freire 1970). Despite its many drawbacks – not least the fact that it privileges compliance, uniformity and predictability over creativity, individuality and subjectivity – students continued to experience a content heavy, information-rich and industriously assessed curriculum (Araya & Peters 2010; Kemmis & Smith 2008; Higgs et al 2013).

This is not, of course, to suggest that physiotherapy educators are deliberately perpetuating out-of-date archetypes or actively discouraging students from being critical, mindful or humanistic. I would argue, however, that the traditional physiotherapy curriculum favoured by schools all over the world – including those that have moved to masters- and doctoral-entry – ensures that all of the conditions are in place for this to happens. And perhaps this is not surprising, after all it is not part of the profession's culture for its teachers to engage in the lengthy study of educational theory and practice, and the profession's practice ideology is based more on traditional modes of learning than radical alternatives. Opportunities for experiences 'outside' of physiotherapy are rarely encouraged and policy frameworks that emphasise safety and freedom from risk are privileged over those that encourage innovation and creativity. Physiotherapy educators naturally draw on their own experience of learning to frame the development of new curricula. These experiences consistently emphasise the reductive and abstracted image of the body-as-machine, normalisation and objective detachment. At the same time, physiotherapy academics and educators are considered to be leaders in their specialist fields and they are rewarded with some of the highest levels of pay within the profession. Physiotherapy courses are often heavily over-subscribed and the popularity of their programmes within the university is often unmatched. Given all of this, it is perhaps not surprising that physiotherapy educators stick with a formula that seems to have worked well for them in the past.

There are exceptions, however, and a number of physiotherapy educators are now promoting radically different and interesting approaches to education that move away from the kinds of educational approaches familiar to traditional physiotherapy programmes (Patton et al 2013; Dahl-Michelsen 2015; Hammond 2013; Kell 2013; Mooney 2012; Eisenberg 2012; Trede et al 2010; Nicholls 2016; Trede & McEwan 2016; Horobin & Thom 2015)[1]. What is true of most of these educators though, is that they have had to leave physiotherapy for a short time to study subjects like educational theory, history, philosophy and sociology in order that they can come back and argue for other ways to engage students in learning.

One of the greatest challenges now facing physiotherapy educators is the instability and ready accessibility of knowledge that was once considered privileged. Physiotherapy curricula are based on truths that have been thought to be stable and largely immutable (how the body can be analysed, how it functions, what it is capable of etc.). This knowledge has traditionally been held in academic journals and weighty textbooks or in the minds of clinical specialists, whose elite social status is based on their ability to cut through the subject's manifest complexities and translate it into language that students can then absorb. For some years now, however, traditional knowledges have been widely available, in multiple formats, to anyone and everyone who chooses to look for them. The mysteries of how to perform Grade V manipulations on the cervical spine, or the detailed anatomy of semimembranosus, are no longer beyond people's reach. They are literally at people's fingertips, in formats that are engaging, transportable and endlessly repeatable. The classical lecture on the physiology of muscle activation, or the dreary talk on the surface anatomy of the median nerve, is now almost redundant given the accessibility of countless online videos and downloadable mobile applications and these new modes of engagement are finding audiences a long way beyond the lecture theatres and tutorial rooms of physiotherapy training schools. These new modes of engagement are challenging the traditional status of training schools, accrediting universities and experts and making knowledge that was once highly regulated and sanctioned available to millions of others.

Rather than embracing the ambiguity and uncertainty of knowledge today, however, physiotherapy educators have largely focused on ways to show that their knowledge still holds truth value (Håkstad et al 2016). Evidence-based practice has played a key role here and most graduate programmes now mandate that the students not only understand but also actively participate in evidence-based decision making in answering assignment questions and justifying their clinical decisions. The pursuit of evidence is seen by many as the bulwark against the kinds of ambiguity and uncertainty that threaten the profession's future. It does, however, risk replacing the real messiness, complexity and innate subjectivity of practice with an abstracted image of objective, value-free, detached practice (Law & Mol 2002): a tension that is being played out every day now in physiotherapy training programmes around the world.

In an illustration of this tension, a few years ago, I was part of a small project that analysed how students were being assessed during their period of clinical education. Prior to the study, our clinical educators' approach to the assessment of the students' clinical performance had been traditional, with the students' competence tested objectively against established standards. Clinical skills were broken down into instrumental tasks and each component was assessed discretely. Students passed the particular competence if they successfully completed all of the requirements of each task. We raised questions about this model of assessment, however, because although it worked well for technical skills, it seemed the wrong way to test the humanistic capabilities that the clinicians said were vitally important and, all-too-often deficient. (Tellingly, these are also the capabilities demanded most often by employers, who argue that they are often poorly developed in new graduates (Øien et al 2011; Prictor & Hill 2011; Wloszczak-Szubzda & Jarosz 2013; Runyan et al 2013; Winther et al 2014; Mendick et al 2015; Trede & Haynes 2009).) Giving some thought to the way assessment moderates behaviour, the project team began by looking at the way these capabilities were assessed and developed a different approach.

The clinical educators who supervised our students were asked to identify three capabilities that mattered to them in their work location. These would be particularly personal approaches to their work that they could then explore with the student, model and then test as the clinical education experience progressed. We assumed that each clinician would have their own idiosyncratic approach and that each location would be different. So, two physiotherapists working on a spinal cord injury rehab unit, for example, might define three quite distinctive capabilities. Some might argue that they wanted the students to learn to motivate their patients, others that they needed to develop strengths in active listening and empathy. We asked the clinicians to use these capabilities instead of the instrumental measures they had used before. We then collected all of the various capabilities together to see what they chose.

In the first year alone, 50 clinical educators gave us nearly 200 different capabilities that they wanted the students to demonstrate: flexibility; adaptability; compassion; commitment to caring; being perceptive of body, mind and spirit; sensitivity; authenticity; engagement; warmth; rapport; assertiveness; hope; fairness and so on. What we realised was that the phrases were more than just desirable capabilities for the student: they were really expressions of the breadth and complexities of practice for the therapist; things that were not often assessed or validated; essential elements to successful, deliberate, meaningful practice that set them apart from others. These were the expressions of the kinds of craft knowledge of the health professions that Joy Higgs and others had written about some years ago (Higgs 2008; Higgs & Edwards 1999; Higgs et al 2001, 2004, 2013; Higgs & Titchen 2008; Titchen & Higgs 2001; Laitinen-Väänänen et al 2008; Delany 2009). What was also clear was that our traditional physiotherapy curricula made little or no allowance for these capabilities and that it was assumed that the physiotherapist would learn to be enabling, creative and cognisant of power imbalances *despite* their curriculum rather than because of it.

The problem of how to make space in an already corpulent curriculum remains a major barrier for physiotherapy educators, however. Many recognise the necessity to give students more than just a battery of assessment tests and treatment techniques, but the ever-growing demands of new material, evidence-based practice and the old problems of teaching a linear programme with few opportunities for deviation or disruption remain. New educational approaches, technologies and tools, like interprofessional collaborative education; technology-mediated communication; inquiry-based, situated and embodied learning are starting to be utilised within physiotherapy programmes, but these new approaches to learning do not, in themselves, resolve the problem of how to blend the best of the old and the new in a way that makes sense in an already packed physiotherapy curriculum (see, e.g. Vuoskoski 2014).

As I have argued throughout the book, the virtues of the body-as-machine have been manifest in the long history of the profession's growth and this is perhaps no more evident than in the field of education where the picture at present looks rosy. Physiotherapy is one of the most popular university programmes and applications for training in many countries far exceed the number of available places. It remains a large, trusted and highly valued profession and it is supported by government funding and protected by profession-specific legislation. Physiotherapists have access to patients who often have their fees subsidised and it is one of the most visible and active health professions internationally. So, what could possibly be a rationale for moving away from an educational model that has served the profession so well for the last century or more? The answer, of course, is the very focus of this book.

Firstly, physiotherapy has to meet many new demands created by a rapidly ageing, chronically ill populations. Added to this, the rising prevalence of preventable lifestyle illnesses is causing a huge drain on depleting public health services. These problems are being met by a professional practice population built around a 20th century healthcare model that privileged expensive, highly trained specialists with considerable power, treating people in regional centres remote from their communities, homes, schools, care centres and workplaces.

Secondly, people's understandings of health have changed. Not only are people much more sceptical of orthodox healthcare and more open to holistic and embodied (alternative and complementary) health experiences, they are increasingly encouraged to spend their disposable income on a rapidly diversifying market for healthcare services, products and technologies. Orthodox medicine (to which physiotherapy is wedded) no longer holds a monopoly on how people can experience or think about health and wellbeing.

Thirdly, traditional forms of knowledge, and the ways people engage with them, have been disrupted by digital technologies. Subjects that were once considered specialised and obtainable only to those with special privileges are now widely available and accessible in myriad ways and appealing new forms. Higher education is no longer the default location for learning about anatomy, physiology, biomechanics, kinesiology, research methods, assessment and treatment techniques. The primary role for educational institutions is increasingly to teach students to discriminate between true and false knowledge claims; to assess and accredit their learning and to teach those things that cannot be learnt remotely. This is especially true of the humanistic skills of inter-personal relations, the skills needed to cope with the complexity of clinical care and teamwork.

And fourthly, there appears to be a growing separation between the aspirations of established orthodox professions like physiotherapy and needs of the population. Health professionals have traditionally needed to demonstrate their *difference* from others to justify governmental support, today the emphasis has shifted to interprofessional collaboration. The quest for elite status has continued in physiotherapy with the development of masters- and doctoral-entry programmes and the pursuit of specialisation, but government health priorities have shifted towards low-cost care in the community, prevention and health promotion, and the lowest level of specialisation needed to manage the greatest number of people.

Given these tensions, I would argue that physiotherapy education is at a point of flux; still enjoying prestige and social capital, but perhaps relying too heavily on approaches to learning and teaching that are at odds with the cultural shifts in healthcare and society at large. In 2003, the New Zealand's Health Workforce Advisory Committee stated that 'simply doing more of the same is not an option (p. 21) . . . A major culture change (or paradigm shift) is required (p. 2) . . . Some totally new roles and ways of working will emerge'. (p. 5) (Health Workforce Advisory Committee 2003). This message has been increasingly repeated by governments, health funders and policy advisers in most developed countries in recent years.

Liam Donaldson, Chief Medical Officer for England between 1998 and 2010, reinforced this message when he stated that, 'The need for health services to give priority to developing health professionals equipped to practice in new ways and thrive in new organisation environments requires a rapid response to reshape curricula training programmes' (Alexander et al 2004, p. 7). Since then, calls for reform have only grown louder. A recent report by the UK's Department of Health titled *Equity and Excellence: Liberating the NHS* (Department of Health 2010) called for much greater patient choice, shared decision making and individualised healthcare, even to the point of the development of personal health budgets (Foot 2014). The Global Financial Crisis of 2008 has further accelerated calls for health reforms, with many countries experiencing significant pressure to reduce public funding for healthcare (including healthcare education). Given this, one would have to conclude that, if the education of the next generation of physiotherapists continues to follow the model of the past, it would be hard to imagine how future practitioners will be equipped to meet the radical changes now unfolding in 21st century healthcare.

Practice

I would argue that when physiotherapists refer to practice, they are most often thinking about the application of assessment and treatment techniques to patients with particular physical disorders. There is often a close link between theory and practice, but here theory is that which explains the clinical work of diagnosing and treating those disorders that are familiar – and sometimes unfamiliar – to physiotherapists. Practitioners are generally much less concerned with the meaning of assessment itself, the nature of their therapeutic spaces or the systems and structures that help to define their practice. Perhaps this is a function of the profession's characteristic pragmatism? Physiotherapists are known for being practical people who prefer to work physically on clinical problems and they are characteristically less comfortable thinking about why they do what they do (Shaw & DeForge 2012; McCombie et al 2015). But there are some significant structural features to physiotherapy practice that are often hiding in plain sight, which play a very big part in defining the therapist's subjectivity. Some of these features make it possible to communicate trust and respectability to patients without it needing to be stated. Others are important tools in defining where physiotherapy practices begin and end and how treatment sessions are conducted. As physiotherapy changes, these structural features change too. In many situations, they need to change *before* the more visible surface effects can take hold so it is worthwhile considering how these practice structures operate if we are then to imagine physiotherapy otherwise.

Perhaps it is easiest to explain this way of thinking with an analogy. Imagine driving to visit your relatives without a reliable car, a good road network, traffic lights and intersections. Simple customs like driving on the same side of the road, signalling turns and driving at a safe speed are part of a vast infrastructure of rules, practices and cultural beliefs that become familiar and almost invisible to us until an accident happens and we question what went wrong. The same is true of physiotherapy and all other professions and occupations. Physiotherapy would be unidentifiable today if it were not for its own deep-seated and largely invisible infrastructure: its well-established curricula; its treatment beds and clinical spaces; its particular ways of assessing and treating; its conferences, research papers and journals. In many ways, physiotherapy is defined by these things and communicated to its patients, colleagues and competitors through myriad tiny gestures and practices that embody these systems and structures. Maintaining a consistent, stable professional image, therefore, becomes akin to maintaining one's balance, whereby the profession has to react and adapt to the fluid and constantly evolving environment; adjusting minute-by-minute to the variable needs of others; always testing what retains its integrity and what might cause it to fall.

The kinds of physiotherapies that we see today and, by extension, those that have gone before, are the *effects* of all of these influences, pressures and systems. Contrary to the way many people conventionally think about practice, physiotherapy does not begin at the point when the therapist first encounters the patient and begins assessing and treating, because the systems and structures that define what is possible are already in place. Therapies derive *from* the systems and structures that already exist. So, to understand day-to-day practices and understand why physiotherapists practice in particular ways and not others, I would argue that it is necessary to give some thought to the things that make practice possible.

These things are perhaps best illustrated by examining aspects of practice that are the most every day and ordinary. Consider the humble treatment bed, for example. Most physiotherapists think little of the innocuous bed, couch or plinth that sits in almost every physiotherapist's treatment rooms, but it plays a hugely significant role in defining practice[2]. Imagine being a patient, entering the physio-therapist's rooms to find a bed from home in the middle of the treatment area. The bed – perhaps a double bed – looks clean and tidy, dressed in soft fabrics, expensive linen and loose cushions but, all the same, it looks entirely out of place. It conveys entirely the wrong impression of the kind of 'therapeutic' experience the patient is about to receive.

This is obviously a trite example, but it points to the fact that the kind of bed chosen by physiotherapists does more than just provide a surface for assessment and treatment; it conveys a great deal about the professional's respectability and professionalism. So, when a patient walks into a clinical space, the presence of a traditional mechanical bed, with its vinyl cover and exposed machinery, reminds them that the therapist fits into a conventional picture of a clinically-minded professional. Certainly, treatment beds have mechanisms to take them up and down, and sections to allow the therapist to passively position the patient, but these ergonomic considerations are much less significant than the bed's ability to convey a reassuring sense that the practitioner is orthodox and trustworthy, and that the therapist is looking to treat you, not seduce you (Nicholls 2012b)[3].

Like the treatment bed, everything in the physiotherapist's clinic rooms serves a dual purpose, having a surface effect that is often taken-for-granted and obvious, but also having a deeper significance that conveys a powerful symbolism to the patient. Physiotherapy clinic spaces are often painted white, for example. Of course, white is a simple shade that is unlikely to offend anyone, but it is also the colour of clinical work; it conveys cleanliness, honesty and authenticity. White walls are not necessarily any cleaner than sludgy green walls, but they convey the idea of health, hygiene and innocence much better than walls the colour of sputum. Physiotherapists often display anatomical charts on their walls rather than pictures of sunny fields and beaches. Is this because they need to be reminded of the location of the rectus femoris or rather because it conveys a message to the patient about the way the therapist views their body? Uniforms, street signage, preformatted assessment sheets and clinical notes, images on the clinic's website, the design of the waiting area, the topics covered in the subjective assessment, therapeutic equipment, body language, terminology and ways of explaining things to patients are the same: vital functions of physiotherapy, not merely because they serve a practical purpose, but because they also silently and subtly define the nature of the clinical encounter and convey powerful messages about the practitioner and their practices.

Some of the most powerful hidden functions of things like treatment beds, electrotherapy equipment and assessment techniques, are based on their ability to define the proper relationship between the therapist and patient. The therapist's role is often to be active: asking questions; probing for the cause of the patient's complaint; managing the timing of the appointment; directing the patient through a series of procedures often performed *on* them or by them, under instruction[4]. Such practices convey power and authority and function in important and interesting ways. For the therapist to be paid for their services, they must show that they can offer something that patients cannot understand or do for themselves; they must elevate their practice above mere 'common sense' and demonstrate the benefits of lengthy training in the manner of their diagnostic insights and technical skills. They must show that they can both relate to the person's concerns, at the same time as retaining an objective, dispassionate distance from them. They must juggle empathy and detachment, proximity and separation. Although the ability to do all of these things takes many years of training (often without the therapist being consciously aware that they are learning to do it), it is the power to be able to be the one that decides how these complexities are managed that is really critical. The ability to decide *how* to engage in a professional relationship with a patient is far more significant than the technical skills required to do so. This is a power held by the therapist and rarely, if ever, is it held by the patient. Even in today's language of clients and consumers (see chapter endnotes), the power to govern the conduct of a therapeutic encounter still resides firmly in favour of the practitioner.

In some healthcare encounters – particularly those involving life-threatening illness or injury – people are often willing to hand over their bodies to trusted health professionals. Notwithstanding an array of complex ethical issues, most people accept being passive in the face of unremitting pain or critical illness. Thankfully, however, such moments of acute suffering are rare. What is much more common are the kinds of everyday health disruptions and disturbances that affect our ability to go about our daily lives. For these health problems, people have a reasonable expectation that they will be involved, in some way, in decisions about their care[5]. While we accept that encounters with health professionals involve us disclosing personal information, exposing parts of our bodies to scrutiny and a degree of surveillance, confession and sensitive documentation, we also expect to be a partner in healthcare decisions affecting us, rather than passive recipients of whatever it is the therapist deems necessary (Varul 2010; Taylor & Bury 2007; Donaldson 2003).

As with some aspects of emergency care, there are some physiotherapy encounters that rely on the patient being treated passively. Given physiotherapy's innate sensuality (meaning that it engages our body's senses; can be painful or pleasurable; can bring sudden relief, hope and reassurance), it is entirely appropriate that the therapist's attitude sometimes involves a degree of affective detachment. For people to experience the relief and sheer joy that sometimes comes with effective treatment, they must feel safe in the hands of their therapist. For people to expose themselves and parts of their body, it is sometimes helpful to know that the practitioner is focusing on the body-as-machine. So, the constructive indifference to the sensual body learnt by the physiotherapists is important because it can be a powerful analytical tool *and* an important way to communicate the practitioner's indifference to their patient's sensuality. The difficulty comes, however, when these practices, ethical principles, professional rules, systems and structures, prevent therapists from seeing *beyond* the body-as-machine.

Throughout this book, I have argued that there have been some significant benefits to physiotherapists' archetypal approach to practice, but there are also some significant drawbacks. These drawbacks are not immediately obvious in the daily practices of the therapist and reside in the deeper challenges now being faced by the profession. Indeed, looking at the educational structures, therapeutic practices and treatment spaces used by physiotherapists today one might be mistaken for believing that little has changed in physiotherapy over the last 100 years. Despite some superficial technological variations, clinical practice is still based on the same four key modalities; it still develops from the same basic curriculum structure; physiotherapists still use many of the same approaches to assessment and treatment and the profession's relationship with its patients is still based on the idea that treatment is directed at the management of largely acute, mechanical interventions, delivered to a passive body-as-machine. And yet, the tensions facing professional practitioners today are radically different to those experienced in the early 20th century.

As I have argued throughout this book, I believe the remarkable consistency (or possibly intransigence) shown by physiotherapists throughout the profession's history has been made possible by both a focus on the individual body in front of them and an indifference towards the wider cultural, economic, philosophical, political and social conditions that influence people's experience of health and illness. For example, physiotherapists rarely consider the patient's cultural context. They rarely engage with questions of gendered power, disability rights, the importance of diversity and inclusiveness, social justice or the politics and ethics of patient choice. Physiotherapists are infinitely more interested in understanding the differences between competing practice theories (Maitland or McKenzie; motor control or Bobath, for instance) than they are about grand philosophies and theories of the self and other; of being and becoming; of social control and resistance. There are library shelves full of books devoted to explaining the myriad ways of manipulating the spine, but very little of this has been written by physiotherapists, for physiotherapists, about the professionalisation of the physiotherapy; the social organisation of care; the nature of practice; the meaning practitioners give to the body, function, movement and therapy; the role of discipline, coercion and compliance in everyday work and voices of rage and dissent about the profession's historic (mis)treatment of vulnerable people.

Physiotherapists' recent turn towards subjects like chronic pain, health promotion, cognitive behavioural therapy and rehabilitation in critical care point to a subtle shift in the discourses now influencing practitioners, teachers, researchers and regulators. It appears that physiotherapists are increasingly open to the idea that these new clients and service users are enabling the profession to embrace a more humanistic approach to practice. Embracing this change is leading to new approaches to assessment, treatment and evaluation that reflect a broader professional perspective. Studies now openly discuss a biopsychosocial approach to physiotherapy (Brunner et al 2015; Roush & Sharby 2011; Jones et al 2002), notions of complexity and embodiment are more common (Sivertsen & Normann 2014; Sviland et al 2012; Dahl-Michelsen 2015) and there is a greater focus on long-term health conditions that cannot be cured or managed with an acute care model (Øien et al 2009; Pike 2008; French 2013).

Of course, physiotherapists have always had an interest in long-term and complex health problems like chronic neurological disorders and lung diseases, arthritis and cerebral palsy, but in the past therapy was impairment based and the presence of pathology defined the role of the practitioner. The focus was on reme-diating the condition, and other determinants like the patient's wishes, people's cultural values and the particular social context, were often relegated behind the specific aetiology, the clinician's expertise and experience and the availability of suitable resources. Today, many physiotherapists are beginning to see that their knowledge and skills need not be defined by a traditional biomechanical approach to practice. Even the idea that physiotherapy is for people with an existing organic disease or disorder is beginning to come into question, with physiotherapists now working with people to enhance their wellbeing rather than simply treating their illness and injury (Nicholls et al 2009b). Much is beginning to change, then, and as new bleeding edge practices emerge that are challenge the conception of what physiotherapy is and might become (Kleinke 1998).

Implicit in the new focus on patient-centred care, for example, is a willingness by the profession to relinquish its power to treat patients passively. The logic of patient-centred care states that in a world where patients are considered people, the body cannot be seen as a machine made up of semi-independent parts that can be replaced or repaired (Bleakley 2014; Cushing 2015; McWhinney 1985). This logic demands that healthcare professionals embrace the idea that they share deci-sion making is shared with their patients and *clinical* decision making no longer takes precedence by default. Professions like physiotherapy have approached patient-centred care with some caution, however, perhaps because handing some of their power over to patients comes with the possibility that the patient will not want the kinds of physiotherapy being offered. It may also be because physiother-apists have yet to develop an approach to practice that does not privilege the expert practitioner treating the passive body-as-machine (Gzil et al 2007; Trede & Flowers 2014; Mudge et al 2013).

Physiotherapists are increasingly being asked to embrace new approaches to care that emphasise the need to share power, move beyond the traditional health/illness binary, coordinate service delivery and rationalise health resources (Eisenberg 2012; Praestegaard et al 2014; Mooney 2012). However, in recent years, we have seen the growth of standardised care pathways, interprofessional collaborative and evidence-based practice, which all emanate from the manageri-alism and bureaucratisation of healthcare that has developed over the last 40 years (and discussed in Chapter 5) (Gabe et al 2015; Dutta 2015; Robertson 2001). These approaches serve to shift the power away from the autonomous professional (whose actions are variously seen as risky, overly subjective, inconsistent and even self-serving) (Schunk & Thut 2003; Morden et al 2015; Mingardi 2015) and putatively concentrate power in the hands of service users and managers. Importantly, physiotherapists and others have willingly adopted many of these approaches, perhaps seduced by the available research funding or swayed by the rhetoric of patient rights and best practice.

Physiotherapy practice is, therefore, experiencing some significant existential tensions, particularly surrounding its traditional power and authority. On the one hand, it still needs to promote its expertise and distinctive professional identity, but it is increasingly being asked to democratise its practice and share power with those it once treated quite passively. It demands autonomy, but is dependent on service users, policy makers, funding agents, insurance companies and individual patients and service users for support in order to retain its status. All of these tensions have their effects in the day-to-day practices of the therapist, but lacking a sophisticated understanding of the things going on beyond the limits of the body-as-machine many physiotherapists feel a sense of frustration at their perceived impotence. One of the places where it is possible to see these tensions being played out most clearly is in the field of professional regulation.

Regulation

When people think about regulation, they often think about it in negative terms. They think it is restrictive, constraining, bureaucratic and boring, it is designed to stifle creativity and constrain growth or it is a brake on progress and a hurdle to be overcome (Gordon 2009; Field 2006). In professional practice, regulation is seen as a necessary way to manage the risks inherent when people operate – in both the literal and metaphorical sense – on others. Because physiotherapy is such a practical field and its practitioners such pragmatic people, regulation is recognised as a necessary condition of existence. Perhaps because of this, it is rarely analysed or critiqued and remains under-theorised in physiotherapy (Miles-Tapping 1989; Higgs et al 2001; Swisher & Page 2005). Historically, little has been written about how key regulatory functions of physiotherapy are defined, how innovation and change are addressed and how important issues like autonomy and the ethical governance are viewed in practice.

In recent years, however, there has been increased interest in some of these fields and a number of researchers and theorists are giving thought to the ethical challenges of physiotherapy practice; how to teach regulatory issues like standards of practice and professionalism in education; the relationship between self and other; the profession's history; the challenge of professional encroachment and interprofessional practice and physiotherapists' responses to the broader changes taking place in healthcare around the world (Praestegaard et al 2014; Pretorius et al 2015; Kumar et al 2013; Dutton 2014; Guenther et al 2014; Noronha et al 2016; Grignon et al 2014; Thille et al 2014).

What is striking about this nascent body of work is that it is beginning to reveal some of the complexities and subtleties of physiotherapy thought and practice: aspects of practice that have always been there, but largely unacknowledged. It is challenging the traditional view of professional regulation in which professional autonomy and independence are seen as desirable and inherently good, and that practitioners are best served by having a clear, marketable professional identity, underpinned by evidence-based practice and a close collaborative relationship with orthodox medicine (Praestegaard et al 2014; Gibson et al 2010; Trede 2008).

Although regulatory authorities are commonly unappreciated today, the establishment of a State-sanctioned professional board was once considered a mark of success for a health profession and in some jurisdictions this is still the case. To be considered big enough, important enough or even *dangerous* enough for the State to want to regulate you was a clear indication that the profession had 'arrived' (Palmer 1930). It did, of course, come with some obligations: to review graduate competence; to abide by a particular scopes and standards of practice and to do the work of the State by constantly monitoring ethical or professional boundaries. But regulation also came with privileges that were denied to those who were not considered large enough or 'mainstream' enough to warrant professional registration: it conferred orthodoxy and respectability on the profession; it provided protective legislation and marginalised competing professions and it gave registered practitioners privileged access to individuals and groups eligible for subsidised healthcare (Mingardi 2015; Einhorn & Logue 2003; Bertilsson 1990). There has always been a tension, therefore, for health professions, because they operate in a shifting space that lies between opportunity and cost, freedom and constraint, autonomy and dependence, orthodoxy and heterodoxy and this tension often plays out in disputes around regulation.

Historically, physiotherapists appear to have been quite happy with their regulatory legislation. When the 1949 *Physiotherapy Act* was repealed in New Zealand in 2003, for example, it was the oldest single piece of profession-specific legislation in the country's history. The Act gave physiotherapists some extraordinary protections, including making it illegal to practice therapeutic massage unless one was registered as a physiotherapist[6]. Notwithstanding the years of work that went into gaining control of national physiotherapy boards and councils from doctors who had traditionally dominated the profession and disputes over pay rates (Bentley & Dunstan 2006; Murphy 1995; Barclay 1994; Anderson 1977), regulatory authorities seem to occupy a largely benign space in the physiotherapy profession; neither offending nor provoking, they are seen as necessarily bureaucratic organisations that protect the profession's most basic 'vital' functions. Regulatory authorities are far from benign, however, and their systems and structures are important to interrogate *because* they sometimes appear to be merely procedural. On the contrary, physiotherapy boards and councils play a hugely significant role in shaping the culture of the profession and demand consideration.

Regulatory authorities emerged with the worker's guilds that began to form in 16th century Europe and present day physiotherapy regulatory authorities bear many similarities to the organisations that formed in 16th century Europe. Guilds were collections of skilled artisans who came together to secure better terms of trade, provide protection for members and regulate their craft. They catered for bespoke tradespeople who were otherwise independent practitioners. Artisans could be distinguished from artists because of their more limited freedom of expression but equally, their work required skill to be replicated and could not be easily manufactured by a machine (Smith 2004). Artisanal work often required a great deal of physical labour (i.e. blacksmiths, carpenters and stonemasons) or fine dexterity (goldsmiths, hatters and tailors) (Crossick 1997). Artisans gave us the modern apprenticeship, the idea of learning at the 'elbow of the master', the 'master-piece' as a test of the craftsman's right to be called an artisan and be part of a guild[7] and the 'trade-mark'. Artisan guilds were the forerunner of the trade unions (Farr 1997) and the professional bodies that now regulate artisanal crafts like physiotherapy (Nicholls 2016).

Since World War II, there has been a growing interest in the work of professionals in society and the role that regulatory mechanisms like boards and societies play in defining the work of practitioners (Abbott & Meerabeau 1998; Evetts 2006; Larkin 2002; Saks 2010; Evetts 2003; Elston 1991). Much of the early sociological literature on professional regulation focused on the tasks that distinguished professions from each other and from 'lay' members of society (Durkheim 1933; Carr-Sanders & Wilson 1933; Parsons 1951). This 'functionalist' way of understanding professional roles was heavily criticised in the 1960s and 1970s, with critical theorists arguing that it failed to account for the role that professional power, market 'closure' and elitism played in the aspirations and histories of professions like doctors and physiotherapists (Wilensky 1964; Etzioni 1969; Freidson 1970). Over time, these 'structuralist' critiques have, themselves, come into question and scholars working in the field of what is now called the sociology of professionalisation provide more nuanced and complex analyses of the role of regulation and practice in shaping healthcare practice today (Allsop & Saks 2002; Johnson et al 1995; Evetts 1999, 2003; Saks 2010; Kuhlmann & Saks 2008; Saks 1995; Light 1995; Beach & Davies 2013; Freshwater et al 2013; Larkin 2002; Nancarrow & Borthwick 2005; Davies 2007; Williams & Lawlis 2014).

Some of this thinking permeated physiotherapy and provided fertile territory for the first wave of university-based educators and practice philosophers in the 1980s and 1990s. People like Barbara Richardson (1999), Joy Higgs (Higgs et al 2001; Higgs & Titchen 2001), Julius Sim (1985), Sally French (2013) and others began to ask questions about the profession's roles and functions in society and, in so doing, created the possibility for the academic study of professionalisation applicable to physiotherapy. Intriguingly, a body of non-physiotherapy scholars has also begun to ask questions about the physiotherapy's culture, history and social capital. Valerie Fournier, for example, has written about the ways that physiotherapists have protected their professional margins from alternative and complementary therapists (Fournier 1999, 2000, 2002), Kevin Dew has written about boundary disputes between physiotherapists and chiropractors (Dew 2003). This work is adding to a growing body of physiotherapy scholarship that is challenging traditional notions of physiotherapy's professional identity and professionalisation project (Oliveira & Nunes 2015; Hammond et al 2015; Owen 2014; Sanders et al 2014; Praestegaard et al 2014; Aguilar et al 2013; Shaw & DeForge 2012; Eisenberg 2012; Nicholls 2012a; Trede et al 2010; Gibson et al 2010; Ramklass 2009; Kell & Owen 2008; Anderson et al 2005).

Following through with the balance metaphor I used earlier, these studies challenge the professional body and cause momentary instability. They demand myriad tiny actions, checks, nudges, routines and refinements from practitioners, educators, legislators and regulators, which either bring about a new rebalancing or force the profession to step onto new ground (Praestegaard et al 2014; Nicholls 2012b). These are all forms of regulation designed to police the profession's vulnerable margins and maintain its professional integrity. So when Trede et al argued that a 'crisis in clinical practice across healthcare professions including physiotherapy' challenged the professional identity of clinicians (Trede et al 2010, pp. 1–2), or when Eisenberg (2012) saw fault lines in the traditional power asymmetry between physiotherapists and patients, and when Kell and Owen argued that physiotherapy's traditional political ambivalence posed significant threats to its professional future (Kell & Owen 2008), the authors were articulating disruptions that could provoke a regulatory response. Rarely, if ever, do these stimuli result in the kinds of top-down, heavy-handed regulation that are often associated with boards and legislating authorities, however. Instead, we see a matrix of microscopic, interconnected actions, techniques and tactics, designed to restore balance and consistency, allowing the profession to return to its previous position or find a new stable standpoint.

What might be understood now about regulation is that it cannot succeed if it is *only* top-down. The regulatory boards of most countries are simply too small to police every clinician at every moment. And so, regulatory authorities have had to learn ways to get health professionals to remain within the confines of good conduct without needing to monitor their every action. This is an imperfect science and no board can even have total command over a profession, so the task becomes how to get doctors, nurses, physiotherapists and other health professionals to behave appropriately *without* force. Most authorities use a combination of normalisation (codes of conduct, standards of practice), surveillance (annual registration renewals, practice audits, practice portfolios) and discipline (tribunals and hearings, often led by the profession's own members) to provide assurance to the State and the public that social rights afforded to the group are being met by its responsibilities.

The most powerful regulatory practice, however, is the regulation that practitioners do to themselves. Physiotherapists govern their conduct every day in practice. They do so based on their own internal construction of what good physiotherapy means, which derives, in part, from the way they have been socialised to think about their practice (Martin et al 2013; Hammond 2007; Richardson et al 2002). Rather than grand gestures, self-governance is usually made up of myriad microscopic, performative acts that, taken together, provide the necessary evidence that the physiotherapist is legitimate, orthodox and responsible. It is the design of their clinic spaces; the way they organise patient assessments; the way they use their hands when they touch (Bjorbækmo and Mengshoel 2016); in their note-writing; in their advertising and promotional websites; their communications with others; the way they regulate their own bodily form and function and their reflections on themselves.

Awareness of the power of self-governance has helped to make reflective practice an important regulatory mechanism in recent years. Operating at the intersection of modern managerial practices and a growing confessional culture (Gubrium & Holstein 2002), reflective practice occupies a difficult position in contemporary regulation, particularly in professional fields like physiotherapy (Donaghy & Morss 2000; White 2004; Ward & Gracey 2006; Clouder 2000). Lacking a strong educational focus on critical self-scrutiny, physiotherapists have, in the past, found reflective practice quite alien and bewildering. Regulatory authorities have also found that using reflection as part of a review of continuing professional development can be fraught with difficulties. Not knowing what the Board wants from its annual reflective portfolio, for example, practitioners often bombard the authority with questions: 'how much should I write here?', 'what do you want me to say in this section?', 'what constitutes evidence of learning?' and so on. In an attempt to manage the clinician's questions, the regulatory authority provides the clinician with guidelines to make the task as straightforward as possible. Consequently, the board no longer receives 'honest' self-reflections from the clinician. Instead, they receive evidence of how well the clinician has worked out what it is that the Board wants them to say. It then becomes the *Board's* role to do the reflective practice work in defining what it is that it wants from the clinicians in order that it can answer the practitioner's myriad questions and avoid dissent (Rolfe & Gardner 2006; Gilbert 2001).

Fortunately, reflective practice is only one tool in the regulatory authority's armoury and there are many other techniques and mechanisms that are used by boards to show that physiotherapists are safe to practice and fit for purpose: Auditing school curricula, setting standards for entry from overseas applicants, holding hearings into complaints, annual audits of members' fitness for practice, defining professional standards and codes of conduct, establishing definitions of physiotherapy and lobbying for legislation to protect professional scopes, are all devices used by boards to protect the profession's social capital. Because of the nature of physiotherapy practice, Boards are particularly concerned with the profession's licence to touch, particularly its intimacy and implied sensuality. Perhaps no other subject poses such great reputational risk to physiotherapy as a loss of faith in its dispassionate use of touch. And so mechanisms to protect the profession and the public must be sophisticated and extensive.

The particular way physiotherapists have chosen to discipline touch in practice appears to work well, given the astonishingly low rates of complaint internationally (Hudon et al 2014; Praestegaard & Gard 2013; Ingham et al 2013; Roush et al 2015). It does, however, come at some cost, not least to the practitioner's ability to see people as embodied, innately sensual, living beings with feelings, desires and needs (McIntosh 2005; Lauterstein 2004; Juhan 1987; Williams 1998a, 1998b). In a recent paper I wrote with Dave Holmes, we discussed the necessity for physiotherapy to transgress its traditional approach to touch in order that we might better understand the advantages *and* disadvantages of the profession's current approaches to regulation and professional discipline (Nicholls & Holmes 2012). In the article, we argued that touch was innately linked to sensuality, but that this was often confused with sexuality (both in the mind of therapists and the public) and that this historical confusion mediated its current approach to the body's 'leaky fluids . . . overflowing desires and voracious appetites' (Williams 1998b, p. 438) making 'this potentially confusing and highly charged situation safe for our clients and for ourselves by maintaining professional boundaries' (McIntosh 2005, p. 1). While on the surface this seems a desirable outcome, it also places significant constraints on how practitioners might engage with people in more holistic, embodied ways when dealing with things like chronic illness, long-term pain and the humanistic dimensions of care. Juhan articulated the dilemma in this way:

> In a culture that is as starved for touch as ours, I suspect there may be some healthful benefits to pleasant tactile stimulations in almost any form whatever. But in order to discuss the kind of bodywork I mean, I strongly feel the need for a word [other than massage] that in no way implies contact that is merely sensual, or that is sexual in any shape or form.
>
> The term 'physical therapy' avoids these associations, but it is too narrow in the scope of its normal use. It refers to an official medical discipline, one which is licensed only after protracted and highly specific studies, prescribed only by physicians, and applied through fixed procedures. Such academic rigor certainly does not count against it as a responsible therapeutic practice, but it does effectively partition 'physical therapy' off from many other useful kinds of touching and manipulation. In particular, it typically eliminates a good deal of the intuitive element which seems to be such an important part of other approaches and which is fact many physical therapists have confessed to me that they wish they could use more freely in the clinical practice.
>
> (Juhan 1987, p. xx, original emphasis preserved)

This heavily regulated approach to touch spills over into the profession's entire approach to treatment, which, in turn, becomes a double-edged sword. On the one hand, it means therapists can exploit their professional access to patients with existing organic disease, treating them in quite mechanistic ways until the particular acute episode that prompted the referral or appointment has been resolved. On the other hand, it often means that physiotherapists cannot easily use their hard-earned abilities to help people who just need careful, thoughtful, caring touch: the depressed and self-harming teenager; the patient with end-stage lung cancer; the middle-aged businesswoman worrying for her job, children, elderly parents and so on. Physiotherapy's disciplinary logic mandates that there has to be a physiological rationale for physiotherapists to touch patients; it cannot be performed simply because it temporarily relieves discomfort or simply feels nice. Such associations between touch and sensuality have been taboo in physiotherapy for years, and this means that a huge swathe of contemporary healthcare practice is now being left in the hands of others, in much the same way as male patients were ignored by the founders of physiotherapy in the years before WWI.

This is not to say that some therapists are not now venturing into this marginal therapeutic territory, where physiotherapy's traditional absolutism around touch is being tested, but those wishing to practice in new and innovative ways may find themselves pitched against regulatory authorities, whose instincts and responsibilities are more attuned to preventing boundary breaches than encouraging them. Operating at the margins of orthodox practice comes with significant risks of censure and discipline, therefore, and so bleeding edge practitioners often operate quietly and in isolation (Nicholls et al 2009b). But it is here, at the outer margins of what is considered legitimate and orthodox, that the template for innovative new practices and growth in physiotherapy is being forged. And so, it is here at the margins of orthodox practice that it is possible to encounter an inherent tension in the nature of professional regulation and the question of professional autonomy becomes particularly interesting.

For their part, authorities need to show that the profession's boundary is stable and intact, but they also need to recognise that the profession must adapt if it is to survive. Adaptation implies deviation from accepted norms that, in turn, tests the regulatory authority's abilities to police the profession's margins. Practitioners who reach too far into practices that are perceived to be potentially hazardous, ineffective or unsupported by conventional reason must be disciplined because they represent a reputational risk to the profession, but the board cannot be too heavy-handed because it governs a profession that is putatively autonomous. Not surprisingly then, much of the debate around the future of professions like physiotherapy has revolved around what, exactly, autonomy means and how autonomous physiotherapy practitioners really are.

Questions of professional autonomy have been central to physiotherapy practice since a critical mass of therapists began to be concerned with medical and State oversight of the profession in the 1930s and 1940s (Ovretveit 1985). Wanting the support, patronage and funding from doctors and the government, while, at the same time, not wanting to be *controlled* by them has resulted in decades of conversations, resolutions, disputes and minor acts of resistance that have shaped the profession's identity (Barclay 1994; Murphy 1995; Bentley & Dunstan 2006). The first true marker of physiotherapists' professional autonomy was achieved, for many, after the 1970s, with the recognition of physiotherapy as a first-contact profession, which brought enormous opportunities for growth in size and social capital to the profession (Bury & Stokes 2013).

Physiotherapists have increasingly realised, however, that the separatist language of professional autonomy, freedom and distinctiveness causes as many problems as it resolves, and educators, practitioners and researchers are increasingly recognising the need for new ways of expressing the inter-relationships and positive dependencies they have with others (Gibson et al 2012; Gibson 2006). These ideas of 'connectivity', in contrast to autonomy, extend beyond just the relationship between physiotherapists and other healthcare providers, they also explore practitioner's relationships with patients, communities, ideas, objects (assessment tools, prostheses etc.), systems and structures. As I have noted elsewhere, they are particularly significant move because they open up 'radically different ways of engaging in health-care practice' (Nicholls et al 2016, p. 2):

> These approaches are particularly exciting for physiotherapists, because they center around the body and the ways we are challenging traditional beliefs about what our bodies can do, where bodies begin and end, and how we might relate to other people, objects, technologies, and ideas in the future.
>
> (Nicholls et al 2016, p. 2)

One of of the challenges now facing physiotherapists, is how to envisage a future professional practice that resists the isolationist language of autonomy, independence and freedom, and focuses instead on connectivity, collaboration and sharing. To achieve such a shift, physiotherapists will rely on new forms of regulation that open up the possibility of different ways of thinking and practising, rather than constraining and limiting opportunities for growth beyond a predefined and somewhat 'Victorian' notion of what physiotherapy has been in the past. Of all the locations and sites where this debate will take place, touch is perhaps the most radical and significant because, if physiotherapists can embrace a different attitude towards touch – one that preserves the profession's heritage and respectability but also allows for a more mature engagement with its innate sensuality – then the profession may indeed have found a model of practice that can serve the profession into the future.

Pivotally important here is the practitioner's understanding of the role regulation plays in her practice. Many aspects of the present regulatory regime constrain more than they enable, but regulation itself can be a very positive force for change. Regulation is not something necessarily done by 'others' – including members of our own professions – and imposed on us from afar. Often it involves actions practitioners willingly, positively and sometimes even knowingly, apply to ourselves. Regulation cannot, therefore, only be seen as negative, because to do so misses the point that practitioners rely on regulation, as much as they rely on our attitudes, knowledge and skills, to define their professional subjectivity. The question is not how to subvert regulations, but rather how to make them serve the function of creating an 'otherwise' physiotherapy. The final dimension of physiotherapy thinking and practice I want to address in this chapter is, in many ways, similar to the question of regulation. Given its ubiquity, research has the potential to constrain growth and development in physiotherapy as much as, if not more than, regulation. So, to conclude this chapter, I want to explore how research today is shaping the possibilities for present and future physiotherapy thinking and practice.

Research

Perhaps the most significant influences on the growth and development of physiotherapy over the last 40 years has been in the amount and quality of research now being conducted not only *on* physiotherapy, but also *by* physiotherapists. The fact that research has only become a significant preoccupation for physiotherapists since the 1980s is perhaps a little surprising, given that the profession has always been so closely tied to medicine. Despite the fact that physiotherapy had been awarding degrees in America since 1927 (Murphy 1995, p. 83), and in Australia since 1950 (Bentley & Dunstan 2006, p. 136); that it had established journals like the *Journal of the Incorporated Society of Trained Masseuses* in 1915 (Barclay 1994, p. 54) and that it had been publishing profession-specific research findings since Lucile's Grunewald's influential 1928 survey of physiotherapy as a profession (Grunewald 1928), little physiotherapy-specific research was available to readers until university programmes became the norm. This is explained, in part, by the fact that there were few postgraduate research training programmes before 1980; few career opportunities for researchers and – not being a first-contact profession – barely any demands for physiotherapists to test the efficacy of their interventions.

Having an inherent focus on the body-as-machine, I would argue that physiotherapists have placed a great deal of value in objective measurement and so when research began to develop, it is perhaps not surprising that it quickly became dominated by quantitative designs. In recent years, clinical trials, experimental and other quantitative empirical studies have come to dominate the physiotherapy literature. Demands to be evidence-based, have combined with competitive market pressures to demonstrate that *our* treatment 'X' are better and more cost-effective than *their* treatment 'Y'. These demands have been superimposed on a desire to be seen as an objective and value-neutral clinical science, which have all lead to a dramatic increase in the consumption and production of quantitative research in physiotherapy in recent years.

Adopting quantitative research methodologies has perhaps given physiotherapists the satisfying sense that they are cementing their intimate relationship with the medical profession; a pattern they had followed since the first moments of the profession's conception. But it has also repeatedly thrown up the question of how best to upskill physiotherapists so that they can communicate in biomedical research terms, in the same way that physiotherapists learnt anatomical, physiological and pathological language over a century ago. How, for instance, should the profession prepare practitioners in the complexities of research designs; hierarchies of evidence; study methods and statistical tests; applications for competitive funding and ethical reporting; presentations and academic publishing and latterly, knowledge translation and economic impacts (Nast et al 2015; Dannapfel et al 2013; Rankin et al 2012)?

Eager to take advantage of the possibilities now available to them, physiotherapists have tackled these challenges with with enthusiasm and invested enormous energy and professional capital in the idea of physiotherapy as a science (Stevens et al 2016; Hammond et al 2015; Scurlock-Evans et al 2014; Aguilar et al 2013; Kell & Horlick-Jones 2012). Since Moseley et al's 2002 survey of the Physiotherapy Evidence Database (PEDro) (Moseley et al 2002), which showed that there had been an exponential growth in the number of physiotherapy clinical trials and reviews since the first published trial in 1955, the pace of chance in research publishing has only grown faster and the quality of research now being produced in physiotherapy is now quite remarkable. Stevens et al, for example, recently reported that there are now more than '33,000 reports of randomised controlled trials, systematic reviews and evidence-based clinical practice guidelines about the effects of physiotherapy interventions' (Stevens et al 2016).

Unfortunately, a number of recent studies have shown that physiotherapists are reluctant to make use of the vast volumes of research that they now have available to them; that clinicians are defaulting to experiential knowledge, peers and trusted sources, rather than the findings of experimental studies and that they are finding the volume of evidence more paralysing than enabling (Condon et al 2016; Dannapfel et al 2013; Scurlock-Evans et al 2014). Perhaps most significantly, practitioners are becoming increasingly aware that research and evidence-based approaches to practice will not, on their own, convince the public that physiotherapy is preferable to other physical therapies like chiropractic, osteopathy, massage and exercise therapies. The public, it seems, have an appetite for these alternatives to orthodox medicine, despite attempts of professionals like doctors, physiotherapists and the institutions that support them to convince them of their concerns (Marchione & Stobbe 2009; Mizrachi et al 2005; Holmes et al 2006).

Some of the reasons for this contrary public behaviour lie in the problem now emerging with evidence-based medicine (EBM), with Greenhalgh et al recently arguing that it places too much emphasis on experimental evidence at the expense of clinical experience and tacit knowledge; appears removed from real patients and 'seldom fit[s] the textbook description of disease and differ[s] from those included in research trials' (Greenhalgh et al 2014, p. 1). Spence recently described EBM as a 'a loaded gun at clinicians' heads', leading to evidence-based justifications for overtreatment (Spence 2014). Practitioners themselves are also more willing to challenge the institutional power of EBM, which increasingly appears to project the health professional as socially neutral, objective and politically disinterested (Goldenberg 2006), or places overwhelming demands and de-skilling possibilities upon clinicians (Murray et al 2007).

Underpinning much of this criticism, is the philosophical privilege that medicine (and physiotherapy) has traditionally given to a biomedical view of health and illness. Medical science, and the research that has grown from it, follows Enlightenment principles that research must be verifiable, repeatable, objective, free from bias and falsifiable. While this works well as a tool for evaluating whether one pharmaceutical intervention achieves better physical effects than another, it works less well for studies in which randomisation and control become practically or ethically challenging, or when we move beyond physiological variables to consider humanistic and social dimensions of life. Fortunately, medicine has come to recognise and even embrace the essential subjectivity of its practice and so new epistemologies approaches to research have followed in its wake (Nicholls 2009a, 2009b, 2009c; Petty et al 2012a, 2012b).

Unfortunately, many of these alternative epistemologies remain subordinate in medicine and approaches that could offer liberating new ways to think about practice are being weakened by the desire to retain the same positivist, quantitative principles at all cost. The much lauded biopsychosocial (BPS) model, for example, has been trumpeted as evidence of a holistic approach to medical practice.

Based on General Systems Theory (Braziller & Grinker 1967), George Engel developed the biopsychosocial model as a 'unified concept of health and disability' (Engel 1960). The approach was always based on a desire to develop a systematic, reductive, psychologically-informed, scientific view of people's behaviour and social relations and was never meant to embrace subjective, qualitative or socially constructed understandings of health and illness (Malmgren 2005; Horton-Salway 2002; Ghaemi 2010). In a similar way, attempts by the medical community to establish an international classification of functioning, disability and health (ICF) relied on the classic biomedical tools of normalisation and external appraisal as tools of objective verification (see Chapter 8). The ICF and other putatively 'humanistic' outcome measures and classification systems subtly project a sense of holism, but practice very traditional approaches to medical positivism.

Within a specific research context, we have even seen the co-option of quantitative approaches to biomedical research pervading *qualitative* research in recent years. Elizabeth Adams St. Pierre wrote recently of the troubling trend in qualitative research to focus almost exclusively on methodological rigour (St. Pierre 2014). Remembering qualitative research at its inception in the 1980s, Adams recalls how methods were secondary to more critical and radical questions about the necessity to emancipate marginalised voices; expose power asymmetries operating to suppress women, people of colour, disabled people and other social minorities and challenge hegemonic systems like biomedicine – from which professions like physiotherapy gained enormous social privilege (St. Pierre 2014). Slowly, however, over the 1990s and 2000s, qualitative research gained the attention of the orthodox medical community, which began to critique its lack of scientific rigour. Qualitative researchers responded by focusing on methods of verification, including developing new terms to replace generalisability, reliability and validity (see, e.g. Denzin & Lincoln 1994; Morse et al 2002; Tong et al 2007), systematic approaches to data collection and analysis (Morse et al 2002) and arguments in support of the very forms of objectivity and external falsifiability that the founders of the qualitative research movement had fought so hard against. Adams argued that qualitative research has now become corrupted by a focus on the methods of sampling, rigorous data collection and largely descriptive, thematic analysis that lacks the true animating power of critical humanistic and social inquiry (St. Pierre 2014).

Certainly, in physiotherapy, the vast bulk of research is quantitative and what qualitative research is being undertaken is dominated by the kinds of philosophically-limited but methodologically verifiable and objective approaches that Adams and others are increasingly decrying. In many ways, the kinds of research most physiotherapists undertake betrays, as much as any other practice associated with the profession, the values and beliefs, tensions and complexities that the profession now faces. Physiotherapists tacitly know that they must retain an affinity with biomedicine, but do not want to be seen as hand-maidens to the medical profession; they want to benefit from their alliance with the State, but want to retain their autonomy and distinctiveness; they want to show the full breadth and value of their work, but also want to ally themselves with the perception that they are a scientifically-informed practice. Physiotherapists want to keep abreast of the latest best practice, but recognise that this is impossible, given the volume of competing and, sometimes, conflicting literature now demanding their attention. Physiotherapists also want to treat each of their patients as unique individuals living in a specific cultural context, with unique histories and personalities, but at the same time, they want to be able to normalise, measure and objectify them in order that they can fulfil others' expectations of how physiotherapists should practice.

Research, then, fulfils a critical and contested role in defining physiotherapy's professional subjectivity. It is perhaps not surprising, given these tensions, that many physiotherapy leaders see the future for the profession as increasingly research intensive. Moving to post-baccalaureate qualifications in the 1990s, and later to full doctoral-entry in the North America and elsewhere, has put pressure on others to follow suit (Pagliarulo 2016). This has, in turn, increased the requirement for students to be consumers, and in some cases producers, of publishable quality research. Most regulatory authorities now mandate continuing professional development and many clinicians are engaging in post-qualification courses at universities, which assume that research is a fundamental constituent of critical inquiry. Clinicians themselves are increasingly being asked to undertake, or at least participate in, applied research studies as part of their everyday work. And the requirement to engage in research-informed debate on social media, through peer support networks, weekend study courses and almost every event at which physiotherapy practice is discussed, has become ubiquitous. Whether this emphasis and pressure to engage in research leads, ultimately, to physiotherapists asking critical questions about the past, present and future of the profession, however, remains to be seen.

Closing words

This chapter is the first of two that looks to take the historical and theoretical ideas built up in the previous nine chapters and answer the question 'so what?' How does an understanding of the ways physiotherapy has historically approached the body, touch, movement, function, posture and rehabilitation inform practice today, and what might this mean for the profession's future? The present tensions facing the teaching, practice, registration and research fields are many and varied, and these sites provide fertile territory for thoughtful consideration of the ways in which physiotherapy is enabling certain ways of thinking while constraining others.

There are a number of ways in which physiotherapy might grow and develop, and some pointers can be seen in the choices the profession is making about how it wants to educate its students, deliver its care, regulate its conduct and research its practice. With a few very notable exceptions, current evidence would suggest that physiotherapy is taking the second option that I listed at the opening of the chapter. Considering the weight of biomedical, quantitative research now being conducted by physiotherapists; the ongoing primacy of biomedical approach, even in supposedly 'holistic' tools like the BPS and ICF; the moves to specialisation and elite doctoral-entry graduating status; the regulation of any form of practice that threatens the traditional biomechanical margins of the profession and the distinct lack of any comprehensive discussion of the cultural, economic, historical, philosophical, political and social determinants of current physiotherapy practice, it would suggest that physiotherapy has chosen to return to what it knows best and enhances the idea of body-as-machine.

There are countervailing powers at work, however (Light 2000), and a number of academics, clinicians, researchers, students and teachers are raising dissent. In 2014, for example, a tentative inquiry among a handful of international colleagues with a shared interest in critiquing physiotherapy led to the formation of the Critical Physiotherapy Network (CPN). At the time of writing, the CPN has nearly 500 members spread across four continents and more than 30 countries. Similarly, journals like *Physiotherapy Theory and Practice* are being challenged to restructure their operations because of the weight of new critical material crossing the editor's desk. The diversity of approaches, philosophies and ways of engaging with physiotherapy across the world are now offering a serious challenge to physiotherapy's biomechanical traditional[8]. This book also represents an expression of a growing critical attitude towards the profession's past, present and future. In the final chapter, I return to the beginning of the book and bring together all of the arguments made thus far to answer the question of whether we are, in fact, experiencing the end of physiotherapy.

Notes

1   One of the most unusual and interesting alternative approaches to physiotherapy education can be found in Norwegian Psychomotor Physiotherapy (NPMP) (Sviland et al 2014; Dragesund 2012; Øien et al 2007; Sviland 2014; Dragesund & Råheim 2008). NPMP offers a radical alternative physiotherapy curriculum, emphasising the hermeneutic embodiment of practice. It has been in the instigator for some of the most interesting new thinking about physiotherapy's relationship to the body and the patient, and the ways in which physiotherapy practice can be taught and thought.

2   Everything about the treatment bed is problematic and needs to be thought through by the therapist. Even its name is problematic: do you call it a 'bed', or is this too reminiscent of the thing you have at home; is it a couch, or is this what psychotherapy patients lie on; is it a plinth, or does this sound too much like an altar?

3   It is a common medical practice for treatment beds to be quite austere and uncomfortable. Physiotherapists drew on this in adopting beds that were also very basic and functional. Because therapists wanted to desensualise their practice – particularly where touching was involved – beds were designed to offer minimal comfort. For the same reason, physiotherapist rarely dress their beds with expensive linens and soft furnishings. Of course, vinyl bed coverings are hygienic and practical, but it is the austerity of the bed that is its most powerful and enduring feature and the one that conveys the therapist's intentions without it needing to be repeatedly restated.

4   Terms like client and consumer have come into more common use in recent years as people have felt more able to express their personal preferences and have demanded that their investment in their own health be respected and mobilised by health professionals (Sharf & Street Jr 1997; McLaughlin 2009; Chamberlin 1990). As outlined in the Glossary, unless otherwise indicated, I have used the more traditional word 'patient' throughout the book, partly to indicate physiotherapy's traditional approach to treating the body-as-machine.

5 I am not suggesting here that people who are critically ill, in unremitting pain, or otherwise unable to communicate their needs and wishes, abdicate their right to safe, fair and ethically sound treatment, only that that their situation can sometimes makes it more difficult for them to take an active role in these discussions. Indeed, being unable to communicate ones beliefs, desires, preferences and values makes ethical care all the more important.

6 It is an interesting quirk of the *1949 Physiotherapy Act* that it stated that only registered physiotherapists could practice therapeutic massage. The alternative option for masseurs who had not passed through one of the country's two physiotherapy school was to register their practice under the 1978 *Massage Parlours Act* – the legislation that covered brothels and prostitutes.

7 Note here, the subtle but powerful gendering of language that excludes many women who were skilled craftspeople in their own right. There is a notable history of the gendering of trades that highlights how women were specifically excluded from trade guilds, working 'men's' clubs, trade unions and other industrial institutions as anxieties about women's emancipation and suffrage became more pronounced (Smith 2004). It is possible, perhaps even likely, that rules established by early massage organisations like the STM, which deliberately excluded men, were a reaction to this isolation and separation.

8 At the time of writing, for example, members of the CPN are collaborating on the first book to compile critical studies of physiotherapy spanning the performing arts, ethics and moral theory, object oriented ontology, critical disability studies, education, human/animal based therapy and gender studies. The book will be published by Cappelen Damm and will be avaible for free download in 2017.

References

Abbott, P. & Meerabeau, L., 1998, Professionals, professionalization and the caring professions, in L. Meerabeua (ed.), *The sociology of the caring professions*, University College London Press, London, pp. 1–19.

Aguilar, A., Stupans, I., Scutter, S. & King, S., 2013, Exploring the professional values of Australian physiotherapists, *Physiotherapy Research International*, 18(1), pp. 27–36.

Alexander, J.A., Ramsey, J.A. & Thomson, S.M., 2004, Designing the health workforce for the 21st century, *Medical Journal of Australia*, 180(1), pp. 7–9.

Allsop, J. & Saks, M., 2002, *Regulating the health professions*, Routledge, Abingdon, Oxon.

Anderson, E.M., 1977, *New Zealand society of physiotherapists: Golden Jubilee 1923–1973*, New Zealand Society of Physiotherapists, Wellington, New Zealand.

Anderson, G., Ellis, E., Williams, V. & Gates, C., 2005, Profile of the physiotherapy profession in New South Wales (1975–2002), *The Australian Journal of Physiotherapy*, 51(2), pp. 109–16.

Araya, D. & Peters, M., 2010, *Education in the creative economy: Knowledge and learning in the age of innovation*, Peter Lang, New York.

Barclay, J., 1994, *In good hands: The history of the Chartered Society of Physiotherapy 1894–1994*, Butterworth Heinemann, Oxford.

Beach, A. & Davies, C., 2013, *Interpreting professional self-regulation: A history of the United Kingdom Central Council for Nursing, Midwifery and Health Visiting*, Routledge, Abingdon, Oxon.

Bentley, P. & Dunstan, D., 2006, *The path to professionalism: Physiotherapy in Australia to the 1980s*, Australian Physiotherapy Association, Melbourne, Australia.

Bertilsson, M., 1990, The Welfare State, the professions and citizens, in M. Burrage & R. Torstendahl (eds.), *The formation of professions*, Sage, London, pp. 114–33.

Bjorbækmo, W.S. & Mengshoel, A.M., 2016, "A touch of physiotherapy" – the significance and meaning of touch in the practice of physiotherapy. *Physiotherapy Theory and Practice*, 32(1), 10–19.

Bleakley, A., 2014, *Patient-centred medicine in transition: The heart of the matter*, Springer, Wien.

Braziller, G. & Grinker, R.R., 1967, *Toward a unified theory of human behavior: An introduction to general systems theory*, Basic Books, New York.

Brunner, E., Herdt, A.D., Minguet, P., Baldew, S.-S. & Probst, M., 2015, Can cognitive behavioural therapy based strategies be integrated into physiotherapy for the prevention of chronic low back pain?: A systematic review, *Disability and Rehabilitation*, doi: 10.3109/09638288.2012.683848.

Bury, T.J. & Stokes, E.K., 2013, Direct access and patient/client self-referral to physiotherapy: A review of contemporary practice within the European Union, *Physiotherapy*, 99(4), pp. 285–91.

Carr-Sanders, A.P. & Wilson, P.A., 1933, *The professions*, Oxford University Press, Oxford.

Chamberlin, J., 1990, The ex-patients movement: Where weve been and where were going, *Journal of Mind and Behavior*, 11(3–4), pp. 323–36.

Clouder, L., 2000, Reflective practice: Realising its potential, *Physiotherapy*, 86, pp. 517–22.

Condon, C., McGrane, N., Mockler, D. & Stokes, E., 2016, Ability of physiotherapists to undertake evidence-based practice steps: A scoping review, *Physiotherapy*, 102(1), pp. 10–19.

Crossick, G., 1997, *The Artisan and the European town, 1500–1900*, Scholar Press, Aldershot.

Cushing, A.M., 2015, Learning patient-centred communication: The journey and the territory, *Patient Education and Counseling*, 98(10), pp. 1236–42.

Dahl-Michelsen, T., 2015, Curing and caring competences in the skills training of physiotherapy students, *Physiotherapy Theory and Practice*, 31(1), pp. 8–16.

Dannapfel, P., Peolsson, A. & Nilsen, P., 2013, What supports physiotherapists' use of research in clinical practice?: A qualitative study in Sweden, *Implementation science: IS*, 8(1), p. 31.

Davies, C., 2007, The promise of 21st century professionalism: Regulatory reform and integrated care, *Journal of Interprofessional Care*, 21(3), pp. 233–9.

Delany, C. & Watkin, D., 2009, A study of critical reflection in health professional education: 'learning where others are coming from', *Advances in Health Science Education Theory Practice*, 14(3), pp. 411–29.

Denzin, N.K. & Lincoln, Y.S., 1994, *Handbook of qualitative research*, Sage Publications, Thousand Oaks, CA.

Department of Health, 2010, *Equity and excellence: Liberating the NHS*, Department of Health, London.

Dew, K., 2003, *Borderland practices: Regulating alternative therapies in New Zealand*, University of Otago Press, Dunedin, New Zealand.

Donaghy, M.E. & Morss, K., 2000, Guided reflection: A framework to facilitate and assess reflective practice within the discipline of physiotherapy, *Physiotherapy Theory and Practice*, 16(1), pp. 3–14.

Donaldson, L., 2003, Expert patients usher in a new era of opportunity for the NHS, *British Medical Journal*, 326(7402), p. 1279.

Dragesund, T., 2012, *Development of a self-report questionnaire in the context of Norwegian Psychomotor Physiotherapy (NPMP)*, doctoral thesis, University of Bergen, Bergen.

Dragesund, T. & Råheim, M., 2008, Norwegian psychomotor physiotherapy and patients with chronic pain: Patients' perspective on body awareness, *Physiotherapy Theory and Practice*, 24(4), pp. 243–54.

Durkheim, 1933, *The division of labor in society*, Free Press, New York.

Dutta, M.J., 2015, *Neoliberal health organizing: Communication, meaning, and politics*, Left Coast Press, Walnut Creek, CA.

Dutton, L.L., 2014, The informal and hidden curriculum in physical therapist education, *Journal of Physical Therapy Education*, 28(3), p. 50.

Einhorn, E.S. & Logue, J., 2003, *Modern welfare states: Scandinavian politics and policy in the global age*, Praeger, Westport, CN.

Eisenberg, N.R., 2012, Post-structural conceptualizations of power relationships in physiotherapy, *Physiotherapy Theory and Practice*, 28(6), pp. 439–46.

Elston, M.A. 1991, The politics of professional power: Medicine in a changing health service, in G. Gabe, M. Calnan & M. Bury (eds.), *The sociology of the health service*, Routledge, London, pp. 58–88.

Engel, G.L., 1960, A unified concept of health and disease, *Perspectives in Biological Medicine*, 3, pp. 459–85.

Etzioni, A., 1969, *The semi-professions and their organization*, Free Press, New York.

Evetts, J., 1999, Professions: Changes and continuities, *International Review of Sociology*, 9, pp. 75–85.

Evetts, J., 2003, The sociological analysis of professionalism, *International Sociology*, 18(2), pp. 395–415.

Evetts, J., 2006, Short note: The sociology of professional groups: New directions, *Current Sociology*, 54(1), pp. 133–43.

Farr, J.R., 1997, On the shop floor: Guilds, artisans, and the European market economy, 1350–1750, *Journal of Early Modern History*, 1(1), pp. 24–54.

Field, R.I., 2006, *Healthcare regulation in America: Complexity, confrontation, and compromise*, Oxford University Press, Oxford.

Foot, C., Gilburt, H., Dunn, P., Jabbal, J., Seale, Goodrich, J., . . . Taylor, J., 2014, *People in control of their own health and care – The state of involvement*, The King's Fund, London.

Fournier, V., 1999, The appeal to "professionalism" as a disciplinary mechanism, *Sociological Review*, 47(2), pp. 280–307.

Fournier, V., 2000, Boundary work and the (un)making of the professions, in N. Malin (ed.), *Professionalism, boundaries and the workplace*, Routledge, London, pp. 67–86.

Fournier, V., 2002, Amateurism, quackery and professional conduct, in M. Dent & S. Whitehead (eds.), *Managing professional identities: Knowledge, performativities and the 'new' professional*, Routledge, London, pp. 116–37.

Freidson, E., 1970, *Profession of medicine: A study of the sociology of applied knowledge*, Dodd Mead, New York.

Freire, P., 1970, The banking concept of education, in A.S. Canestrari & B.A. Marlowe (eds.), *Educational foundations: An anthology of critical readings*, Sage, Los Angeles, CA, pp. 99–111.

French, S., 2013, *Physiotherapy: A psychosocial approach*, Butterworth Heinemann, London.

Freshwater, D., Fisher, P. & Walsh, E., 2013, Revisiting the panopticon: Professional regulation, surveillance and sousveillance, *Nursing Inquiry*, 22(1), pp. 3–12.

Gabe, J., Harley, K. & Calnan, M., 2015, Healthcare choice: Discourses, perceptions, experiences and practices, *Current Sociology*, 63, 623–35.

Ghaemi, S.N., 2010, *The rise and fall of the biopsychosocial model: Reconciling art and science in psychiatry*, Johns Hopkins University Press, Baltimore, MD.

Gibson, B.E., 2006, Disability, connectivity and transgressing the autonomous body, *Journal of Medical Humanities*, 27(3), pp. 187–96.

Gibson, B.E., Nixon, S.A. & Nicholls, D.A., 2010, Critical reflections on the physiotherapy profession in Canada, *Physiotherapy Canada, Physiothérapie Canada*, 62(2), pp. 98–100, 101–3.

Gibson, B.E., Carnevale, F.A. & King, G., 2012, 'This is my way': Reimagining disability, in/dependence and interconnectedness of persons and assistive technologies, *Disability and Rehabilitation*, 34(22), pp. 1894–9.

Gilbert, T., 2001, Reflective practice and clinical supervision: Meticulous rituals of the confessional, *Journal of Advanced Nursing*, 36(2), pp. 199–205.

Goldenberg, M.J., 2006, On evidence and evidence-based medicine: Lessons from the philosophy of science, *Social Science & Medicine (1982)*, 62(11), pp. 2621–32.

Gordon, C., 2009, *Dead on arrival: The politics of healthcare in twentieth-century America*, Princeton University Press, Princeton, NJ.

Greenhalgh, T., Howick, J., Maskrey, N. & Evidence Based Medicine Renaissance Group, 2014, Evidence based medicine: A movement in crisis?, *BMJ (Clinical Research Ed.)*, 348:g3725, doi: 10.1136/bmj.g3725.

Grignon, T.P., Emma Henley PT, D.P.T., Lee, K.M., Abentroth, M.J. & Jette, D.U., 2014, Expected graduate outcomes in U.S. physical therapist education programs: A qualitative study, *Journal of Physical Therapy Education*, 28(1), p. 48.

Grunewald, L.R., 1928, A study of physiotherapy as a vocation, *The Physiotherapy Review*, 8(4), pp. 37–49.

Gubrium, J.F. & Holstein, J.A., 2002, *Handbook of interview research: Context & methods*, Sage, Thousand Oaks, CA.

Guenther, L.A., McGinnis, P., Romen, M. & Patel, K., 2014, Self assessment of professional core values among physical therapists, *HPA Resource*, 14(3), pp. J15–J24.

Gzil, F., Lefeve, C., Cammelli, M., Pachoud, B., Ravaud, J.F. & Leplege, A., 2007, Why is rehabilitation not yet fully person-centred and should it be more person-centred?, *Disability and Rehabilitation*, 29(20–21), pp. 1616–24.

Håkstad, R.B., Obstfelder, A., & Øberg, G.K., 2016, Parents' perceptions of primary health care physiotherapy with preterm infants: Normalization, clarity, and trust. *Qual Health Res*, 26(10), 1341–50.

Hammond, R., 2007, Editorial — Individuation through socialization, *Physiotherapy Research International*, 12(3), pp. 123–5.

Hammond, R., Cross, V. & Moore, A., 2015, The construction of professional identity by physiotherapists: A qualitative study, *Physiotherapy*, 102(1), 71–7.

Hammond, J.A., 2013, *Doing gender in physiotherapy education: A critical pedagogic approach to understanding how students construct gender identities in an undergraduate physiotherapy programme in the United Kingdom*, doctoral thesis, Kingston University, London.

Health Workforce Advisory Committee, 2003, The New Zealand health workforce: Future directions: Recommendations to the Minister of Health 2003, Ministry of Health, Wellington, New Zealand.

Higgs, J. & Edwards, H., 1999, *Educating beginning practitioners: Challenges for health professional education*, Butterworth-Heinemann, Oxford.

Higgs, J. & Titchen, A., 2001, *Practice knowledge and expertise in the health professions*, Butterworth-Heinemann, Oxford.

Higgs, J. & Titchen, A., 2008, *Professional practice in health, education and the creative arts*, John Wiley & Sons, Chichester.

Higgs, J., Refshauge, K. & Ellis, E., 2001, Portrait of the physiotherapy profession, *Journal of Interprofessional Care*, 15(1), pp. 79–89.

Higgs, J., Richardson, B. & Dahlgren, M.A., 2004, *Developing practice knowledge for health professionals*, Butterworth-Heinemann, Edinburgh.

Higgs, J., Jones, M.A., Loftus, S. & Christensen, N., 2008, *Clinical reasoning in the health professions*, Elsevier Health Sciences UK, London.

Higgs, J., Barnett, R., Billett, S., Hutchings, M. & Trede, F., 2013, *Practice-based education: Perspectives and strategies* (Vol. 6). Sense, Rotterdam.

Holmes, D., Murray, S.J., Perron, A. & Rail, G., 2006, Deconstructing the evidence-based discourse in health sciences: Truth, power and fascism, *International Journal of Evidence Based Healthcare*, 4(3), pp. 180–6.

Horobin, H. & Thom, V., 2015, Starting with transitions: Internationalisation for a post graduate physiotherapy course, in W. Green & C. Whitsed (eds.), *Critical perspectives on internationalizing the curriculum in disciplines: Reflective narrative accounts from business, education and health*, Sense, Dordrecht, pp. 249–60.

Horton-Salway, M., 2002, Bio-psycho-social reasoning in GP's case narratives: The discursive construction of ME patients' identities, *Health*, 6(4), pp. 401–21.

Hudon, A., Drolet, M. & Williams-Jones, B., 2014, Ethical issues raised by private practice physiotherapy are more diverse than first meets the eye: Recommendations from a literature review, *Physiotherapy Canada. Physiothérapie Canada*, 67(2), pp. 124–32.

Ingham, D., Mohr, T., Walker, J.R. & Mabey, R., 2013, Ten year history of physical therapist disciplinary reports, *HPA Resource*, 13(3), pp. 11–25.

Johnson, T., Larkin, G. & Saks, M., 1995, *Health professions and the state in Europe*, Routledge, London.

Jones, M., Edwards, I. & Gifford, L., 2002, Conceptual models for implementing biopsychosocial theory in clinical practice, *Manual Therapy*, 7(1), pp. 2–9.

Juhan, D., 1987, *Job's body: A handbook for bodywork*, Station Hill Press, New York.

Kell, C., 2013, Placement education pedagogy as social participation: What are students really learning? *Physiotherapy Research International*, 19(1), pp. 44–54.

Kell, C. & Horlick-Jones, T., 2012, 'Disciplining witnesses' in the teaching of physiotherapy: Some insights into the practical accomplishment of a science-based healthcare profession, *Communication Medicine*, 9(3), pp. 253–68.

Kell, C. & Owen, G., 2008, Physiotherapy as a profession: Where are we now? *International Journal of Therapy and Rehabilitation*, 15(4), pp. 158–67.

Kemmis, S. & Smith, T.J., 2008, *Enabling praxis: Challenges for education*. Sense Publications, Rotterdam.

Kleinke, J.D., 1998, *Bleeding edge: The business of healthcare in the new century*, Jones and Bartlett, Boston, MA.

Kuhlmann, E. & Saks, M., 2008, *Rethinking professional governance: International directions in healthcare*, The Policy Press, London.

Kumar, S.P., Sisodia, V. & Jacob, E., 2013, Levels of professionalism among physical therapists in India – A national cross-sectional survey. *Journal of Sports Medicine & Doping Studies*, 3(123), doi: 10.4172/2161-0673.1000123.

Laitinen-Väänänen, S., Luukka, M.-R. & Talvitie, U., 2008, Physiotherapy under discussion: A discourse analytic study of physiotherapy students' clinical education, *Advances in Physiotherapy*, 10(1), pp. 2–8.

Larkin, G. 2002, The regulation of the professions allied to medicine, in J. Allsop & M. Saks (eds.), *Regulating the health professions*, Routledge, Abingdon, Oxon, pp. 120–33.

Lauterstein, D., 2004, Touching heaven: Bodywork and the realm of the incredible: A therapist's viewpoint, *Massage & Bodywork Magazine*, December/January.

Law, J. & Mol, A. (eds.), 2002, *Complexities: Social studies of knowledge practices*, Duke University Press, Durham, NC.

Light, D.W., 1995, Coutervailing powers: A framework for professions in transition, in T. Johnson, G. Larkin & M. Saks (eds.), *Professions and the state in Europe*, Routledge, London, pp. 25–44.

Light, D.W., 2000, The medical profession and organisational change: From professional dominance to countervailing power, in C.E. Bird, P. Conrad & A.M. Fremont (eds.), *Handbook of Medical Sociology*, Prentice Hall, Upper Saddle River, NJ, pp. 201–16.

Malmgren, H., 2005, The theoretical basis of the biopsychosocial model, in P. White (ed.), *Biopsychosocial medicine*, Oxford University Press, Oxford, pp. 21–35.

Marchione, M. & Stobbe, M., 2009, *Americans spend $34 billion on alternative medicine*, American College of Traditional Chinese Medicine, accessed from www.actcm.edu/news/americans-spend-34-billion-on-alternative-medicine/, retrieved 20 March 2015.

Martin, G.P., Leslie, M., Minion, J., Willars, J. & Dixon-Woods, M., 2013, Between surveillance and subjectification: Professionals and the governance of quality and patient safety in English hospitals, *Social Science & Medicine (1982)*, 99, pp. 80–8.

McCombie, R.P., O'Connor, S.S. & Schumacher, S.D., 2015, A comparative investigation of personality traits between two allied health professions: Occupational therapy and physiotherapy, *International Journal of Therapy and Rehabilitation*, 22(8), pp. 377–84.

McIntosh, N, 2005, *The educated heart: Professional boundaries for massage therapists, bodyworkers, and movement therapists*, Lippincott, Williams & Wilkins, Philadelphia, PA.

McLaughlin, H., 2009, What's in a name: Client, patient, customer, consumer, expert by experience, service user – what's next? *British Journal of Social Work*, 39(6), pp. 1101–17.

McWhinney, I.R., 1985, Patient-centred and doctor-centred models of clinical decision-making, in M. Sheldon, J. Brooke & A. Rector (eds.), *Decision-making in general practice*, Macmillan Education UK, London, pp. 31–46.

Mendick, N., Young, B., Holcombe, C. & Salmon, P., 2015, How do surgeons think they learn about communication? A qualitative study, *Medical Education*, 49(4), pp. 408–16.

Miles-Tapping, C., 1989, Sponsorship and sacrifice in the historical development of Canadian physiotherapy, *Physiotherapy Canada, Physiothérapie Canada*, 41(2), pp. 72–80.

Mingardi, A., 2015, Healthcare and the slippery slope of state growth: Lessons from the past, *Journal of Medicine and Philosophy*, 40(2), pp. 169–89.

Mizrachi, N., Shuval, J.T. & Gross, S., 2005, Boundary at work: Alternative medicine in biomedical settings, *Sociology of Health & Illness*, 27(1), pp. 20–43.

Mooney S., 2012, *Physiotherapy clinical education: Power interplay examined through the lens of Bourdieu*, doctoral thesis, Auckland University of Technology, Auckland, New Zealand.

Morden, A., Jinks, C. & Ong, B.N., 2015, Risk and self-managing chronic joint pain: Looking beyond individual lifestyles and behaviour, *Sociology of Health & Illness*, 37(6), pp. 888–903.

Morse, J., Barrett, M., Mayan, M., Olson, K. & Spiers, J., 2002, Verification strategies for establishing reliability and validity in qualitative research, *International Journal of Qualitative Methods*, 1(2), pp. 1–19.

Moseley, A.M., Herbert, R.D., Sherrington, C. & Maher, C.G., 2002, Evidence for physiotherapy practice: A survey of the physiotherapy evidence database (PEDro), *Australian Journal of Physiotherapy*, 48(1), pp. 43–9.

Mudge, S., Stretton, C. & Kayes, N., 2013, Are physiotherapists comfortable with person-centred practice?: An autoethnographic insight, *Disability and Rehabilitation*, doi: 10.3109/09638288.2013.797515.

Murphy, W., 1995, *Healing the generations: A history of physical therapy and the American Physical Therapy Association*, Greenwich Publishing, Lyme, CN.

Murray, S.J., Holmes, D., Perron, A. & Rail, G., 2007, No exit?: Intellectual integrity under the regime of 'evidence' and 'best-practices', *Journal of Evaluation in Clinical Practice*, 13(4), pp. 512–16.

Nancarrow, S.A. & Borthwick, A.M., 2005, Dynamic professional boundaries in the healthcare workforce, *Sociology of Health & Illness*, 27(7), pp. 897–919.

Nast, I., Tal, A., Schmid, S., Schoeb, V., Rau, B., Barbero, M. & Kool, J., 2015, Physiotherapy research priorities in Switzerland: Views of the various stakeholders. *Physiotherapy Research International*, 21(3), pp. 137–46.

Nicholls, D.A., 2009a, Qualitative research: Part one – philosophy. *International Journal of Therapy and Rehabilitation*, 16(10), pp. 526–34.

Nicholls, D.A., 2009b, Qualitative research: Part two – methodology. *International Journal of Therapy and Rehabilitation*, 16(11), pp. 586–92.

Nicholls, D.A., 2009c, Qualitative research: Part three – methods. *International Journal of Therapy and Rehabilitation*, 16(12), pp. 638–47.

Nicholls, D.A., 2012a, Postmodernism and physiotherapy research, *Physical Therapy Reviews*, 17(6), pp. 360–8.

Nicholls, D.A., 2012b, Foucault and physiotherapy. *Physiotherapy Theory and Practice*, 28(6), pp. 447–53.

Nicholls, D.A., 2016, Parrhésia, artisans and the possibilities for deliberate practice, in F. Trede & C. McEwan (eds.), *Educating the deliberate practitioner*, Springer, Amsterdam, pp. 91–106.

Nicholls, D.A. & Holmes, D., 2012, Discipline, desire, and transgression in physiotherapy practice, *Physiotherapy Theory and Practice*, 28(6), pp. 454–65.

Nicholls, D.A. & Larmer, P., 2005, Possible futures for physiotherapy: An exploration of the New Zealand context, *New Zealand Journal of Physiotherapy*, 33(2), pp. 55–60.

Nicholls, D.A., Reid, D.A. & Larmer, P.J., 2009a, Crisis, what crisis? Revisiting 'possible futures for physiotherapy', *New Zealand Journal of Physiotherapy*, 37(3), pp. 105–14.

Nicholls, D.A., Walton, J.A. & Price, K., 2009b, Making breathing your business: Enterprising practices at the margins of orthodoxy, *Health: An Interdisciplinary for the Social Study of Health, Illness and Medicine*, 13(3), pp. 337–60.

Nicholls, D.A., Atkinson, K., Bjorbækmo, W.S., Gibson, B.E., Latchem, J., Olesen, J., Ralls, J. & Setchell, J., 2016, Connectivity: An emerging concept for physiotherapy practice, *Physiotherapy Theory and Practice*, 32(3), pp. 159–70.

Noronha, S., Anderson, D., Lee, M.M., Krumdick, N.D., Irwin, K.E., Burton-Hess, J., Ciancio, M., Wallingford, M. & Workman, G.M., 2016, Professionalism in physician assistant, physical therapist, occupational therapist, clinical psychology, and biomedical sciences students, *Journal of Allied Health*, 45(1), pp. 71–8.

Øien, A.M., Iversen, S. & Stensland, P., 2007, Narratives of embodied experiences – Therapy processes in Norwegian Psychomotor Physiotherapy, *Advances in Physiotherapy*, 9(1), pp. 31–9.

Øien, A.M., Råheim, M., Iversen, S. & Steihaug, S., 2009, Self-perception as embodied knowledge-changing processes for patients with chronic pain, *Advances in Physiotherapy*, 11(3), pp. 121–9.

Øien, A.M., Steihaug, S., Iversen, S. & Råheim, M., 2011, Communication as negotiation processes in long-term physiotherapy: A qualitative study, *Scandinavian Journal of Caring Sciences*, 25(1), pp. 53–61.

Oliveira, A.L. & Nunes, E.D., 2015, Physiotherapy: A historical analysis of the transformation from an occupation to a profession in Brazil, *Brazilian Journal of Physical Therapy*, 19(4), pp. 286–93.

Ovretveit, J., 1985, Medical dominance and the development of professional autonomy in physiotherapy, *Sociol Health & Illness*, 7(1), pp. 76–93.

Owen G., 2014, *Becoming a practice profession: A genealogy of physiotherapy's moving/touching practice*, doctoral thesis, University of Cardiff, Cardiff.

Pagliarulo, M.A., 2016, The profession of physical therapy: Definition and development, in M.A. Pagliarulo (ed.), *Introduction to physical therapy*, Elsevier, St. Louis, MO, pp. 3–22.

Palmer, M., 1930, Editorial, *Journal of the Chartered Society of Massage and Medical Gymnastics* (April), p. 261.

Parsons, T., 1951, *The social system*, Free Press, New York.

Patton, N., Higgs, J. & Smith, M., 2013, Using theories of learning in workplaces to enhance physiotherapy clinical education, *Physiotherapy Theory and Practice*, 29(7), pp. 493–503.

Petty, N.J., Thomson, O.P. & Stew, G., 2012a, Ready for a paradigm shift? Part 1: Introducing the philosophy of qualitative research. *Manual Therapy*, 17(4), pp. 267–74. doi: 10.1016/j.math.2012.03.006.

Petty, N.J., Thomson, O.P. & Stew, G., 2012b, Ready for a paradigm shift? Part 2: Introducing qualitative research methodologies and methods. *Manual Therapy*, 17(5), pp. 378–84. doi: 10.1016/j.math.2012.03.004.

Pike, A.J., 2008, Body-mindfulness in physiotherapy for the management of long-term chronic pain, *Physical Therapy Reviews*, 13(1), pp. 45–56.

Praestegaard, J. & Gard, G., 2013, Ethical issues in physiotherapy – Reflected from the perspective of physiotherapists in private practice, *Physiotherapy Theory and Practice*, 29(2), pp. 96–112.

Praestegaard, J., Gard, G. & Glasdam, S., 2014, Physiotherapy as a disciplinary institution in modern society – A Foucauldian perspective on physiotherapy in Danish private practice, *Physiotherapy Theory and Practice*, 31(1), pp. 17–28.

Pretorius, A., Karunaratne, N. & Fehring, S., 2015, Australian physiotherapy workforce at a glance: A narrative review, *Australian Health Review*, 40(4), pp. 438–42.

Prictor, M. & Hill, S., 2011, Does communication with consumers and carers need to improve?, in S. Hill (ed.), *The knowledgeable patient: Communication and participation in health – A Cochrane Handbook*, Wiley Blackwell, London.

Ramklass, S.S., 2009, An investigation into the alignment of a South African physiotherapy curriculum and the expectations of the healthcare system, *Physiotherapy*, 95(3), pp. 216–23.

Rankin, G., Rushton, A., Olver, P. & Moore, A., 2012, Chartered Society of Physiotherapy's identification of national research priorities for physiotherapy using a modified Delphi technique, *Physiotherapy*, 98(3), pp. 260–72.

Richardson, B., 1999, Professional development: 1. Professional socialisation and professionalisation, *Physiotherapy*, 85(9), pp. 461–7.

Richardson, B., Lindquist, I., Engardt, M. & Aitman, C., 2002, Professional socialization: Students' expectations of being a physiotherapist, *Medical Teacher*, 24(6), pp. 622–7.

Robertson, A., 2001, Biotechnology, political rationality and discourses on health risk, *Health*, 5(3), pp. 293–309.

Rolfe, G. & Gardner, L., 2006, 'Do not ask who I am?': Confession, emancipation and (self)-management through reflection, *Journal of Nursing Management*, 14(8), pp. 593–600.

Roush, S.E. & Sharby, N., 2011, Disability reconsidered: The paradox of physical therapy, *Physical Therapy*, 91(12), pp. 1715–27.

Roush, S.E., Cox, K., Garlick, J., Kane, M. & Marchand, L., 2015, Physical therapists' perceptions of sexual boundaries in clinical practice in the United States, *Physiotherapy Theory and Practice*, 31(5), pp. 327–36.

Runyan, A., Ellington, K. & Wershof Schwartz, A., 2013, A compelling practice: Empowering future leaders in the medical humanities, *Journal of Medical Humanities*, 34(4), pp. 493–5.

Saks, M., 1995, *Professions and the public interest*, Routledge, London.

Saks, M., 2010, Analyzing the professions: The case for the neo-Weberian approach, *Comparative Sociology*, 9(6), pp. 887–915.

Sanders, T., Ong, B.N., Sowden, G. & Foster, N., 2014, Implementing change in physiotherapy: Professions, contexts and interventions, *Journal of Health Organization and Management*, 28(1), pp. 96–114.

Schunk, C. & Thut, C., 2003, Autonomous practice: Issues of risk: How PTs can ensure that hard-won freedoms don't literally become liabilities, *PT – Magazine of Physical Therapy*, 11(5), pp. 34–8.

Scurlock-Evans, L., Upton, P. & Upton, D., 2014, Evidence-based practice in physiotherapy: A systematic review of barriers, enablers and interventions, *Physiotherapy*, 100(3), pp. 208–19.

Sharf, B.F. & Street Jr, R.L., 1997, The patient as a central construct: Shifting the emphasis, *Health Communication*, 9(1), pp. 1–11.

Shaw, J.A. & DeForge, R.T., 2012, Physiotherapy as bricolage: Theorizing expert practice, *Physiotherapy Theory and Practice*, 28(6), pp. 420–7.

Sim, J., 1985, Physiotherapy: A professional profile, *Physiotherapy Practice*, 1, pp. 14–22.

Sivertsen, M. & Normann, B., 2014, Embodiment and self in reorientation to everyday life following severe traumatic brain injury, *Physiotherapy Theory and Practice*, pp. 1–7.

Smith, P.H., 2004, *The body of the artisan: Art and experience in the scientific revolution*, University of Chicago Press, Chicago, IL.

Spence, D., 2014, Evidence based medicine is broken, *BMJ (Clinical Research Ed.)*, 348:g22.

Stevens, M.L., Moseley, A.M., Elkins, M.R., Lin, C.C. & Maher, C.G., 2016, Evidence-based physiotherapy and the use of PEDro, *Physiotherapy*, doi: 10.1016/j.physio.2016.07.004.

St. Pierre, E.A., 2014, A brief and personal history of post qualitative research: Toward 'Post Inquiry', *JCT (Online)*, 30(2).

Sviland, R., Martinsen, K. & Råheim, M., 2014, To be held and to hold one's own: Narratives of embodied transformation in the treatment of long lasting musculoskeletal problems, *Medicine, Healthcare and Philosophy*, 17(4), pp. 609–24.

Sviland, R., Råheim, M. & Martinsen, K., 2012, Touched in sensation – moved by respiration, *Scandinavian Journal of Caring Sciences*, 26(4), pp. 811–19.

Sviland R., 2014, *Norwegian psychomotor physiotherapy and embodied narrative identity, A theory generating study*, doctoral thesis, University of Bergen, Bergen.

Swisher, L.L. & Page, C.G., 2005, *Professionalism in physical therapy*, Elsevier, St. Louis, MO.

Taylor, D. & Bury, M., 2007, Chronic illness, expert patients and care transition, *Sociology of Health & Illness*, 29(1), pp. 27–45.

Thille, P., Ward, N., & Russell, G., 2014, Self-management support in primary care: Enactments, disruptions, and conversational consequences. *Social Science & Medicine*, May(108), pp. 97–105.

Titchen, A. & Higgs, J., 2001, Towards professional artistry and creativity in practice, in J. Higgs & A. Titchen (eds.), *Professional practice in health, education and the creative arts*, Blackwell Science, Oxford, pp. 273–90.

Tong, A., Sainsbury, P. & Craig, J., 2007, Consolidated criteria for reporting qualitative research (COREQ): A 32-item checklist for interviews and focus groups. *International Journal for Quality in Health Care*, 19(6), pp. 349–57.

Trede, F., 2008, *A critical practice model for physiotherapy practice: Developing practice through critical transformative dialogues*, Vdm Verlag, Saarbrücken.

Trede, F. & Flowers, R., 2014, Patient-centred context of health practice relationships, in J. Higgs, A. Croker, D. Tasker, J. Hummell & N. Patton (eds.), *Health practice relationships*, Sense, Rotterdam, pp. 37–46.

Trede, F. & Haynes, A. 2009, Developing person-centred relationships with clients and families. In J. Higgs, M.S. Smith, G.W. Webb, M.S. Skinner & A.C. Croker (eds.), *Contexts of physiotherapy practice*. Churchill Livingstone, Sydney, Australia, pp. 246–59.

Trede, F., Higgs, J., Jones, M. & Edwards, I., 2010, Emancipatory practice: A model for physiotherapy practice, *Focus on Health Professional Education*, 5(2), pp. 1–13.

Trede, F. & McEwan, C. (eds.), 2016, *Educating the deliberate professional*, Sense, Amsterdam.

Varul, M.Z., 2010, Talcott Parsons, the sick role and chronic illness, *Body & Society*, 16(2), pp. 72–94.

Vuoskoski, P.H. 2014, *Work-placement assessment as a lived-through educationally meaningful experience of the student: An application of the phenomenological descriptive approach*. Doctoral thesis, Macquarie University, North Ryde, Australia.

Ward, A. & Gracey, J., 2006, Reflective practice in physiotherapy curricula: A survey of UK university based professional practice coordinators, *Medical Teacher*, 28, pp. e32–9.

White, R., 2004, Using reflective practice in the physiotherapy curriculum, in S. Tate & M. Sills (eds.), *The development of critical reflection in the health professions*, Academy of Higher Education, London, pp. 24–31.

Wilensky, H.L., 1964, The professionalization of everyone?, *American Journal of Sociology*, 70, pp. 137–58.

Williams, L. & Lawlis, T., 2014, Jostling for position: A sociology of allied health, in J. Germov (ed.), *Second opinion: An introduction to health sociology*, Oxford University Press, South Melbourne, Australia, pp. 439–63.

Williams, S.J., 1998a, Bodily dys-order: Desire, excess and the transgression of corporeal boundaries, *Body & Society*, 4(2), pp. 59–82.

Williams, S.J., 1998b, Health as moral performance: Ritual, transgression and taboo, *Health*, 2(4), pp. 435–57.

Winther, H., Grøntved, S. N., Kold Gravesen, E. & Ilkjær, I., 2014, The dancing nurses and the language of the body: Training somatic awareness, bodily communication, and embodied professional competence in nurse education, *Journal of Holistic Nursing*, 33(3), pp. 182–92.

Wloszczak-Szubzda, A. & Jarosz, M.J., 2013, Professional communication competences of physiotherapists – Practice and educational perspectives, *Annals of Agricultural and Environmental Medicine*, 20(1), pp. 189–94.

10 The end of physiotherapy

Introduction

I have been working as a physiotherapist now, in one form or another, for nearly 30 years, and during that time, I have seen some amazing physiotherapists do some incredible things with patients. I have seen a woman sit up and drink a cup of tea half-an-hour after being in acute respiratory failure. I have seen a man rigid with spasticity move like a ballerina and another melt in relief as his chronic back pain subsided. I have seen patients regain years of life from slow, steady rehabilitation and psychotic, violent offenders calmed with massage. All of these things, and more, have been brought about by physiotherapists: by people who have learned, through long years of patient observation and thoughtful study, how the body works and how to use their hands to greatest effect. But for all the wonderful things I have seen, I have also spent much of my professional life wondering why we, as physiotherapists, do not make more of the experiences, skills and manifest opportunities available to us. Why is it that we have chosen to focus on the biomechanical body at the exclusion of more holistic view of people? Why have we long claimed that physiotherapy is about 'movement', but only really engaged with the physical movement of discrete body parts? Why is it that we have willingly embraced quantitative research, but not qualitative? Why have we shown such an abiding passion for complex anatomical and pathological ideas, but turned our professional 'nose' up at philosophy and sociology? Why have we focused so much on technical skills and discounted individual therapists' individual values and beliefs? Why do we think physiotherapy is so complicated that the public does not understand what we do? Why is it that we have never really understood that the limits on how we think and practice are largely self-imposed? And why have we shown so little propensity for critical self-scrutiny and change? With its mix of powerful human experiences of trauma and recovery; its insights into lives lived with tragedy, suffering and profound grace under pressure and its challenges to find personal and profession meaning in the face of sometimes overwhelming complexity, it is perhaps not surprising that physiotherapy has given me a lifetime of rich and rewarding experiences and provided the substrate for this extended case study of a discipline with a very particular history and philosophy of practice.

In the opening chapter of the book, I wrote about what I called the 'physiotherapy paradox' – the idea that it was in the very nature of physiotherapy to overlook the forces that are at the heart of the profession's present problems. I argued that the profession's fixation on the body-as-machine, causes physiotherapists to disregard cultural, historical, economic, philosophical, political and social discourses that are now vital if the profession is to understand the changing economy of healthcare. I have tried to give evidence to this idea over the course of the book and explored not only how this came about, but also what it might mean for the profession into the future. The book has been directed to the problem posed by Gwyn Owen, when she wrote recently that, 'What is currently unclear in the historic literature is how and why physiotherapy practice . . . has evolved to become what it is' (Owen 2014, p. 5). My argument has been that physiotherapy has benefitted hugely from its biomechanical approach to the body, its affinity with medicine and its relationship with 'the State' and has consequently grown into one of the world's largest and most established orthodox health professions. It has done so in the face of scandal, war, epidemic disease, healthcare reorganisation, competition, technological revolution and globalisation, and has quietly and assuredly established itself as a popular, trusted and respected health profession. But that the very same influences that once nurtured physiotherapy might now be working against it, and that the principles that once gave physiotherapists confidence and security might now be undermining their efforts to progress.

Once physiotherapists turned to the body-as-machine to show that they could touch bodies without fear of licentiousness or scandal. Now people seemingly want more from their therapist than cold, technical touch and detached depersonalisation. Once it was enough that physiotherapists distinguished themselves with their knowledge of the patho-anatomical knowledge of movement. Now that knowledge is widely available to anyone with an Internet connection and people are demanding more empathy and humanistic engagement from their therapist. Once physiotherapists benefitted from the protection of the State and patients lay in hospitals and clinics waiting for their treatment. Now, care is moving inexorably into much more dispersed and competitive locations and people are weighing up the full cost of physiotherapy against myriad other options available to them.

Fortunately, physiotherapists know how to adapt. Throughout its history, the profession has responded to the call for more masseuses, better training and the needs of ever-more complex clinical problems by finding ways to fashion relatively simple techniques of massage, mobilisation and manipulation of tissues, electrotherapy, hydrotherapy and remedial exercise, into practices that are both contemporary and yet redolent of the past. My argument in this book, however, is that the challenges faced by the profession today are of a different order to the ones posed in the past. Where physiotherapists were once asked to take their newfound legitimacy and apply it to the flood of injured servicemen that arrived in field hospitals and embryonic rehabilitation centres during World War I, they are now being asked to relinquish patients, traditional disorders and treatment sites, and hand over care to less-well trained and less expensive carers; where once the doctor, nurse and physiotherapist constituted the three practitioners most patients saw when they became ill, now people are overwhelmed by the variety of care options available to them and where once the idea of a 'normal' body was sufficient, now no-one truly knows what the body is capable of or able to be adapted to.

In essence, the entire history of the profession has been one of growth and expansion. In the last few decades, however, a neoliberal ideology of healthcare has slowly and inexorably replaced the model that nurtured physiotherapy for much of the 20th century. Safe in its belief that what had worked in the past would work in the future, physiotherapists have continued to educate their students in much the same way; practice as if the same ideology would be sufficient for the future needs of the public and promote the same relationships between the therapist and the patient, doctor, legislator and third-party payer, despite the fact that the entire economy of healthcare has changed. And it has done so with a mixture of confident belligerence, hopeful expectation and cautious optimism, tinged with just a little anxious awareness that things might not, after all, be the same tomorrow as they were yesterday.

So, this book attempts to tackle the questions posed by the changing economy of healthcare head on and critically analyse the reasons how physiotherapy 'has evolved to become what it is'. At the same time, isn't everyone claiming that it is the end of something-or-other these days? Isn't it just part of the postmodern zeitgeist to prophesy the end of 'the good years'; to encourage a kind of nihilistic despondence in the face of climate change, global financial crisis and random acts of terror? Yes, certainly, there is some justification for this argument. One could easily be forgiven for thinking that this book takes a negative view of the profession's future, after all the book is called *The End of Physiotherapy*. But to view this book – and its deliberately provocative title – as nihilistic or negative would be to misunderstand my intentions. In many ways my hope is that the book points to a much more interesting, diverse, inclusive, critically deliberate, exciting and satisfying role for physiotherapists in the future. My belief is that if physiotherapists can transcend the ideology that once did so much to nurture the profession, but now threatens to strangle it, then patients, legislators and funders will find new reasons to turn to physiotherapy and that whole new vistas will open up to practitioners. Certainly, we live in a time when myriad opportunities are available to a profession that has established its legitimacy and orthodoxy, proven its trustworthiness and efficacy and shown its ability to serve diverse communities of need. So, over the course of the next few pages I want to explore some of these challenges and opportunities in more detail and point to ways that physiotherapy might choose to become something other than it is today.

The changing economy of healthcare

No-one practicing as a physiotherapist today, whether they work in a large hospital or out in the community, can fail to be aware of some of the seismic changes now taking place in the broader economy of healthcare. As I explained in the first chapter, I use the term 'economy of healthcare' to refer to more than just the exchange of goods and services. Economy, in the sense I use it, refers to the day-to-day exchanges between therapists and patients, the human experiences of care, the social systems that make practices like physiotherapy possible, the political economy and the legal and ethical contracts established between professions and the public. It is a deliberately broad term, but also one that focuses attention on the fact that phys-iotherapy, like all professions, is fundamentally political. If, for instance, the government of a particular state decides to shift its priorities away from funding centralised, specialised care and focus, instead, on facilitating care in the community – as has been seen in many developed countries over the last 40 years – the organi-sation, design and distribution of physiotherapy would have to change, or the State would look to other providers who were better suited to its new priorities. Thus, I would argue that one cannot undertake a critical history of a profession like physiotherapy without considering how it has been shaped by the changing econ-omy of healthcare.

Today, we all live in a time of profound disruption and disordering where many of the basic tenets of healthcare are being dismantled and replaced by far more complex, manifold and dispersed systems and structures. A recent report by the UK King's Fund argued that 'The NHS faces unprecedented financial and opera-tional challenges as a result of a rising demand for services and constrained resources' (Ham et al 2016). Ham argues that 'NHS providers recorded a record deficit in 2015/16, general practice is in crisis and mental health and community services are under huge pressure' (ibid). Significantly, 'Performance is suffering, with targets for waiting times being missed. These challenges are amplified by cuts to social care and public health and by the requirement for the NHS to deliver £22 billion of productivity improvements by 2020/21' (ibid).

What is more, '[t]he UK has the highest public spending since 1983, the lowest tax burden since 1961 and the highest borrowing since World War II. The newly elected Government's first priority is to reduce the deficit and restore economic growth' (Hughes 2011). For its part, 'The U.S. healthcare system remains in a state of crisis. Despite incremental efforts at reform, the number of uninsured continues to grow, the cost of care continues to rise, and the safety and quality of care are questioned' (American Nurses Association 2008, p. 1). In 2006, at the height of the pre-global financial crisis economic boom, 17%, or just over 50 million people, had no health insurance. At the same time health expenditure in the United States rose to nearly $2 trillion, 'accounting for approximately 16% of the coun-try's gross domestic product' (American Nurses Association 2008, p. 3). Perhaps not surprisingly, there is a growing appetite for analysis and reform with attention turning to ways of 'sustaining existing services and standards of care, developing new and better models of care, and tackling these challenges by reforming . . . "from within"' (Ham et al 2016).

Radical new models of care have involved a raft of changes, particularly to social welfare systems that are increasingly labelled as overly-centralised, bureau-cratic and unaffordable. The antithesis of the principles of social welfare have emerged in recent years in the shape of the idea of telemedicine (Taylor et al 2012), lifestyle monitoring (Hargreaves 2014) and, perhaps even more strikingly, the idea of personal health budgets where each individual is allocated funds that might otherwise have been used for State-based services like pensions and allow-ances, benefits and services (Sorman 2016). At the heart of many of these innovations lie coordinated care plans, 'developed in partnership with a healthcare professional, for instance a community nurse, or someone from a voluntary or community organisation' (Department of Health 2012, p. 48). These plans place case manag-ers at the centre of care planning, mediating between traditional service providers and patients, affording extraordinary powers to those who become service com-missioners. New initiatives like the idea of the 'Medical Home' follow on from this, and shift the traditional power base from the orthodox health professionals, to a diverse group of variously qualified local 'actors', including health profes-sionals, family members and community support workers (Schoen et al 2007, pp. w730–1; Gilfillan et al 2010).

The new health workforce

One of the most significant disruptions to the established model of orthodox healthcare, therefore, has been the move to deconstruct traditional medical hierar-chies and share the power of healthcare decision-making and delivery among a much wider (and cheaper) group of people. As the power of orthodox health pro-fessionals has come under increasing scrutiny (see McCullough 2016 and Philip 2015, for example), radical new proposals for the democratisation of health care have emerged. A recent study from the Royal Society for Public Health in the UK suggested that 'unpaid volunteers, social care providers, police and fire officers, housing and education staff' are now 'an instrumental part of the new public health landscape', promoting 'healthy messages and initiat[ing] or embed[ding] behaviour change' through having a 'healthy conversation' with a customer, client or patient, or signposting someone to a relevant service (Centre for Workforce Intelligence 2015a). There is little doubt that 'demand for lower 'levels' of skill – such as those associated with unpaid care, support carers' are projected to 'substantially outstrip growth in demand for higher skill levels associated with medical and dental pro-fessionals' in the coming years (Centre for Workforce Intelligence 2015b).

The Centre for Workforce Intelligence recently argued that 'there are approxi-mately 5 million people providing unpaid care and support to family or friends due to disability, illness or poor mental health' in the UK alone (Centre for Workforce Intelligence 2015a, and that these 'lay' carers represent a significantly misunder-stood, underutilised and under-represented workforce. It is estimated that 70% of the additional workforce required by 2035 in the UK will come from unpaid carers, volunteers and people with no formal training in healthcare (Centre for Workforce Intelligence 2015a). A very similar picture is emerging across mainland Europe, North America and Australasia with community health workers (CHWs) operat-ing as 'barefoot doctors' (Kangovi et al 2015), sometimes in quite taxing situa-tions that were once the sole province of trained, experienced and regulated health professionals.

Alongside measures to share the burden of care throughout the community, many have cautiously embraced health promotion messages that have encouraged individuals to take more personal responsibility for their own present and future wellbeing. Conscious, perhaps, of the unsustainable cost of specialised healthcare, some have argued that greater consumer empowerment offers some opportunities for a transformation in the traditional therapist/patient relationships. As Baxter and Nall argue,

> Perhaps one of the most salient characteristics of the contemporary health care environment is the prevalence of empowered or activated patients, who increasingly expect to be treated as equal partners in their care and have a voice in health policy.
>
> (Baxter & Nall 2009, p. 23)

A recent study of Canadian physiotherapists' attitudes to healthcare trends and reform showed that:

> While some may find this informed patient/consumer to be a threat and even a potential hazard, it is clear to many that the informed patient is better equipped to become a collaborator in their own healthcare, rather than just a passive patient looking to a doctor for a panacea. Given the growing trend of physiotherapists having to 'do more with less', embracing the potential power of today's informed patient/consumer only makes sense in enabling effective, collaborative care.
>
> (Jones et al 2014, p. 25)

Increasingly, new hybrid healthcare worker roles are emerging. Here, health policy makers and funders are looking to leverage everyday social connections and engagements as low-cost ways to affect people's healthcare decisions (Ihle et al 2014). One such initiative has seen 'hairdressers, retail staff and librarians [encouraged] to have "healthy conversations" with people' (Kangovi et al 2015, p. 2). Such conversations, it is argued, are about '[e]mpowering people in pain, or with significant functional impairments to take greater control over their own therapy' (ibid). As with all such approaches, however, there is the risk that they not only undermine the complex of skills required to deliver health improvements, but also bypass the 'trust, authority, reputation and confidence in the support and advice being given' (ibid).

Another initiative emerging in the space between the traditional healthcare professional and patient, is the healthcare assistant (HCA). Neither a clinical specialist nor a lay service-user, the HCA has met with a mixed response from practitioners (Somerville et al 2015). Jones, for instance, argued in a recent study, that 'Across the board, our interviewees expressed concern about the increasingly consultative role played by physiotherapists and their greater reliance on support staff' (Jones et al 2014, p. 19). Jones's study showed that 'Some [respondents] indicated that there was a perceived or real decrease in service level when physiotherapy assistants (PTAs) were used to implement the treatment plan prescribed by the physiotherapist' (ibid). However, 'limitations on funding and a shift in payment models suggest that the use of PTAs is on the rise and shows no signs of abating' (ibid).

Many physiotherapists naturally feel 'uneasy in letting go of the work that has historically been very hands-on' (Jones et al 2014, p. 21), and that 'using PTAs will diminish the quality of the treatment' (Jones et al 2014, p. 41). Most physiotherapists understand, however, that their role is subtly changing 'from being expert "fixers" to becoming coaches and enablers' (Department of Health 2012, p. 32). Despite this, there is still a real reluctance for physiotherapists to delegate more routine and technical tasks to support workers:

> For AHPs [Allied Health Professionals] to evolve to meet future demands, it is necessary to reallocate lower-level tasks to a support workforce in order to create capacity to concentrate on complex tasks only an AHP can do. Qualitative data indicated that nearly half (55.5%) of AHPs withheld delegation of clinical tasks to assistants.
>
> (Somerville et al 2015, p. 269)

The predicted future shortages of skilled healthcare workers may, on their own, force professions like physiotherapy to adapt and change (Baxter & Nall 2009). In developed countries, demand for formal healthcare continues to rise as populations age, with the WHO estimating a 'global deficit of about 12.9 million skilled health professionals [not including physiotherapists and other allied health professionals] by 2035' (Centre for Workforce Intelligence 2015b, p. 5). Consequently, the 'supply of healthcare workers is unlikely to keep pace with this demand as the workforce itself ages' (Salsberg 2003, p. 1). Increasing demand has revealed shortages and ever-present rationalisation around politically contingent responses, such as the call for greater 'front-line' practitioners (Patel 2014). Added to the growing shortage of practitioners, the distribution of the skilled workforce is vastly skewed towards urban population centres of wealth and away from less affluent areas of cities, rural and remote regions. A recent report suggests that in countries like Australia, the unequal distribution of health resources is creating a two-tier healthcare system, separating those who can afford 'luxuries' such as physiotherapy, from those who cannot (Mason 2013). According to the WHO, although an 'estimated 650 million people worldwide experience some form of disability and [are] in need of health and rehabilitation services' and densities of physiotherapists remain highly variable (WHO 2009).

Changing boundaries

Faced with such pressure to reform, many health professions have, perhaps understandably, retrenched somewhat; looking to secure their professional identities in the face of profound uncertainty. In Jones, Norman and Saunder's recent Canadian report on 'Trends and Drivers of Change in Physiotherapy in Ontario in 2014', the authors argue that 'the truth is that the healthcare sector still operates in silos' (Jones et al 2014, p. 32). The system 'is defined by institutions that effectively operate in isolation to each other; and where care providers are focused on disease management for individual patients and not health and wellness' (ibid). Organisations like Health Workforce Australia, whose mandate is to deconstruct and redesign traditional healthcare hierarchies, have flourished in recent years. These centrally funded organisations are aggressively pursuing workforce boundary reform; the overhaul of profession-specific legislation; recommending new approaches to workforce flexibility; promoting efforts to achieve an optimal distribution of the workforce and the removal of unnecessary, profession-specific nomenclature, demarcations and restrictions on health professionals working up to, and beyond, their existing scopes of practice (Health Workforce Australia 2015, p. 10).

Because physiotherapists do not 'own' massage, mobilisation and manipulation techniques, exercise, hydro- and electrotherapy, regulation does not exclude others from practicing these techniques, the profession is particularly vulnerable to horizontal and vertical encroachment. The diffuse nature of these practices makes it difficult to define physiotherapists' point of difference and most of the techniques used by physiotherapists are being delivered, in one form or another, by variously trained and registered others. Electrotherapy, massage and hydrotherapies have long been a staple of beauty therapies and the burgeoning spa industry; techniques of tissue mobilisation and manipulation are now so diffuse that there is no longer a single professional entity for physiotherapists to challenge and exercise- and activity-based interventions have become ubiquitous. At the root of much of this competition for authority and market 'share' is a profound disruption in consumer expectations about care. As Jones et al blithely point out; 'we are no longer the Canada we were when "Medicare was born"' (Jones et al 2014, p. 32);

> We are changing as a society; and we are changing as patients and consumers of care, increasingly expecting to be stakeholders in our own care journey. As a result, healthcare is becoming more 'personal', and delivery models will need to change to reflect this transformation. While it will take time to implement, there is potential and desire to create a 'bottom up' integrated system, as opposed to the 'top down' fragmented, siloed system that has historically been the case.
>
> (Jones et al 2014, p. 32)

The profound change now taking place in the cultural fabric of society – not only in developed countries, but throughout the world – cannot be ignored. Fundamental beliefs about such seemingly obvious and taken for granted assumptions about what is right and wrong, good and bad, normal and abnormal, able-bodied and disabled, male and female, even alive and dead, are now open for debate (Robson 2014). Two of the most uncomfortable 'isms' of the last half century – neoliberalism and postmodernism – both celebrate uncertainty, and uncertainty often breeds change (Jolley et al 2014, see especially Figure 2.1 on p. 33), with some of this change foretelling dramatic disruptions to the nature of future work – even for skilled professional practitioners like physiotherapists (Yagi 2015; Hurtado-de-Mendoza et al 2015; Gabe & Calnan 2009).

At the heart of these disruptions is the cultural shift taking place in the democratisation of knowledge, brought about by radical new ways to access, produce and distribute information. This access has profoundly influenced the role of the 'expert' as the one who held special knowledge that was only obtainable after an extensive training. It is also disrupting traditional modes of learning, with much less emphasis now being placed on the ability to retain facts (about the origins and insertions of the inferior peroneal retinaculum, or the normal $PaCO_2$ values, for example) and far more emphasis being given to the co-construction of knowledge. As a result, there is now much greater interest in the voices and priorities of people who have traditionally been marginalised by experts.

Physiotherapists occupy a powerful position here because they can use their orthodox status and social capital to take up positions of advocacy, but such positions rely on them challenging their long-held belief in the idea of a 'normal' body with its historical (and inaccurate) representation of form and function. Physiotherapists can become 'minoritarian' (Deleuze & Guattari 1987) and use their social standing to advocate for those who experience the worst access to quality healthcare, experience marginalisation and discrimination, live in poverty and make healthcare decisions out of necessity rather than choice (Higgs et al 2008; Edwards & Richardson 2008; Øberg et al 2015; Edwards et al 2011; Delany & Golding 2014; Trede & McEwan 2016a). Many of the most complex health problems we are now encountering – and the problems to which governments all over the developed world are most eager to resolve – are those found where there is social disadvantage. The evidence is clear that social determinants of health play an increasingly important role in the consumption of healthcare services, yet orthodox professions like physiotherapy have been slow to recognise their economic, political, social and personal significance (Cleaver, Carvajal and Sheppard 2016). As Carson (2007) makes clear:

> We know health and illness don't exist in a vacuum. Health is intimately connected with access to sanitation, a functional sewerage system, clean water, adequate housing, education, communications and transport, and access to appropriate health facilities and personnel. It just sounds like good common sense. Yet why is it that health is so often talked about in biomedical ways that ignore the social determinants? Why is so much research carried out within narrow disciplinary boundaries that ignore social and cultural factors? Why do government departments of health and housing, education and the environment seem not to talk to each other when looking for solutions to dire national problems like the current state of indigenous health?
>
> (Carson et al 2007, p. xxi)

As Keleher and MacDougall argue, one of the problems with contemporary healthcare is that it focuses on 'soft target' risk factors 'such as physical activity, nutrition and weight control that target individuals rather than environments and structural conditions that in turn, are causal pathways for heart disease, diabetes and cancer' (Keleher & MacDougall 2009, p. 28), often ignoring the evidence that unequivocally points to the fact that:

> [T]he utility of individual prevention strategies is quite weak. In other words, individual high-risk strategies of prevention are costly and not particularly effective. The alternative is a population-based prevention strategy. The theory behind population health is that in order to improve health, we must seek 'to control the determinants of incidence in the population as a whole.
>
> (Marmot 2001, p. 993)

The complexity of the situation is increasingly problematic for educators, practitioners and researchers alike, however. With each side claiming the evidence to support their position. In 2012, for example, Marilyn Moffatt, Professor of Physical Therapy at New York University and then President of WCPT argued that;

> Throughout the world . . . physical therapist education programs continue to spend too many hours teaching students how to mobilize and manipulate joints, conduct research projects with little significance, and spend all too few hours on the development of movement science and exercise expertise.
>
> (*Moffatt 2012, p. 23*)

No doubt, advocates for mobilisation and manipulation would take exception with this view. Uncertainty and instability prevails therefore, with practitioners unsure whether behavioural interventions, traditional treatments or movement science and exercise are the keys to the profession's future.

Technological fantasies

One hope, that many people today hold to, is that technology will be able to reduce the incidence of illness and injury, improve access to services and reduce the cost of and demand for specialised care. We may soon be entering a time, for instance, when driverless cars make traumatic brain injury almost a rarity, where pain management following arthroplasty sees patients returning home on the same day as their operation and improved anaesthetics and surgical techniques see an end to common post-operative complications. New 'transhuman' technologies may soon revolutionise not only disabled people's experiences of function and movement (Istvan 2015), but may also enhance the bodies of what were once called 'able-bodied' people. At Massachusetts Institute of Technology, researchers are 'working on technologies that could enhance normal human function, allowing us to walk or run faster, carry more weight, or climb more easily' (Humphries 2014). Autonomous exoskeletons are already in design that reduce the metabolic cost of walking and everyday tasks (Mooney et al 2014; Knight 2015); there are Functional Electrical Stimulation-enabled devices that blur the boundary between human and machine (see manufacturers like BrainGate, Omron, Cyberdyne and the Phoenix Exoskeleton). At MIT, Hugh Herr recently suggested that we should try to imagine a time in 50 years when, '[if] you want a third arm, you can have a third arm' (Humphries 2014).

Such innovations were once a thing of fantasy, but the advent of consumer-led reconstructive surgery, wearable fitness devices linked to cloud data capture technology, clothing designed to 'police your posture' (https://www.liveathos.com), home-based telemetry and digital surveillance, and thousands of products and consumables designed to enhance our appearance, function, body shape and size, aptitudes and abilities, performance at work and at home, no-one can doubt that if there is a growing interest in the possibilities for body enhancement. Of course, one of the things that is axiomatic about such developments is that they will only be available to those who can afford them, and there are some real concerns about a form of 'digital apartheid' developing around such bodily enhancements (Brown & Czerniewicz 2010).

One of the areas where transhumanism arguably offers the most exciting opportunities is in the management of chronic illnesses, which have remained doggedly resistant to many of the best efforts of orthodox medicine over the last century. Chronic diseases like heart disease, stroke, cancer, depression and diabetes may be characterised 'by their long development period' and 'multiple factors leading to their onset, and a prolonged course of illness' (Mason 2013, p. 64). And these may still lead inexorably to 'other health complications such as functional impairment or disability' (ibid). Carl May called chronic illnesses 'the great epidemic of our time' (May et al 2009). Defined by their impermeability to cost containment, their reliance on palliating technologies, and the crises of eligibility frequently expressed by their sufferers, long-term conditions will represent over 80% of the additional demand for future healthcare in the UK (Centre for Workforce Intelligence 2015b, p. 1), with a significant percentage of this demand arising from physical disability. According to the UK's Department of Health, people with long-term conditions account for 50% of all General Practitioner appointments, 64% of all outpatient appointments, 70% of all inpatient bed days and, in total, 'around 70% of the total health and care spend in England' (Department of Health 2012, p. 3). Not surprisingly, governments throughout the world are looking at ways to manage the immensely challenging problems now being posed by complex and multidimensional health problems: turning their attention to systems that were designed over a century ago to manage acute, linear health problems, when it was sufficient to operate in binaries and talk of people as healthy or sick, able-bodied or disabled, mad or sane. It is now evident that 'doing more of the same will not be good enough' (ibid) and that we are only just beginning to see the kinds of radical healthcare reforms that may emerge in the coming decades.

Whether such alternatives have a significant impact on the future of physiotherapy remains an open question, but one thing is clear: if physiotherapy continues to operate with the same ideological focus on the body-as-machine; delivering largely short-term episodic care for acute, largely self-limiting conditions, with an emphasis on doing things *to* patients rather than working *alongside* people, we may well find ourselves replaced by less-well qualified, cheaper or more technologically sophisticated healthcare providers. And yet, who can doubt that there will continue to be a need for *some* aspects of physical therapy in the future? People have sought out physical therapies for their pain and suffering for millennia and it is unlikely that we will cease to enjoy embodied healthcare experiences now, even if society does become saturated with technology. People will always value the ability of some skilled practitioners to diagnose complex health problems and use an understanding of bodies to facilitate relief and recovery. And it is likely that people will always be needed who can thoughtfully manage patients with multiple comorbidities and complex multidimensional health problems, particularly where their remedies make use of low-cost, transportable and freely available resources like touch, mobilisation and exercise.

Health service users have long called for more of these kinds of embodied, personalised experiences of healthcare, but physiotherapists and others have found it difficult to shift from their traditional approach to assessment and treatment:

> Patients universally say that they wish to be treated as a whole person and for the NHS to act as one team. Despite this, those people who have more than one condition, particularly older people, face an increasingly fragmented and 'specialised' response. It is clear that [long term condition] 'needs' transcend the organisational boundaries of social, primary, community and secondary care.
>
> (Department of Health 2012)

The challenge remains, therefore, to find an economic model that will provide the necessary support for physiotherapists to move away from its traditional ideologies, associations, practical and theoretical limitations, and into the brave new world of 21st century healthcare. Fortunately, in this regard, things are far from bleak and despite all of the dire warnings about the future for professions like physiotherapy, we may well be living through the most fertile, creative and opportune moment in the history of modern healthcare. Before now, physiotherapy has either been too small and politically insignificant; too wedded to a biomechanical ideology; or too secure in its tenure, to want to break free from its past. There is a climate of change emerging, however, and a growing appetite to think differently about the role physical therapies can play in future healthcare. Clearly, the model inherited from the profession's predecessors is in transition, and new opportunities are emerging, but as Jones et al argue; 'while these changes can contribute to an environment that is at times confusing, challenging and even frustrating, they also create conditions that are ripe with opportunity' (Jones et al 2014, p. 1).

Emerging opportunities for an 'otherwise' profession

One of the first question physiotherapists might ask themselves about their future role in the changing economy of healthcare, is whether there is currently anyone better placed to take advantage of the changing economy of healthcare? Who else can claim to be a highly respected, orthodox, first-contact diagnostician; with a focus on the whole body and skills in the assessment, treatment and rehabilitation of activity, movement and functional disorders; with discretion in day-to-day practice and a long history of working within today's health priorities, and the delivery of highly personal, low-cost skills; in a manner that the public trusts, and sits comfortably alongside the work of doctors, nurses and other allied health professionals? Physiotherapy is, in many ways, perfectly positioned to be a major force in the healthcare services of the future. To explore this opportunity, however, the profession must be able to move beyond its self-imposed constraints and find a way to transcend many of the orthodoxies that it spent the first century of its professional life establishing. Physiotherapists need to rehabilate themselves and their professional subjectivity in the same way that they learned to rehabilitate others. They need to turn the assessment techniques they learned in the intensive care units, orthopaedic wards and private practices to diagnose the problems now facing the profession and use their treatment skills in service of professional reform.

The pain and functional limitations now being experienced by physiotherapists are the result of long periods spent working in adverse conditions. Their (professional) body is ageing and showing signs of being ill-equipped for the rigours of 21st century living. Physiotherapists have parts of their professional body rebelling and protesting about the stresses we are experiencing (Gill 2016). Analogies like this, hopefully, remind us that physiotherapy is the way it is because, rather than being a sovereign, autonomous, self-determining entity, it is a contingent response to a set of complex social problems and survives and prospers because it offers the best available response to those problems. If the problems being posed by society change but the profession tries to remain the same then, inevitably, dysfunction will gain a foothold, and it becomes conceivable that a once buoyant profession will disperse and become diminished. The challenge, then, for any profession that wants to remain relevant in the face of profound social change, is not to stick doggedly to its long-held traditions, defiantly holding to ways of working that served past problems, but to assess the need, diagnose what needs to change and prepare the body better for the changing world it lives within.

Throughout the profession's history, physiotherapists have shown remarkable plasticity in the way they have adapted to the changing economy of healthcare. Only recently in the UK, the advent of enterprise bargaining resulted in sudden and dramatic restrictions on doctors' working hours (Morris et al 2014). Almost overnight, new opportunities emerged for physiotherapists and other health professions to take on traditionally restricted medical and surgical roles. Physiotherapists were trained to perform invasive procedures like cannulation and bronchoscopy, read advanced images and prescribe and administer some medications. And although these were treated as 'emergency measures' and restricted to the locations where the training had occurred, it showed that physiotherapists were both willing and able to take on these new practices.

Myriad new roles and opportunities for diversification now exist just beyond the limits of present-day physiotherapy practice. Almost all of the difficulties and challenges currently perplexing governments, health policy analysts, academics, other health professionals and the general public today are amenable to new forms of physiotherapy. From the rising costs of long-term illness and the increased reliance on low-cost activity-based interventions to keep people active into old age; to people's desire for more holistic, embodied healthcare experiences and our need to engage in life-long self-care; to the body 'projects' that enhance our sense of self-fulfilment and improve our home and working lives, improve the welfare of dependent populations and provide a focus for community development and greater collective wellbeing; physiotherapy may, in the future, offer some profoundly important and valuable responses.

Moving beyond the present

To take advantage of these opportunities, however, physiotherapists will have to do more than simply offer new wine in old bottles. Moving beyond the margins of the profession's current ideology may require physiotherapists to embrace modes of thought and practice that detach them from many of their traditional moorings. Having spent much of their professional history anchored to biomedicine, they may find that the reductive objectivity offered by mainstream medicine constrains more than it enables. They may find that they need a new vocabulary of terms; a new language, in effect, to help them define new ways of thinking and being. They may find that they need to explore territory occupied by others – neighbours in the arts, humanities, physical and social sciences, for example – in order that they can bring back new ideas and new ways to develop their practice. And they may need to ask difficult ethical and moral questions of ourselves. Would we, for instance, abandon the century-long project that is the physiotherapy profession, if it was in the best interests of their patients? Would the profession be prepared to relinquish their social standing and authority to allow patients to take centre-stage in designing the future of healthcare?

Such questions are hugely challenging for a profession that has little or no history of critical self-inquiry. Fortunately, steps in the right direction need not depend solely on radical reflexivity and deep epistemological analysis, which is significant because physiotherapists are largely unfamiliar with these approaches. Merely opening the profession to greater diversity may be one way to begin the profession's transformation: accepting that there can never be only one definition of physiotherapy and embracing the idea of a *thousand* physiotherapies might give individual practitioners the confidence to explore new modes of expression. Considering the kinds of activities, bodies, functions and movements that are now available to physiotherapists – without prejudicing that exploration by imposing a requirement to remain fixated by the body-as-machine – might allow physiotherapists to recognise the multiplicity of locations, centres and 'nodes' of activity that physiotherapists could be engaged in the future (Setchell et al 2017). And embracing heterogeneity over homogeneity, plurality over monoculture, dispersal over regulated constraint, difference over sameness and inclusiveness over isolation may offer radical opportunities and new ways to think about the education, practice, regulation and research of, and by, physiotherapists in the future.

But, to be clear, I am not talking here of relatively superficial gestures that appear to deviate from tradition but, in reality, leave long-established physiotherapy approaches and ideologies intact. For example, offering digitally enhanced ways of learning anatomy will not displace the body-as-machine as a central tenet of physiotherapy practice; becoming smoking cessation advocates and anti-fat campaigners will do little to challenge our authoritarian position in health care; and adopting biopsychosocial models or 'mind-body' practices will not be sufficient for physiotherapists holistic if we do not, at the same time, challenge the persistent primacy of biomedical approaches to healthcare in the profession.

Instead, I am arguing that physiotherapists need to embrace the full potential of ideas like movement, touch, activity, function and ability, and challenge our traditional restrictions on how we allow ourselves to think about these concepts. I am encouraging practitioners to think about new practice locations, clients, communities, agencies and funders; new epistemologies that do not rely on the biomedical, reductive and normative notions of what bodies are and can achieve. I am saying that physiotherapists need to explore new practice definitions that embrace diversity and inclusiveness and encourage a thousand expressions of physical therapy to emerge; new modes of engagement with clients that allow us to work alongside people and communities and move away from authoritarian, dominant relations of power; new epistemologies that allow for more than merely measurable, value-free, supposedly objective evaluations of efficacy and new ways of becoming physiotherapists that embraces the complexity, ambiguity and uncertainty inherent in real-world practice.

Physiotherapists should not be complacent in thinking that change will be easy, however. A recent study by Sanders and colleagues showed that physiotherapists had concerns about how to work 'with' patients, when they were more used to 'doing things to them' (Sanders et al 2014, p. 106). As one participant in the study put it; '[P]hysios are trained to do things and if they're sitting and talking . . . they're not doing something . . . that's quite challenging I think, you know, people sitting talking to patients, rather than doing things to them' (quote from participant in Sanders et al 2014, p. 107). Finding new ways to work with people from diverse communities of need may be challenging for traditional physiotherapy practitioners, but it is becoming increasingly necessary.

Being able to adapt to changing needs may well be one of the characteristic features of health professional education in the future and the ability to work *with* people and all of their attendant subjectivities, perspectives and diverse needs may well be vital for the long-term health of professions like physiotherapy. It is telling that the 'shift from dealing with "patients" to interacting with *people* (before they actually become patients) is a trend that is *just beginning to emerge*' (Jones et al 2014, p. 8, my emphasis). Given the volume of criticism levelled at the orthodox health professions over the last half century for exactly this disregard for patients as people first, it is concerning that physiotherapists are only now realising that 'this is where healthcare is going: driven not by the institutions and services themselves but by the people who use them' (Jones et al 2014, pp. 8–9).

Greater recognition of the person-as-patient, and not just the body-as-machine, may be one the most profound influences on future physiotherapy practice. Most mature, experienced physiotherapists learned long ago, that you cannot survive and prosper as a health professional without acknowledging people's innate subjectivity: their unique histories and personal perspectives; the family ties and social networks that sustain them; their emotions, passions and quirks. And yet most practitioners have had to acquire this understanding *despite* their training and scope of practice, rather than *because* of it. Many physiotherapists I have known have felt decidedly uncomfortable about exploring therapeutic approaches that extend even a little beyond the prevailing orthodoxy – so pervasive is the rhetoric around the body-as-machine (Nicholls et al 2009). Clearly, for a change to come, physiotherapists must be encouraged to break the mould, challenge convention, experiment – and fail – in the knowledge that they will be encouraged to try again.

For physiotherapy to prosper, they may need to embrace a much broader idea of embodied humanity and in recognising the humanity of others, encourage greater personal self-expression in ourselves. It would be nice to think that physiotherapy in the future not only values and embraces other people's unique cultural values, gender expressions, political opinions and spiritual beliefs, but also makes space for these in professional training and daily practice. As Franziska Trede and Celina McEwan recently argued, the challenge is to develop 'moral, thoughtful, purposeful and agentic stances that enable practitioners to counterbalance one-dimensional and instrumental practices' (Trede & McEwan 2016b, p. 7).

The advent of patient-centred care – interesting in itself, in that it suggests that previous forms of healthcare were something other than 'patient-centred' – is forcing health professionals to confront the power that they have held and the ways in which they have been authoritarian, rather than merely authoritative. At the heart of the question posed by patient-centred care is power: the power to decide, literally and metaphorically, how you want to be treated; the power to have your personal proclivities respected, even if they deviate from best evidence or best practice; the power to choose. People are increasingly sensitive to the fact that health professions, as agents of the State, have long held too much power and commanded too much responsibility for the wellbeing of the population. Today, people expect to have much more say in their healthcare and expect to be active participants in clinical decisions. The challenge, then, for health professionals is how to share power and relinquish some of the authority that once equated to social responsibility and status while still providing meaningful care. There are enormous risks here, because to truly embrace patient-centred care assumes that patients may decide they do not actually want the services physiotherapists offer. Perhaps this risk explains, to some extent, why traditional orthodox health professions like physiotherapy have engaged far more in proclaiming the virtues of evidence-based practice as mechanisms to mediate between the profession and the public than in riskier power-sharing mechanisms like patient-centred care?

Perhaps the welcome embrace given to evidence-based practice speaks more to the physiotherapy profession's relationship to the State than it does to its relationship with healthcare consumers. In the face of an ever expanding demand for healthcare and controls on healthcare spending, the use of 'evidence' has become a main vehicle for funders and policy makers to justify the investment. Once it was a profession's proximity and alignment with medicine that provided the best chance for a profession to acquire state support. Today, funders require more than just a symbiotic relationship with medicine to support clinical interventions and clinical evidence has become the main vehicle to discriminate between what will be funded and what will not. Evidence, therefore, plays a crucial role in the development of physiotherapy. Physiotherapists would be wise, however, to understand that evidence-based practice is, perhaps, more relevant for the profession's changing relationship with central funders than it is for the consumers of its services who continue to show an interest in an ever widening market for healthcare products and services, regardless of whether there is evidence of the intervention or not. Added to this, no efforts on the part of orthodox healthcare professions – including medicine – appears to be changing that, which further points to the fact that it is will be the broader political and social economy of healthcare that will determine the future for professions like physiotherapy and traditional hierarchies and hegemonies.

Possibilities for radical change

In many ways, the future direction for the profession has been anticipated for many years. As long ago as 1964, E.M. Stewart, then the Principal of the School of Physiotherapy at King's College Hospital in London, argued that rapid developments in medical knowledge, preventative medicine, and growing populations of aged and disabled, would lead to some traditional treatments going into decline and a rise in physiotherapy delivered away from large hospital centres (Stewart 1964, p. 230). In a similar piece predicting physiotherapy in 2094, Wise and Hemmings (1994) argued that the very young and the very old would probably make up most of the profession's clients; that medical advances would mean that physiotherapists focus more on prevention and the maintenance of health than treatment and we would have physiotherapists working in 'information centres for health' (ibid, p. 11A); community based care would increase (although they did believe that hospitals were 'here to stay, at least for the next hundred years' (ibid, p. 100A)); remuneration would be negotiated locally; practitioners would become 'doctors' and demand more research; and most of our core skills would survive (ibid). The authors conclude, reassuringly, that;

> So long as human beings are on this earth and going about their business and pleasure, interacting with each other, nicely and nastily, there will continue to be ample requirement for the services of Chartered Physiotherapists.
>
> (Wise & Hemmings 1994, p. 101A)

Ultimately, then, the 'end' of physiotherapy – its purpose and reason for existing – will be determined by how physiotherapists themselves respond to the changing economy of healthcare. Whether it is the challenge of an increasingly ageing, chronically ill population; complex patients with multiple comorbidities; the restructured healthcare system with its emphasis on lay carers and HCAs; skilled workforce shortages; people's growing scepticism towards traditional authority figures and orthodox professionals; the growing popularity of 'alternative' thera-pies, 'body projects' and embodied health experiences; the growing discrepancies between the 'worried well' and the 'precariat'; power sharing in healthcare and consumer rights; the demands for evidence and accountability; global political, economic and environmental instability or the challenges of transhumanism and the possibilities for bodies that no longer conform to conventional notions of 'normal'. More than anything, physiotherapy is a fortunate position because it has a vested interest in the outcome of *all* of these tensions. So, rather than seeing these tensions as problems, physiotherapists might think about how they can draw on their social capital; extensive training; access to the people from the full spec-trum of the population; knowledge of the body, movement and function; highly developed interpersonal skills and history of service, to transform their practice as the needs of the population change.

After all, it was physiotherapists that decided how they wanted physiotherapy to be more than a century ago. It was physiotherapists themselves that decided they wanted to focus on the body-as-machine so that they could legitimise their touch and gain the support of the medical profession, the public and the State. It was physiotherapy practitioners that decided they wanted to sidestep 'other' ways of thinking about health and illness and concentrate, instead, on the body of the person in front of them. So, I would argue, it is entirely up to physiotherapists if they now want to change this, and embrace a different professional subjectivity. Of course, they must do this with a very close eye on their funders and patrons, and they will be successful only if they align their aspirations for a fulfilling professional identity with the needs of the public at large. But what should be absolutely clear by now is that perpetuating the professional practices of yesterday, in the hope that they will be valued and accepted tomorrow, will only lead to the profession becoming increasingly marginalised and positioned as, literally, out of touch.

Expressed in this way, change sounds a relatively straightforward process: physiotherapists simply accept that their future requires them to change, and then begin the process of drafting a new professional constitution. The reality is, how-ever, somewhat different, and the task for physiotherapy is made doubly difficult by the fact that they have no history of engaging in the kinds of thinking that would make change easier. They are not schooled in cultural studies, the arts or the humanities, so perhaps struggle to see how they can embrace more completely people's individual experiences of health or the possibilities for a more social engagement in wellbeing; they have little experience of critical or political theory, economics, anthropology, philosophy or sociology and so struggle with the language and possibilities of critique and they have little or no sense of their own history, so find it hard to see how physiotherapy has been historically or socially possible. Without some of these skills, it will be difficult for physiotherapists to imagine a different future, beyond minor disruptions and selective shifts.

Evidence suggests that physiotherapists are beginning to engage in some of these debates, however. Thanks to the move into higher education, there is now a critical mass of thinkers, practitioners and writers in and around physiotherapy, who have supplemented their professional training with study in other, more diverse disciplines. These people are now starting to have a stronger voice in the profession, offering supportive critique of the physiotherapy's past, present and future possibilities. Unfortunately, for the vast majority of physiotherapists, the emphasis remains firmly on the body-as-machine and the need to strengthen the profession's traditional scientific base. Scan the current editions of leading physiotherapy journals, the abstracts submitted to national and international conferences or the textbooks produced for students and you would probably conclude that the profession wants to consolidate its affinity with biomechanical thinking and the body-as-machine rather than challenge it. Examine the reports emanating from professional societies, however, and you will see a different picture. Bodies like WCPT, the CSP, the APTA and other organisations around the world, are pushing for the profession to recognise the realities of changing economy of healthcare and accelerate their reforms. The picture is complex, fluid and highly dynamic, therefore, and physiotherapists will need to have a strong sense of their professional subjectivity if they are to make a meaningful contribution to it.

Ironically, practitioners continue to complain that the public and many of our sister professions do not know what physiotherapists are or what they do (Paul & Mullerpatan 2015; Vincent-Onabajo et al 2014; Varghese et al 2012; Pagliarulo 2007). They complain that physiotherapists do not have a clear 'brand identity' or market themselves well and that the profession lacks its own distinctive ideology. My argument in this book is that the very approach that has been so important in establishing the profession's legitimacy and orthodox status, is the cause of these deficiencies. (After all, if physiotherapy was actually as vague and non-specific as some physiotherapists claim, it could not have been reproduced so successfully year-on-year for more than a hundred years?) Perhaps it is that physiotherapy is anything but opaque, but that physiotherapists have lacked the vocabulary to explain it? Returning to the quote that opened the book, it is the nature of majority cultures not to know themselves and physiotherapy has been dominant in the physical therapies for over 100 years.

In the past, there was no need to think about the ways in which cultural, existential, interpersonal, philosophical, political or social discourses affected people's sense of health and wellbeing: other people would take care of these. There was no need to interrogate these things because the profession was growing and becoming more established. Even today, with all the manifest tensions surrounding their practice, it is hard to be critical. Are physiotherapists not one of the most respected health professions? Do they not have oversubscribed graduate courses and a ready market for their practitioners? Are they not protected by legislation and given privileged access to patients in the public health system? Physiotherapy has never really needed to interrogate itself. Almost every major social event that changed the nature of healthcare over the course of the 20th century has worked in the profession's favour. Physiotherapy grew with war, epidemic, political and social reform, and accumulated credit and kudos along the way.

So why now challenge all of this and argue that we may be experiencing the *End of Physiotherapy*? The answer to this is laid out in the pages of this book, but ostensibly it is because the changing economy of healthcare is now creating conditions that work against the model of physiotherapy created in the 20ᵗʰ century. For the first time, the future for physiotherapy looks decidedly uncertain and the profession is being asked questions about its practice that physiotherapy clinicians, educators, researchers and students are ill-equipped to answer. So, the reason for undertaking a critical history of the profession's past, present and future is to better understand the causes of these tensions and the reasons for their present struggles. What is clear from this work is that if the profession is to meet the challenge of 21ˢᵗ century healthcare, physiotherapists will need to know themselves better and embrace the idea that tomorrow may look decidedly different to yesterday.

Closing words

After the long journey through a wealth of ideas and evidence, it is proper that I return to the beginning and ask about the end of physiotherapy. As I mentioned in the introduction, the title is a deliberate play on two different meanings of 'the end'. The first is teleological, in that it deals with the *purpose* of physiotherapy: how it came to be the way it is; what the profession it *for*; what 'ends' does it serve. My hope is that this book has provided a detailed critique of the profession's history of the present. I fully appreciated that there are enough qualifications and exceptions to the arguments set out in this book to constitute another book, and I hope that readers feel motivated to critique the arguments presented here and offer their own conclusions. There will be huge regional variations in people's experiences, for example, and only some, perhaps even only a few, of the arguments set out here will be relevant to everyone. The book concentrates heavily on the experiences of physiotherapists in the Commonwealth countries, especially the United Kingdom, and physical therapists in North America. There will be therapists in mainland Europe, Scandinavia, Africa, Asia and elsewhere, who will feel that only some of these arguments apply to them. There will also be historians and critical scholars in and around physiotherapy who will draw exception to my focus on certain moments in the history of the profession, and use of certain texts to illustrate my arguments.

I also appreciate that today's readers will look at the most recent history of the profession in Chapter 5 with a more critical eye than perhaps the other chapters, because few will have worked in physiotherapy before 1974. That being said, I hope that they can accept that this was only ever going to be a partial history of the profession and I have had to exclude far more material than I have been able to include. No critical history can ever be complete: they are always partial, subjective accounts. I hope, however, that I have been consistent in my approach and thorough in my methodology. (Interested readers will be able to find a brief outline of the methodological principles employed in developing this book in the Epilogue that follows this chapter.)

The 'end' or *purpose* of physiotherapy is only one of the two main functions for the text, however. The other function is to predicts the beginning of the chronological end of physiotherapy as a professional discipline. Everything I have argued in this book points to the fact that physiotherapy is experiencing profound change, and that the profession is both largely unaware and philosophically unprepared for the changing economy of healthcare. There is no doubt that physiotherapy will need to change, but my argument here is that the very model of practice adopted and sedimented by the profession over its long history will increasingly continue to obstruct its attempts to reform by limiting its ability to engage with the broader discourses of health and wellbeing that are today becoming the currency of exchange in healthcare.

To be clear, I am convinced that people will always need physical therapies: they will always seek out the trusted touch of skilled hands and the ability of people to analyse disabilities and functional impairments; they will always seek out what Nina McIntosh called the 'honest pleasure of sensuality' (McIntosh 2005, p. 100), and the dispassionate gaze of the clinical scientist. People will always need the help of practitioners who can cure and care, work *on* and *with* us, show us how to optimise our sense of health and wellbeing and advocate for us when we are voiceless. People will always demand these things, so the future for the physical therapies is not in question. What is in question, however, is whether the professional subjectivity that we currently understand as 'physiotherapy' can fully meet this challenge and become all of these things. Given all of the arguments set out in this book, my contention is that physiotherapy, as we know it today, is too closely anchored to Victorian ideals of legitimate practice, the 20th century construct of an orthodox profession and the biomedical paradigm of the body-as-machine, to be able to change. I believe that physiotherapists are paradoxically perpetuating a model of practice that is antithetical to many of the demands of 21st century healthcare.

So, what is to be done? If we are, indeed, seeing the beginning of the end of the physiotherapy profession, what should we do and what might the future look like if we decide not to do these things? Firstly, I should say that the purpose of this book is not to provide *the* answer to these questions. My belief is that the future for the profession is much more diverse, inclusive and diffuse. To that end, it would be contradictory to even propose that there can be a simple, single answer. My hope is that the book opens the door for a thousand answers: a thousand debates and discussions; a thousand physiotherapies. Physiotherapists clearly need to invest in a great deal more critical scholarship around culture, history and expend a great deal more energy understanding the philosophy of their profession. They need to follow the example of medical sociology, nursing history, occupational therapy and psychology, in interrogating the nuances and subtleties of their professional culture; creating the space for new ways of thinking and practising. They should do this, however, with the full realisation that this is never a project that can be completed, or one that will bring harmony and synthesis. Experience from its sister professions, who have engaged in these discussions for more than half a century, points to the fact that these discussions only create more uncertainty. But uncertainty itself should be seen as a positive thing: provoking physiotherapists to deeper insights and more radical understandings of the full breadth and depth of their work.

Physiotherapists clearly need to develop their students to be more than technically competent. If future generations are to engage with the full breadth of physiotherapy practice, then they must develop more than just clinical skills. It will be necessary to develop what Trede and McEwan recently called *deliberate* practitioners (Trede & McEwan 2016a). It will be important to find ways of formulating curricula that expose the students to the arts, humanities, philosophy, sociology *and* the biological sciences, and educators must be able to do this without creating an unmanageably large entry qualification. And naturally, educators and existing practitioners who have not necessarily benefitted from the kinds of holistic education that might make radical thinking possible, must be supported to nurture this new breed of graduates as they enter practice.

All health practitioners must embrace difference and the unorthodox if they are to provide creative solutions to new problems. They must be prepared to transgress traditional beliefs and values and embrace deviance, otherness and subversion, if they are going to create spaces for change. They must be prepared to relinquish power and empower others – especially their patients – in full knowledge of the fact that this may lead to them losing control and authority. They must become minoritarian and be prepared to advocate for voices that have traditionally been silenced by mainstream healthcare. And they must be prepared to embrace a wide range of different approaches and practice philosophies. Physiotherapy in the future must be eclectic and diffuse, multidimensional and complex, amoeboid and plastic.

It will be important that practitioners can understand those times when they must continue to practice in the 'old' way, knowing when it is appropriate to treat people's bodies as machines. There will be many times when people will need reductive, biomechanical treatment because they just want to be fixed. So, physiotherapists and others cannot lose the artisanal skills that they have spent a century or more perfecting. But moments when people just want to be passively fixed are becoming increasingly rare and physiotherapy is unlikely to prosper in the future if it cannot also embrace more holistic notions of care and collaboration. Fortunately, there are thousands of other ways to think and practice that are available to physiotherapy now if the profession chooses to reach beyond itself and exceed its current professional subjectivity.

If, in the end, however, physiotherapy finds it too hard to change, or decides that these 'other' ways of thinking and practising are really not what practitioners want, then what can the profession expect to happen? Firstly, it is likely that much of the technical knowledge, and many of the most essential technical skills currently performed by physiotherapists will be taken up by people who either cost less to train or are cheaper to employ. We are already seeing the widespread dissemination of manual techniques across the Internet, and the foundational knowledge that once formed the cornerstone of the science of physiotherapy is increasingly being 'externalised' (i.e. held by powerful personal devices that provide instant recall for facts that were once rote learned and memorised). Physiotherapists can expect that much of the work of fixing short-term, acute, self-limiting conditions – that makes up a considerable proportion of physiotherapists' daily work – will be taken up by others. Similarly, much of the routine activity- and exercise-based rehabilitation that physiotherapists fought so hard to claim will be delivered by people from a much wider cohort of the population. We may even see, in the near future, the full effect of remote technologically-enhanced exercise-based rehabilitation, where the person's 'therapist' may be a computer, or an 'assistant' located in another country.

Increasingly, physiotherapy will focus on complex and specialised healthcare; working with patients with multiple comorbidities in challenging clinical situations. This may suit the drive towards specialisation within the profession, but with a shrinking public healthcare system it is likely that the burden of cost will fall increasingly on individuals themselves. With the cost of prolonged rehabilitation being so high, it is likely that only those who can afford to pay directly, or through their insurance premiums, will eligible for physiotherapy. As a result, the profession will cease to be available to the whole population, and will increasingly become a luxury of the 'worried well'. Because the growing population of people who make up the majority of complex health problems, and feature so prominently in government health priorities, come from communities of social disadvantage, physiotherapy will increasingly be seen a luxury and will gradually be marginalised from government initiatives to improve the health of the wider population.

If this were a welcome prospect for their patients, it would be at least gratifying to know that these changes would improve people's care. But I believe, and I think that most of my colleagues believe, these changes would significantly diminish people's experiences of healthcare and lead to much less satisfactory outcomes. For these reasons alone, we should fight to make sure that physiotherapy does not go down this track. The challenge is ours then. It is for physiotherapists themselves to take up the challenge of becoming truly patient-centred; deciding how they want to adapt to the changing economy of healthcare. It is for physiotherapists to look at their professional culture and ask how they got here and how they can now react. If they leave these conversations to others, or fail to grasp the manifest opportunities now available to them, then we will surely see the end of physiotherapy.

References

American Nurses Association, 2008, *Health system reform agenda*. Silver Spring, MD: American Nursing Association. From www.nursingworld.org/Content/Healthcareand PolicyIssues/Agenda/ANAsHealthSystemReformAgenda.pdf, retrieved 3 July 2016.

Baxter, D. & Nall, C., 2009, Current trends in physiotherapy practice. In J. Higgs, M.S. Smith, G.W. Webb, M.S. Skinner & A.C. Croker (eds.), *Contexts of Physiotherapy Practice*. Churchill Livingstone, Sydney, Australia, pp. 20–32.

Brown, C. & Czerniewicz, L., 2010, Debunking the digital native: beyond digital apartheid, towards digital democracy, *Journal of Computer Assisted Learning*, 26(5), pp. 357–69.

Carson, B., Dunbar, T., Chenhall, R.D. & Bailie, R., 2007, *Social determinants of indigenous health*, Allen & Unwin, London.

Centre for Workforce Intelligence, 2015a, *Understanding the wider public health workforce*. Royal Society for Public Health. From https://www.gov.uk/government/uploads/system/ uploads/attachment_data/file/507752/CfWI_Understanding_the_wider_public_health_ workforce.pdf, retrieved 9 April 2016.

Centre for Workforce Intelligence, 2015b, *Future demand for skills: Initial results*. London: Royal Society for Public Health. From https://www.gov.uk/government/uploads/system/uploads/attachment_data/file/507498/CfWI_Horizon_2035_Future_demand_for_skills.pdf, retrieved 10 February 2016.

Cleaver, S.R., Carvajal, J.K. & Sheppard, P.S., 2016, Cultural humility: A way of thinking to inform practice globally. *Physiotherapy Canada: Physiothérapie Canada*, 68(1), pp. 1–2.

Delany, C. & Golding, C., 2014, Teaching clinical reasoning by making thinking visible: an action research project with allied health clinical educators, *BMC Medical Education*, 14(1), p. 20.

Deleuze, G. & Guattari, F., 1987, *A thousand plateaus — Capitalism and schizophrenia*, Translated by B. Massumi. University of Minnesota Press, Minneapolis, MN.

Department of Health, 2012, *Long term conditions compendium of information*. London: Department of Health. From https://www.gov.uk/government/uploads/system/uploads/attachment_data/file/216528/dh_134486.pdf, retrieved 18 April 2016.

Edwards, I. & Richardson, B., 2008, Clinical reasoning and population health: decision making for an emerging paradigm of healthcare, *Physiotherapy Theory and Practice*, 24(3), pp. 183–93.

Edwards, I., Delany, C.M., Townsend, A.F. & Swisher, L.L., 2011, Moral agency as enacted justice: a clinical and ethical decision-making framework for responding to health inequities and social injustice, *Physical Therapy*, 91(11), pp. 1653–63.

Gabe, J. & Calnan, M. (eds.), 2009, *The New Sociology of the Health Service*, Routledge, Abingdon, Oxon.

Gilfillan, R.J., Tomcavage, J., Rosenthal, M.B., Davis, D.E., Graham, J., Roy, J.A., Pierdon, S.B., Bloom Jr, F.J., Graf, T.R. & Goldman, R., 2010, Value and the medical home: effects of transformed primary care, *The American Journal of Managed Care*, 16(8), pp. 607–14.

Gill, T., 2016, CSP members march in Birmingham for the NHS, *Frontline*, 4 October 2016.

Ham, C., McKenna, H. & Dunn, P., 2016, *Tackling the growing crisis in the NHS*. The King's Fund. From www.kingsfund.org.uk/publications/articles/nhs-agenda-for-action?utm_source=twitter&utm_medium=social&utm_term=thekingsfund, retrieved 19 June 2016.

Hargreaves, S., 2014, A mixed methods exploration of the relationship between activities within the home and health in older people with heart failure: implications for lifestyle monitoring, doctoral thesis, University of Sheffield, Sheffield, UK.

Health Workforce Australia, 2015, *Health workforce 2025: Consumer edition*. Adelaide: Health Workforce Australia. From www.tcen.com.au/sites/newtcen/files/files/CSSP/hwa_health-workforce_2025_consumer-edition.pdf, retrieved 3 February 2016.

Higgs, J., Jones, M.A., Loftus, S. & Christensen, N., 2008, *Clinical reasoning in the health professions*, Elsevier Health Sciences UK, London.

Hughes, L., 2011, *Report to the national allied health professional advisory board on the outcomes of the modernising allied health professional careers programme*. London: Department of Health. From https://www.gov.uk/government/uploads/system/uploads/attachment_data/file/215721/dh_124803.pdf, retrieved 8 July 2015.

Humphries, C., 2014, The body electric, *MIT Technology Review*, 21 October 2014.

Hurtado-de-Mendoza, A., Cabling, M.L. & Sheppard, V.B., 2015, Rethinking agency and medical adherence technology: applying Actor Network Theory to the case study of Digital Pills, *Nursing Inquiry*, 22(4), pp. 326–35.

Ihle, R. & Sudmann, T.T., 2014, Health encounters with minority patients. *FLEKS-Scandinavian Journal of Intercultural Theory and Practice*, 1(2), pp. 1–20.

Istvan, Z., 2015, Future transhumanist tech may soon change the definition of disability, *TechCrunch*, 14 September 2015.

Jolley, G., Freeman, T., Baum, F., Hurley, C., Lawless, A., Bentley, M., Labonté, R. & Sanders, D., 2014, Health policy in South Australia 2003–10: Primary healthcare work-force perceptions of the impact of policy change on health promotion, *Health Promotion Journal of Australia: Official Journal of Australian Association of Health Promotion Professionals*, 25(2), pp. 116–24.

Jones, J., Norman, K. & Saunders, S., 2014, *The state of the union: Trends and drivers of change in physiotherapy in Ontario in 2014*. From http://hdl.handle.net/1974/12616, retrieved 8 July 2015.

Kangovi, S., Grande, D. & Trinh-Shevrin, C., 2015, From rhetoric to reality – community health workers in post-reform U.S. healthcare, *The New England Journal of Medicine*, 372(24), pp. 2277–9.

Keleher, H. & MacDougall, C., 2009, *Understanding health: A determinants approach*, 2nd ed., Oxford University Press, South Melbourne.

Knight, W., 2015, The exoskeletons are coming, *MIT Technology Review*, 16 July 2015.

Marmot, M., 2001, Economic and social determinants of disease, *Bulletin of the World Health Organization*, 79(10), pp. 988–9.

Mason, J., 2013, *Review of Australian government health workforce programmes*. Canberra: Department of Health. From https://www.health.gov.au/internet/main/publishing.nsf/Content/D26858F4B68834EACA257BF0001A8DDC/$File/Review%20of%20Health%20Workforce%20programs.pdf, retrieved 4 May 2016.

May, C., Montori, V.M. & Mair, F.S., 2009, We need minimally disruptive medicine, *BMJ (Clinical Research Ed.)*, 339:b2803.

McCullough, L.B., 2016, Physicians' professionally responsible power: A core concept of clinical ethics, *The Journal of Medicine and Philosophy*, 41(1), pp. 1–9.

McIntosh, N., 2005, *The educated heart: professional boundaries for massage therapists, bodyworkers, and movement therapists*, Lippincott, Williams & Wilkins, Philadelphia, PA.

Moffatt, M., 2012, A history of physical therapy education around the world. *Journal of Physical Therapy Education*, 26(1), pp. 13–23.

Mooney, L.M., Rouse, E.J. & Herr, H.M., 2014, Autonomous exoskeleton reduces metabolic cost of human walking during load carriage. *Journal of Neuroengineering and Rehabilitation*, 11(80), doi: 10.1186/1743-0003-11-80.

Morris, J., Grimmer, K., Gilmore, L., Perera, C., Waddington, G., Kyle, G., Ashman, B. & Murphy, K., 2014, Principles to guide sustainable implementation of extended-scope-of-practice physiotherapy workforce redesign initiatives in Australia: stakeholder perspectives, barriers, supports, and incentives, *Journal of Multidisciplinary Healthcare*, 7, pp. 249–58.

Nicholls, D.A., Walton, J.A. & Price, K., 2009, Making breathing your business: enterprising practices at the margins of orthodoxy, *Health: An Interdisciplinary for the Social Study of Health, Illness and Medicine*, 13(3), pp. 337–60.

Øberg, G.K., Normann, B. & Gallagher, S., 2015, Embodied-enactive clinical reasoning in physical therapy, *Physiotherapy Theory and Practice*, pp. 1–9.

Owen G., 2014, Becoming a practice profession: A genealogy of physiotherapy's moving/touching practice, doctoral thesis, University of Cardiff, Cardiff.

Pagliarulo, M.A., 2007, *Introduction to physical therapy*, 3rd ed., Mosby, St. Louis, MO.

Patel, K., Nadel, J. & West, M., 2014, *Redesigning the care team: The critical role of front-line workers and models for success*. Washington, DC: Engelberg Center for Healthcare Reform at Brookings. From https://www.brookings.edu/wp-content/uploads/2016/06/FINAL-Hitachi-Toolkit-32014-1.pdf, retrieved 23 July 2016.

Paul, A. & Mullerpatan, R., 2015, Review of physiotherapy awareness across the globe. *International Journal of Health Sciences and Research (IJHSR)*, 5(10), pp. 294–301.

Philip, K., 2015, Allied health: Untapped potential in the Australian health system. *Australian Health Review: A Publication of the Australian Hospital Association*, 39(3), pp. 244–7.

Robson, D., 2014, The ultimate comeback: Bringing the dead back to life, *BBC Future*, 7 July 2014.

Salsberg, E., 2003, *Making sense of the system: How states can use health workforce policies to increase access and improve quality of care*. Millbank Memorial Fund, New York. From www.milbank.org/uploads/documents/2003salsberg/2003salsberg.html#executive, retrieved 3 September 2016.

Sanders, T., Ong, B.N., Sowden, G. & Foster, N., 2014, Implementing change in physiotherapy: professions, contexts and interventions, *Journal of Health Organization and Management*, 28(1), pp. 96–114.

Schoen, C., Osborn, R., Doty, M.M., Bishop, M., Peugh, J. & Murukutla, N., 2007, Toward higher-performance health systems: adults' healthcare experiences in seven countries, 2007, *Health Affairs (Project Hope)*, 26(6), pp. w717–34.

Setchell, J., Nicholls, D.A. & Gibson, B.E., 2017, Objecting: Multiplicity in the practice of physiotherapy?, *Health: Health: An Interdisciplinary for the Social Study of Health, Illness and Medicine*. doi: 10.1177/1363459316688519.

Somerville, L., Davis, A., Elliott, A.L., Terrill, D., Austin, N. & Philip, K., 2015, Building allied health workforce capacity: a strategic approach to workforce innovation, *Australian Health Review: A Publication of the Australian Hospital Association*, 39(3), pp. 264–70.

Sorman, G., 2016, The Finnish Model, *City Journal*, 18 March 2016, retrieved from http://city-journal.org/html/finnish-model-14302.html, accessed 18 March 2016.

Stewart, E.M., 1964, Physiotherapy – past, present, and future. *Physiotherapy*, 50(7), pp. 228–30.

Taylor, D.M., Stone, S.D. & Huijbregts, M.P., 2012, Remote participants' experiences with a group-based stroke self-management program using videoconference technology. *Rural Remote Health*, 12, 1947.

Trede, F. & McEwan, C. (eds.), 2016a, *Educating the deliberate practitioner*, Springer, Amsterdam.

Trede, F. & McEwan, C. 2016b, Scoping the deliberate professional, in F. Trede & C. McEwan (eds.), *Educating the deliberate professional*, Springer, Amsterdam, pp. 3–14.

Varghese, B., Kanagaraj, R., Swaminathan, N., Vishal, K., Romer, M. & Cusack, T., 2012, Knowledge and perception of physiotherapy by final year students of various health care professions. *International Journal of Therapy & Rehabilitation*, 19(11).

Vincent-Onabajo, G.O., Mustapha, A. & Oyeyemi, A.Y., 2014, Medical students' awareness of the role of physiotherapists in multidisciplinary healthcare. *Physiotherapy Theory and Practice*, 30(5), pp. 338–44.

WHO, 2009, *Monitoring human resources for health-related rehabilitation services*. Spotlight on health workforce statistics. From www.who.int/hrh/statistics/spotlight_7_en.pdf?ua=1, retrieved 12 August 2016.

Wise, J. & Hemmings, G., 1994, Physiotherapy to 2094. *Physiotherapy*, 80(A), pp. 100A–1A.

Yagi, E., 2015, *Health and healthcare at the crossroads of business and society*, ESSEC Publishing, Cergy Pontoise Cedex, France.

Epilogue
Methodology

Introduction

I made a conscious decision when I set out to write this book to de-emphasise the philosophy and methodology that underpinned it. This is not because I wanted to suggest that my particular analytic lens was unimportant, or that the work was in any way value-neutral and objective. Far from it. I am very comfortable with the idea that this is a subjective, value-laden critical history and I hope it is more meaningful and more engaging as a result. The reality is though that there are very few philosophically-informed critical histories in physiotherapy and most of the people that this book was written for are unused to the kinds of writing now familiar in medical sociology, critical nursing, occupational therapy and critical psychology, disability studies and postmodern qualitative research.

The problem is that if you begin the text making mention of your particular analytic lens it is difficult to then say anything substantive without interlacing your ideas with quite heavy theoretical content and I very much wanted to emphasise physiotherapy and not philosophy in this book. That being said, it should be reasonably obvious that I have made choices all the way through the book about the texts I included, how I analysed the material, which issues I emphasised and which were bypassed. All of these decisions derived from a very particular philosophical foundation that needs to be unpacked a little, if only so that the reader does not fall into the trap of believing that I my goal was to write the last critical word on physiotherapy.

I knew that if I began the study outlining my philosophical and methodological underpinnings, it might discourage many of my colleagues, peers and students from reading it. As I have argued throughout the text, physiotherapists are trained as biomechanical specialists and many are sceptical of historical, philosophical and socio-cultural paradigms. Consequently, most find heavily theoretical works off-putting. Perhaps, as a consequence of this, there are currently few overtly 'critical' long-form works being written by physiotherapists. The situation is better than it was even 20 years ago. We now have a generation of physiotherapists who have studied in the arts and humanities, have gained exposure to critical theory, disability and gender studies, and embodiment philosophy, history and sociology, who have returned to physiotherapy bringing their newfound knowledge with them. A detailed theoretical position would be expected by these people. And so, I have tried to satisfy the experienced and the sceptical theoretician by including an Epilogue that sketches out my philosophical position in what is, I hope, an accessible way.

Key influences

The primary influence on this text has been the work of French philosopher Michel Foucault (1926–1984). Foucault has been a powerful influence in 20th century philosophy and his works can be found in fields as diverse as architecture, art, critical theory, disability studies, ecology, economics, gender studies, history, journalism, management studies, media studies, philosophy, politics, queer theory, qualitative research methodologies, race theory, sociology and even town planning. Foucault was one of a number of now well-known continental philosophers, including Pierre Bourdieu, Simone de Beauvoir, Judith Butler, Jacques Derrida, Gilles Deleuze, Martin Heidegger, Friedrich Nietzsche and Jean-Paul Sartre[1], who radically transformed the philosophical landscape in the 20th century. Many of the approaches now used by qualitative researchers derive from their work and their writings have radically changed how we think about fundamental 'truths', like the nature of power; the subjectivity of knowledge; the instability and fluidity of bodies; the political construction of disability, gender, race and sexuality and the history of ideas.

The writings that I have drawn on most in developing this book include some powerful and, it must be said, 'challenging' works by Foucault, most especially *Discipline and Punish* (Foucault 1977), *The Birth of the Clinic* (Foucault 1973) and Volume I of *The History of Sexuality* (Foucault 1979b). Foucault was notoriously ambiguous about his own methodological approach and argued continually against the kinds of methodological rigour that now beset the field of qualitative research (Pierre 2013; St. Pierre 2014). This has spawned a number of different interpretations of what might be called 'Foucauldian discourse analysis'. Some of these are essentially linguistic and structural in their approach. My preference has always been to focus on what Derek Hook called the 'animating power' of Foucault's writing, which places its emphasis on what people *do* and not on what they *say* they do. This is a critical point, because so much qualitative research in recent years has focused on interviews and other techniques for tapping into the inner tensions, thoughts and motivations of participants. The reader will have noticed, perhaps, that this is not an interview-based study. There are no interviews with current or retired physiotherapists, and the history of the profession has been gleaned from other sources. This is because Foucault argues against such methods, promoting instead the idea that if we want to understand the 'history of the present', or more simply put – how physiotherapy has arrived at this particular point in its history – we should focus on the 'material practices' of everyday life: those things that normally pass unnoticed, hidden in plain sight; the forces that have subtly shaped the profession through appeals to reason, common-sense or morality or have brought about compliance, acceptance, regulation and self-discipline without the need for force (Hook 2001a, 2001b; Tamboukou 1999).

Foucault was interested in how our personal and professional lives had been shaped by particular truths and how we had come to accept certain kinds of knowledge over others. He was fascinated by the way that command of certain truths came with elite social status – think here of the power of doctors, priests, judges, and politicians – and how the ability to control public discourse (what we believe to be true) has shifted over time. Foucault did not believe in absolute truths and argued that everything we know derived from myriad competing interests, discourses and ideas. Our belief in science, God, nature and everyday things like the idea that 'the doctor knows best' are temporary manifestations of a thousand competing interests, all fighting to promote particular truth whilst marginalise the competition. History has taught us that everything we currently take for granted and accept as the truth, is amenable to revision, and that even our most stable ideas are built on shaky foundations.

More than this, Foucault did not believe in the idea of progressive history. He did not believe that we were becoming progressively smarter and more enlightened. As a result, he rejected the traditional approach to historical inquiry, which offered a linear narrative account of the events of the past. Foucauldian histories of the present rarely argue that *this* event led inexorably to *this*, then *this*, then *this* and so on. Rather, Foucault focused on 'ruptures' or moments when the *status quo* was thrown into disarray. Foucault believed that the real animating power governing our day-to-day lives was largely hidden from us and that only when a sudden, disruptive event threw doubt on our everyday understandings would we get to really see how we thought and the ideas that underpinned our actions. Foucault believed that when such events occur, people are forced to take sides and the myriad discourses at play can be more easily seen. People speak up for certain positions and vocally marginalise other competing interests; they use particular techniques, like political lobbying, advertising, organising meetings or writing articles to promote their viewpoint and they work hard to hone their subject position and build alliances. In a physiotherapy context, these moments provide a prime opportunity to see how the profession has positioned itself, how it has made decisions about its beliefs and values, how members of the profession should practice and think and how it has responded to the myriad challenges that have befallen it over the last century.

Foucault was interested in the way new 'truths' replaced old. He was interested in the ways power flowed through society and functioned as a positive force, making things happen, rather than as the more negative idea of power that had become prominent in the post-war era. Foucault was more interested in how people came to do 'the right thing' through coercion, encouragement, training and self-interest than through external force. He was interested in the everyday, microscopic, almost invisible subterranean, micro-political actions that were necessary to make life function in the way it did: our rules, systems and concepts; the roles and positions (or subjectivities) that we adopted; our everyday practices and commonplace objects. He was interested in how power and knowledge made some things possible and denied others; made some truths unpalatable and others powerful and significant. He was fascinated by the reasons why we became more humane around the treatment of the mentally ill (Foucault 1965), how doctors had become powerful figures in society (Foucault 1973); how we had learnt to govern other people's conduct (Foucault 1977); how governments had learnt to rule by coercion, legislation and economic encouragement (Foucault 1979a) and in the years prior to his death, how we had learnt to govern ourselves (Foucault 1985, 1986).

Many authors since have picked up on these themes, and these works have heavily influenced this book. Writings on the 'psy' disciplines by Nikolas Rose (Rose 1993, 1994, 1996a, 1996b, 1997, 1999), on medicine by David Armstrong and Deborah Lupton (Armstrong 1983, 1995, 1998, 2002; Lupton 1997, 2012); works on the critical history of dentistry (Nettleton 1992, 1994), podiatry (Borthwick 1999) and complementary therapies (Dew 2003; Fournier 1999, 2000). Critical histories of physical therapy and rehabilitation cited frequently in this text (Linker 2005, 2007, 2011, 2012; Carden-Coyne 2008, 2009, 2014); nursing (Cheek & Rudge 1994a, 1994b; Price & Cheek 1996; Cheek & Porter 1997; Cheek 1999; Gastaldo & Holmes 1999; Holmes 2001; Holmes & Gastaldo 2002), healthcare (Petersen & Lupton 1996; Petersen & Bunton 1997), government and economics (Dean 1999; Lemke 2002) and many others[2].

Having sketched out the broad terrain of Foucault's writings and ideas, I want to briefly review the particular approach to Foucauldian Discourse Analysis taken in this book. There are five key Foucauldian principles underpinning the way this book was researched and written. These are as follows:

1. A focus on ruptures, discontinuities and contingent history

While the first section of the book traverses the early pre-history of physical therapies, through the massage scandals and WWI, through welfarism to the present neoliberal and postmodern age, I have tried to show that at each historical moment (or *episteme*, as Foucault called it), the actions and conduct of physiotherapists were contingent on the challenges they were faced with, and had little to do with historical progress towards ultimate truth or enlightenment. I write from the basis that physiotherapists today are largely dealing with the cards they have been dealt in much the same way that the profession's forbears did in 1894, 1914, 1944 and 1974. Physiotherapists did not resolve the problem of how to touch people legitimately in 1894. Nor did they form an unbreakable bond with medicine and the State in the inter-war years. In reality, physiotherapists have to renew their relationships and re-establish their core principles every day, through myriad tiny gestures and actions; constantly re-performing (Butler 1997) what it means to be a physiotherapist. Knowledge of the profession's heritage would not rid physiotherapists of the need to be sensitive, respectful or skilful, nor would it take away the need to know the anatomical workings of the body or the pathology of injury. What it would do, however, is give practitioners more options. It would open up the possibility of a thousand new forms of physiotherapy that were previously unknown or unimaginable when practitioners had been trained so carefully to think only of the body-as-machine.

2. A concern with what discourses do, not what people say they do

One of the most noticeable changes in healthcare research over the last 30 years has been the rise of qualitative research and particularly what is called the humanistic 'turn'. Research exploring people's thoughts, feelings and opinions is now commonplace and it would be hard to imagine a qualitative study in physiotherapy that did not include at least some interviews with participants. This 'turn' mirrors a broader societal shift towards public opinion surveys, user focus groups, television interviews, polls, censuses, questionnaires and myriad other devices designed to hear the *vox populi* – the voice of the people. Foucault was very sceptical about this approach, arguing that all of these approaches appeared on the surface to be about giving voice to the people, but were really all confessional (Gilbert 2001; Spitzack 1987; Foucault 1980). He argued that 'Western societies have established the confession as one of the main rituals we rely on for the production of truth' (Foucault 1979b, p. 56), and that:

> It plays a part in justice, medicine, education, family relationships, and love relationships, in the most ordinary affairs of everyday life, and in the most solemn rites; one confesses one's crimes, one's sins one's thoughts and desires, one's illnesses and troubles; one goes about telling, with the greatest precision, whatever is most difficult to tell. One confesses in public and in private, to one's parents, one's educators, one's doctor, to those one loves; one admits to oneself in pleasure and in pain, things it would be impossible to tell to anyone else, the things people write books about. When it is not spontaneous or dictated by some internal imperative, the confession is wrung from a person by violence or threat . . . Western man has become a confessing animal.
> (Foucault 1979b, p. 59)

So if interviews and other common ethnographic and qualitative methods are problematic (Fadyl & Nicholls 2013), what methods are used in this study to explore the ways physiotherapy has been discursively constructed? The focus of the kind of Foucauldian Discourse Analysis used in this book is on what are called material practices – the things people do (for example, writing clinical notes, drafting legislation, lobbying doctors); the objects they use (treatment beds, street signs, referral letters); the subject positions they adopt (fierce masseuse, autonomous practitioner) and the concepts and strategies they deploy (specialisation, the quest for legitimacy, recognition as orthodox). According to Foucault, the most mundane practices are the ones that should attract the greatest attention, because these are the practices that have managed to effectively hide their effective machinery of power.

3. Power as productive

One of Foucault's most controversial principles is that power is productive. Writing in the 1960s and 1970s at the height of the civil rights movement, radical feminism and widespread political activism, Foucault's new ways to analyse the machinery of power gave him instantaneous popularity and notoriety. He provided activists with new tools to critique power structures that oppressed racial minorities, disabled people, women, gay, lesbian and transgender people, but then argued against feminists, Marxists and others, who were promoted the idea that asymmetrical power structures existed in society and needed to be overthrown. Foucault argued that power wasn't like this; that no-one actually ever 'had' power; that power couldn't be possessed and wielded in this way and that power was not at all 'negative'. Rather, he argued that power was an animating force – something entirely positive; it got things done, it created things and made things happen. It was not necessarily oppressive or 'top-down' (although Foucault didn't deny that this sometimes happened), but instead it operated as a network of tiny actions and counter-actions; myriad competitions and contests between people and ideas. Certainly, power marginalised some people and some ideas for some of the time, but he argued that it should never be seen as hegemonic, linear or totalising.

In this book, I have repeatedly tried to show that power has been a highly productive force in physiotherapy and has influenced the profession's decisions about aligning with the medical profession, defining a very restrictive view of the body-as-machine, brutalising injured servicemen, tackling the rehabilitation of polio victims, and so on. While there are gendered questions running through the text, I have tried not to take the position that the women that made up the profession represented a marginalised minority. Similarly, there is a commentary on the power of professionals over disabled people. But I have tried to argue that to view these questions of power as too asymmetrical, risks oversimplifying the vast complexity of discursive networks at play.

4. Postmodern, poststructural research

Foucault is often called a postmodern or poststructural philosopher. This is true in some respects. His approach is certainly sceptical of the kinds of metanarratives that are commonplace in modern biomedicine (that science will find the cure, that medicine has replaced the superstitions of religion, that evidence-based practice vital etc.) (Lyotard 1984). His works are post-structural in the sense that they challenge the belief that power dominates over people and silently situates some in minority positions. But at the same time, he is neither postmodern or poststructural. Foucault rejected being labelled as a particular kind of researcher; resisting the common temptation to want to categorise a body of work in order that we might make sense of it. In the same spirit, I hope this text is somewhat difficult to define. It is, at various times, an historical study. At other times, it is a work of professional philosophy, a series of sociological arguments, and a piece of qualitative research. I hope that by spanning a range of different fields, the work becomes more fluid and available to a wide readership: students looking to understand the history of their profession; clinicians and policy-makers searching for ideas to help them shape the profession's future; teachers and researchers looking for robust resources to help them with their own research.

5. *Not prescribing an answer*

The final Foucauldian principal underpinning this book is perhaps the most counter-intuitive. Readers of Foucault's work will note that he often goes to extraordinary lengths to critique a problem, but never prescribes what he sees as the answer. You will never see in a well-conducted Foucauldian study the argument that 'here is the problem, and here is the solution'. This is different to many kinds of research seen in anthropology, economics, political theory, science and sociology, where the very point of the research is often to try to find the answer. After all, what is the point of studying the reasons why people gamble, smoke, riot or spend too long sitting down, if we are not going to find the solution? Foucault was adamant that he would not be the judge of what was right and wrong. He argued that our role as critics, researchers and scholars was to 're-examine evidence and assumptions, to shake up habitual ways of working and thinking, to dissipate conventional familiarities, to re-evaluate rules and institutions and to participate in the formation of a political will' (Foucault 1989, pp. 462–3). He said:

> I absolutely will not play the part of one who prescribes solutions. I hold that the role of the intellectual today is . . . not proposing solutions or prophesying, since by doing that one can only contribute to the determinate situation of power that must be criticized.
>
> (Foucault 1991, p. 157)

The focus of Foucauldian studies is, therefore, not on prescribing the answer, since Foucault argued that such approaches simply replace one bad hegemony with another. Rather, it is to critique the present in order that we might open a door on a thousand possible alternatives; a myriad responses based on a deeper appreciation for the complexities of the problems facing us, a realisation that any solution we might derive is both temporary and the focus for our next set of inquiries. The fact that there is no end in sight and that our role will always be to critique, interrogate and explore upsets some people. It sounds nihilistic. It sounds as if we will never arrive at the answer. But far from being nihilistic, Foucauldian scholars think this is both realistic and optimistic. It removes the pressure to try to find the last word on the problems facing us; it recognises that no-one ever has, and that our time is better spent working with the conditions we find around us rather than anxiously repeating the mistakes of yesteryear. Perhaps not surprisingly, diversity and inclusiveness are much more comfortable words for Foucauldian scholars than predictability and teleological solutions.

So, in this book, I have used thousands of words to critique the profession and asked how physiotherapy has arrived at this particular point in its history. What I have not done is suggest that if we only did 'x, y and z' our problems would be solved. Others have tried this, and certainly, people seem to want it. But have new definitions of the profession secured our future? Have new scopes of practice resolved our anxieties? Have we found 'the answer' for the daily working challenges that we feel occupy far too much of our time, robbing us of time to do the 'real work' of physiotherapy? Clearly not, and I make no attempt here to add to this work, preferring instead to make it the focus of my next set of critical inquiries.

Closing words

In this chapter, I have tried to provide a brief outline of the methodological and philosophical principles underpinning the book. My hope is that readers with little or no interest in these subjects will be able to find value in the ideas presented here without needing to understand Foucauldian Discourse Analysis. For those interested in why the book focuses on some data on not others, or why it does not prescribe what I think is 'the answer' to physiotherapy's future, will hopefully find this brief chapter instructive. There are many texts that now explore Foucauldian Discourse Analysis in great depth and detail and, hopefully, readers will be encouraged to incorporate some of these ideas into their thinking in the future.

Notes

1 Continental philosophy derives from French, German and Nordic ideas about the nature of existence, being, human experience, power, truth and morality and has been the basis of phenomenology, critical theory, postmodernism and poststructuralism. It contrasts with the Anglo-American tradition of analytic philosophy with its concern for reason and logic, the structure of argument and the foundations of ideas and judgement.

2 Those interested in reading a broad introduction to Foucault's have some excellent resources to refer to, including a number of very good primers (McHoul & Grace 1993; Mills 2003, 2004; Danaher et al 2000). Readers will also be able to find introductions and applications of Foucault's ideas in earlier papers I have written with a number of colleagues (Nicholls 2009; Fadyl et al 2012; Fadyl & Nicholls 2013; Nicholls et al 2009b), these include writings where, like this book, Foucault's methodological and philosophical ideas are not expressed overtly, but underpin the entire study (Nicholls & Larmer 2005; Nicholls & Cheek 2006; Nicholls et al 2009a; Gibson et al 2010; Payne & Nicholls 2010; Nicholls 2012; Werner et al 2004; Nicholls & Holmes 2012).

References

Armstrong, D., 1983, *Political anatomy of the body: Medical knowledge in Britain in the twentieth century*, Cambridge University Press, Cambridge.

Armstrong, D., 1995, The rise of surveillance medicine, *Sociology of Health & Illness*, 17(3), pp. 393–404.

Armstrong, D., 1998, Decline of the hospital: Reconstructing institutional dangers, *Sociology of Health & Illness*, 20(4), p. 445.

Armstrong, D., 2002, *A new history of identity*, Palgrave Macmillan, London.

Borthwick, A.M., 1999, Perspectives in podiatric biomechanics: Foucault and the professional project, *British Journal of Podiatry*, 2(1), pp. 21–8.

Butler, J., 1997, *Excitable speech: A politics of the performative*, Routledge, London.

Carden-Coyne, A., 2008, Painful bodies and brutal women: Remedial massage, gender relations and cultural agency in military hospitals, 1914–18, *Journal of War and Cultural Studies*, 1(2), pp. 139–58.

Carden-Coyne, A., 2009, *Reconstructing the body: Classicism, modernism, and the First World War*, Oxford University Press, Oxford.

Carden-Coyne, A., 2014, *The politics of wounds: Military patients and medical power in the first World War*, Oxford University Press, Oxford.

Cheek, J., 1999, *Postmodern and poststructural approaches to nursing research*, Sage, London.

Cheek, J. & Porter, S., 1997, Reviewing Foucault: Possibilities and problems for nursing and healthcare, *Nursing Inquiry*, 4(2), pp. 108–19.

Cheek, J. & Rudge, T., 1994a, Nursing as textually mediated reality, *Nursing Inquiry*, 1(1), pp. 15–22.

Cheek, J. & Rudge, T., 1994b, The panopticon re-visited?: An exploration of the social and political dimensions of contemporary healthcare and nursing practice, *International Journal of Nursing Studies*, 31(6), pp. 583–91.

Danaher, G., Shirato, T. & Webb, J., 2000, *Understanding Foucault*, Allen and Unwin, Sydney.

Dean, M., 1999, *Governmentality*, Sage, Thousand Oaks, CA.

Dew, K., 2003, *Borderland practices: Regulating alternative therapies in New Zealand*, University of Otago Press, Dunedin, New Zealand.

Fadyl, J.K. & Nicholls, D.A., 2013, Foucault, the subject and the research interview: A critique of methods, *Nursing Inquiry*, 20(1), pp. 23–9.

Fadyl, J.K., Nicholls, D.A., & McPherson, K.M., 2012, Interrogating discourse: The application of Foucault's methodological discussion to specific inquiry, *Health*, 17(5), pp. 478–94.

Foucault, M., 1965, *Madness and civilization: A history of insanity in the age of reason*, Translated by R. Howard. Pantheon, New York.

Foucault, M., 1973, *The birth of the clinic: An archaeology of medical perception*, Tavistock Publications, London.

Foucault, M., 1977, *Discipline and punish: The birth of the prison*, Allen Lane, London.

Foucault, M., 1979a, Governmentality, *Ideology and Consciousness*, 6, pp. 5–21.

Foucault, M., 1979b, *The history of sexuality, Vol. 1: An introduction*, Allen Lane, London.

Foucault, M., 1980, The confession of the flesh, in C. Gordon (ed.), *Power/knowledge: Selected interviews and other writings 1972–1977*, Harvester Wheatsheaf, New York, pp. 194–228.

Foucault, M., 1985, *The use of pleasure: The history of sexuality, Vol. 2*, Translated by R. Hurley. Random House, New York.

Foucault, M., 1986, *The care of the self: The history of sexuality, Vol. 3*, Translated by R. Hurley. Random House, New York.

Foucault, M., 1989, *Interview: The concern for truth, Foucault Live*, Semiotext, New York.

Foucault, M., 1991, Governmentality, in G. Burchell, C. Gordon & P. Miller (eds.), *The Foucault effect: Studies in Governmentality*, Harvester Wheatsheaf, Hemel Hempstead, UK.

Fournier, V., 1999, The appeal to 'professionalism' as a disciplinary mechanism, *Sociological Review*, 47(2), pp. 280–307.

Fournier, V., 2000, Boundary work and the (un)making of the professions, in N. Malin (ed.), *Professionalism, boundaries and the workplace*, Routledge, London, pp. 67–86.

Gastaldo, D. & Holmes, D., 1999, Foucault and nursing: A history of the present, *Nursing Inquiry*, 6(4), pp. 231–40.

Gibson, B.E., Nixon, S.A. & Nicholls, D.A., 2010, Critical reflections on the physiotherapy profession in Canada, *Physiotherapy Canada*, 62(2), pp. 98–100, pp. 101–3.

Gilbert, T., 2001, Reflective practice and clinical supervision: Meticulous rituals of the confessional, *Journal of Advanced Nursing*, 36(2), pp. 199–205.

Holmes, D., 2001, From iron gaze to nursing care: Mental health nursing in the era of panopticism, *Journal of Psychiatric and Mental Health Nursing*, 8(1), pp. 7–15.

Holmes, D. & Gastaldo, D., 2002, Nursing as means of governmentality, *Journal of Advanced Nursing*, 38(6), pp. 557–65.

Hook, D., 2001a, Discourse, knowledge, materiality, history: Foucault and discourse analysis, *Theory & Psychology*, 13, pp. 605–28.

Hook, D., 2001b, The 'disorders of discourse', *Theoria*, 48(97), pp. 41–68.

Lemke, T., 2002, Foucault, governmentality, and critique, *Rethinking Marxism*, 14(3), pp. 49–64.

Linker, B., 2005, Strength and science: Gender, physiotherapy, and medicine in the United States, 1918–35, *Journal of Women's History*, 17(3), pp. 106–32.

Linker, B., 2007, Feet for fighting: Locating disability and social medicine in First World War America, *Social History of Medicine*, 20(1), pp. 91–109.

Linker, B., 2011, *War's waste: Rehabilitation in World War I America*, University of Chicago Press, Chicago, IL.

Linker, B., 2012, A dangerous curve: The role of history in America's scoliosis screening programs, *American Journal of Public Health*, 102(4), pp. 606–16.

Lupton, D., 1997, Doctors on the medical profession, *Sociology of Health & Illness*, 19(4), pp. 480–97.

Lupton, D., 2012, *Medicine as culture: Illness, disease and the body in Western society*, Sage, London.

Lyotard, J., 1984, *The postmodern condition: A report on knowledge*, University of Minnesota Press, Minneapolis, MN.

McHoul, A. & Grace, W., 1993, *A Foucault primer: Discourse, power and the subject*, Melbourne University Press, Melbourne, Australia.

Mills, S., 2003, *Michel Foucault*, Routledge, London.

Mills, S., 2004, *Discourse*, Routledge, London.

Nettleton, S., 1992, *Power, pain and dentistry*, Open University Press, Buckingham, UK.

Nettleton, S., 1994, Inventing mouths: Disciplinary power and dentistry, in C. Jones & R. Porter (eds.), *Reassessing Foucault: Power, medicine and the body*, Routledge, London, pp. 73–90.

Nicholls, D.A., 2009, Putting Foucault to work: An approach to the practical application of Foucault's methodological imperatives, *Aporia*, 1(1), pp. 30–40.

Nicholls, D.A., 2012, Postmodernism and physiotherapy research, *Physical Therapy Reviews*, 17(6), pp. 360–8.

Nicholls, D.A. & Cheek, J., 2006, Physiotherapy and the shadow of prostitution: The Society of Trained Masseuses and the massage scandals of 1894, *Social Science & Medicine*, 62(9), pp. 2336–48.

Nicholls, D.A. & Holmes, D., 2012, Discipline, desire, and transgression in physiotherapy practice, *Physiotherapy Theory and Practice*, 28(6), pp. 454–65.

Nicholls, D.A. & Larmer, P., 2005, Possible futures for physiotherapy: An exploration of the New Zealand context, *New Zealand Journal of Physiotherapy*, 33(2), pp. 55–60.

Nicholls, D.A., Reid, D.A. & Larmer, P.J., 2009a, Crisis, what crisis? Revisiting 'possible futures for physiotherapy', *New Zealand Journal of Physiotherapy*, 37(3), pp. 105–14.

Nicholls, D.A., Walton, J.A. & Price, K., 2009b, Making breathing your business: Enterprising practices at the margins of orthodoxy, *Health: An Interdisciplinary for the Social Study of Health, Illness and Medicine*, 13(3), pp. 337–60.

Payne, D. & Nicholls, D.A., 2010, Managing breastfeeding and work: A Foucauldian secondary analysis, *Journal of Advanced Nursing*, 66(8), pp. 1810–18.

Petersen, A. & Bunton, R., 1997, *Foucault, health and medicine*, Routledge, London.

Petersen, A. & Lupton, D., 1996, *The new public health: Health and self in the age of risk*, Sage, London.

Pierre, E.A.S., 2013, The posts continue: Becoming, *International Journal of Qualitative Studies in Education*, 26(6), pp. 646–57.

Price, K. & Cheek, J., 1996, Pain as a discursive construction, *Social Sciences in Health: International Journal of Research and Practice*, 2(4), pp. 211–17.

Rose, N., 1993, Government, authority and expertise in advanced liberalism, *Economy & Society*, 22(3), p. 283.

Rose, N., 1994, Medicine, history and the present, in C. Jones & R. Porter (eds.), *Reassessing Foucault: Power, medicine and the body*, Routledge, London, pp. 48–72.

Rose, N., 1996a, Governing 'advanced' liberal democracies, in A. Barry & T. Osborne (eds.), *Foucault and political reason: Liberalism, neo-liberalism and rationalities of government*, University of Chicago Press, Chicago, IL, pp. 37–64.

Rose, N., 1996b, Power and subjectivity: Critical history and psychology, in C. Graumann, C. Friedrich & K.J. Gergen (eds.), *Historical dimensions of psychological discourse*, Cambridge University Press, New York, pp. 103–24.

Rose, N., 1997, *Inventing our selves: Psychology, power and personhood*, Cambridge University Press, Cambridge, UK.

Rose, N., 1999, *Powers of freedom: Reframing political thought*, Cambridge University Press, Cambridge, UK.

Spitzack, C., 1987, Confession and signification: The systematic inscription of body consciousness, *Journal of Medicine and Philosophy*, 12(4), pp. 356–69.

St. Pierre, E.A., 2014, A brief and personal history of post qualitative research: Toward 'post inquiry', *JCT (Online)*, 30(2).

Tamboukou, M., 1999, Writing genealogies: An exploration of Foucault's strategies for doing research, *Discourse: Studies in the Cultural Politics of Education*, 20(2), pp. 201–17.

Werner, A., Isaksen, L.W. & Malterud, K., 2004, 'I am not the kind of woman who complains of everything': Illness stories on self and shame in women with chronic pain, *Social Science & Medicine*, 59(5), pp. 1035–45.

Glossary of terms

Body-as-machine   The body-as-machine is a term used to define a particularly depersonalised approach to healthcare. It is based on the long-established medical principal that health professionals should learn to view the body as separate from the mind, personal experience, values and beliefs, cultural and social context, and focus instead on body parts, regions and systems. The body is treated as a machine, such that faulty parts can be repaired or replaced and the person can then return to normal function. The body-as-machine has been one of the defining features of Western healthcare since the Industrial Revolution.

Client, consumer, patient   It is sometimes difficult to decide whether to use the term client, consumer or patient these days. The word 'patient' has become associated with a passive recipient of expert care, but 'client' and 'consumer' come with connotations of financial transaction that many health professionals and service users – another term – find unappealing. Unless quoting directly from another author or referring explicitly to a financial transaction, I have chosen to use the word 'patient' not least because it resonates with a key argument throughout the book that physiotherapists still treat the body-as-machine, and this approach can tend to make patients out of people.

Embodiment   Embodiment is perhaps one of the most fertile areas of new thinking in physiotherapy. It refers to an approach to healthcare that emphasises a broader view of the person. As well as embracing all of the physical aspects of health and illness, it takes into consideration the person's subjective experience, plus all of the cultural, environmental, financial, social, political and spiritual realities of people's lives. It is not truly 'holistic' because it does not aim to be a model or a theory of 'everything', but it certainly represents a broader concept of health and wellbeing than many of the reductive biomedical approach currently operating in Western healthcare.

First contact profession   This term refers to the ability of physiotherapists to treat patient without needing a medical referral. Australian physiotherapists were the first to achieve this hallmark of professional autonomy in 1976 and other countries have since followed suit. First contact status in physiotherapy is still relatively rare worldwide, and is seen by many as a marker of professional maturity and as a statement of public trust in the profession.

New economy of healthcare   This refers to a much broader definition of 'economy' than is conventionally used. In this book, I use the term to refer to the day-to-day exchanges between therapists and patients; the human experiences of care; the social systems that make practices like physiotherapy possible; the political economy and the legal and ethical contracts we establish between professions and the public.

Physiotherapy/physical therapy   I have used the term physiotherapy throughout the book unless referring to countries where physical therapy is the preferred term. Part of the reason for doing this is because the book argues that we may be seeing the end of the profession that has long been associated with a particular notion of physiotherapy constructed in the late 19th century. The distinction between physiotherapy as a *profession* and physical therapy as a range of practices is significant therefore.

The State   It is common to imagine The State as a single monolithic structure run by a few government officials, exerting too much power over passive subjects, but in this book, I have tried to apply a different interpretation. Rather than physiotherapists being seen as pawns in a political game, I view the State as a diffuse network of interconnected agencies, actors, structures and systems. In this approach, power is unevenly distributed among patients, health professionals, regulators, educators, and others, but is more than just oppressive and overbearing. The State is, therefore, more like a 'brain', with a host of nodes and synaptic connections than a pyramid.

Subjectivity vs identity   I have resisted using the word 'identity' when referring to physiotherapy (as in 'physiotherapy identity'), because this term carries connotations of reductive psychology in which particular traits and defined variables are used to codify a complex entity. This approach is problematic and now rather outdated. Subjectivity, on the other hand, allows for a broader, more embodied way of thinking about groups of professionals, and it fits more closely with the ideas expressed later in the book about the future for the profession as a whole.

Index